G000320476

Active Wellness

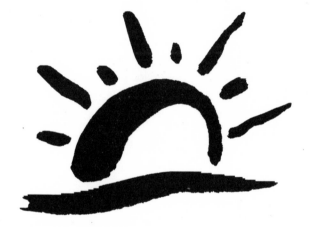

A PERSONALIZED 10 STEP PROGRAMME
FOR A HEALTHY BODY, MIND & SPIRIT

GAYLE REICHLER, MS, RD, CDN
WITH NANCY BURKE

TIME LIFE BOOKS

To Richard, Pat, Beth and Jonathan
for their love, support, and belief in my vision

and to my clients whose efforts and will to grow and
expand their lives is an inspiration.

Author's Note

The Active Wellness programme is an adjunct to, not a substitute for, conventional medical therapy. The nutrition, fitness, and stress management plans discussed in this book are recommendations by a registered dietitian. Before you start your programme, it is important that you consult with your doctor and other health care providers.

I also recommend that you maintain routine medical care and monitor your condition as you proceed in the Active Wellness programme. It is also important that you do not stop taking or make changes in any of your medications without first consulting with the doctor who prescribed them.

One goal of this book is to make you aware of the impact of healthy lifestyle options on your overall well-being. More specifically, I want to help you learn how to reach your personal health goals through satisfying behavioural changes. To that end, this book will introduce you to the strengths of the allied health fields of nutrition, exercise, psychology and alternative health practices such as yoga. Since many of you will be trying these health practices for the first time, please feel free to contact Active Wellness with any questions you may have. If you are unsure about whether the recommendations in this book are right for you, please contact your doctor. Active Wellness can be reached on the Internet at www.activewellness.com.

Published by Time-Life Books, London.

Editorial Staff for *Active Wellness* (US edition):
Cover Design: Frierson Mee + Kraft
Text Design: REDRUTH, Robin Bray, proprietor
Special Contributors:
Celia Beattie, Nancy Burke, Lavonne Carlson,
Judy Davis, Ruth Goldberg, Jeffrey Migdow, M.D.,
Beth Salzer, Susan Stuck, Tipy Taylor, Totally Inc.

Editorial Staff for *Active Wellness* (UK edition):
Managing Editor: Mark Stephenson
Editor: Nancy Duin
Editorial: Kate Cann, Andrew Cartwright
Production Director: Sonia Howie
Production: Mel Vandevelde, Alexia Turner, Gary Stevens
Cover Adaptation: Mark Stephenson

©1998 Gayle Reichler. All rights reserved.

No part of this book may be reproduced in any form or by any electronic or mechanical means, including information storage and retrieval devices or systems, without prior written permission from the publisher, except that brief passages may be quoted for reviews.

First printing.

ISBN: 0 7054 3005 7

TIME-LIFE is a trademark of Time Warner Inc. U.S.A.

CONTENTS

FOREWORD

The publication of this book on Active Wellness by my friend and associate, Gayle Reichler, could not be more timely. A recent issue of the heart journal *Circulation* contains a lead article, written by members of the American Heart Association's Nutrition Committee, which reclassifies obesity as a major risk factor for coronary artery disease. Thus, for the first time, obesity joins the ranks of high cholesterol, cigarette smoking and high blood pressure as a major, modifiable cause of heart disease. It is a little-known fact that obesity is a leading cause of preventable death, second only to smoking. Most disturbing, despite a wealth of information and media attention, and more diets than ever before, obesity and sedentary lifestyle are on the increase. There is such strong concern about the health effects of being overweight that in June 1998 the US National Heart, Lung and Blood Institute updated its weight guidelines to alert physicians and the public to the fact that health problems actually begin at lower ranges of excess weight. Like heart disease, obesity can contribute to health problems such as elevated blood pressure, diabetes, high cholesterol, high triglycerides, low HDL (the 'good' cholesterol) and certain cancers.

I began working with Gayle when she joined the Dr Dean Ornish Lifestyle Program for Reversing Heart Disease at Beth Israel Medical Center in New York City as our nutritionist. Gayle's Active Wellness Program embodied our philosophy of comprehensive lifestyle change as the best way to achieve and maintain good health. Although heredity plays an important role in our risk for diseases, the way we live on a day-to-day basis has an enormous impact on our health, well-being and happiness.

A more healthful lifestyle is something that many desire, but few achieve. Gayle's programme offers more than mere weight management: It is a hands-on healthy lifestyle programme that strives for a more complete state of wellness involving mind, body, and spirit. The Active Wellness Program takes a practical, personalized approach to incorporating wellness into one's life and reflects Gayle's approach to her clients. By responding to each person's unique concerns, she provides the strategies and tools they need to effectively embrace wellness in their lives as a long-term solution. One of Gayle's greatest skills is the ability to incorporate into her programme pleasurable and manageable behaviour changes that lead to a more rewarding, satisfying life. Best of all, once you begin to feel the results, your good feelings will continue to motivate you to achieve your personal goals and improve your level of wellness even further.

If your desire is to stay well, lose weight or prevent illness through lifestyle change, you will find the Active Wellness Program enlightening, enjoyable and rewarding.

Dr. Steven Horowitz
Chief of Cardiology
Beth Israel Medical Center
New York City

Testimonials from Clients

A year ago, at 49 years old, I was 30 pounds overweight. I hadn't exercised in years and I got exhausted just climbing the stairs out of the subway. With two kids and a full-time job, I had decided that life was hard enough without worrying about how I looked.

But somehow, turning 50 like that was just too depressing. For six months I woke up every morning deciding to start my diet—but by lunchtime it was all forgotten.

Then, by total luck, I heard about Active Wellness. The first week, I was inspired by Gayle's approach. The programme didn't seem like a diet—more like a philosophy about feeling good and doing good things for yourself. I could get enthusiastic about that! I lost my first pound. I stuck to the plan, even though I was losing weight slowly at first, because I felt so good. I began walking to work. I felt even better, and patience paid off. I began losing two pounds every week. By my birthday, I had nearly lost the whole 30 pounds. I felt so good, I dyed my hair blond and bought new clothes—even a new bathing suit, which I hadn't done since my son was born, 17 years ago.

I kept going, and a few weeks after my birthday, I reached my weight goal! A year later, Active Wellness remains a very positive part of my life. I never did go on a 'diet'. I fell in love with yoga and find a few minutes for it every morning. At 50, I look better, I feel better, and best of all, I'm truly *younger* than I was before. If Active Wellness could get me going, I know it will inspire you to find the positive, slimmer you!

Laurie Pollock
**Participant in the Active Wellness Programme
at Ogilvy & Mather**

In September 1997, at 57 and 168 pounds, I was heavier than I had ever been and I didn't feel well at all. I put off going to the doctor—I didn't want to ruin my vacation and the holiday season with bad news about my health. At the New Year, I got a reminder from my doctor that it was time for a checkup. My symptoms were getting worse and I knew it was time to take action. I was diagnosed with adult onset Type 2 Diabetes.

The doctor told me to lose 20 pounds, handed me a diet sheet and told me to come back in one month. I gathered information and learned that, to manage my condition, I needed a diet and an exercise plan. I was scared and didn't know if I had the will power or persistence to take control of my health. I hadn't been exercising. I had tried diets before, but they hadn't worked. I needed a solution that would help me get healthy and stay that way.

Then I found Gayle. She started me on the Active Wellness Programme, and I began to feel better and develop more confidence after the first meeting. I was relieved to discover that I could enjoy my life and live healthfully at the same time. I learned to take one day at a time, set short-term, realistic goals, and make better food choices. I began exercising and before I knew it, I was seeing results! At my one-month checkup I had lost 11 pounds, I felt great, and my diabetic symptoms were almost gone! My doctor told me that if I continued, I would no longer be diabetic. I lost another 15 pounds—my weight is now 142, my waist has gone from a 38 to a 33, my blood sugar is normal and I never had to take medication. People say how terrific I look, and I have more energy than when I was a teen! I now know how to take care of myself, so I'm not concerned with 'falling off the wagon'. I was the least likely candidate for this programme, and if I can do it anybody can!

Art Finkelstein

Participant in the Active Wellness Program at NBC

INTRODUCTION

> *The secret of health for both mind and body is not to mourn for the past, not to worry about the future, nor to anticipate troubles, but to live the present moment wisely and earnestly.*
>
> —Buddha

In the late autumn of 1991, I was happily surrounded by loving friends and family, winding down my graduate studies at New York University, and looking forward to my new career as a nutritionist, chef, and healthcare counsellor. As the last golden days of autumn made their appearance in New York, I was filled with excitement and optimism about the future. Little did I know that my life was about to change, and in ways I never could have imagined.

One balmy October afternoon I stepped up to the service line on one of Central Park's public tennis courts, ready for a friendly game of doubles. The sky was cloudless and the sunlight was dazzling, shimmering off the grass and sparkling off our tennis whites. I lifted my racquet and swung and suddenly, pain seared through my spine, doubling me over.

Later that afternoon, my doctor thoroughly examined my back and found nothing wrong there. But during the exam he did notice that my thyroid was enlarged and sent me to have a series of thyroid tests. Two days later I was back in his office for what I thought would be a routine follow-up visit. Instead, I received a shocking diagnosis: I had thyroid cancer.

Me? Cancer? A young, healthy, active woman? I sat there, stunned, as the doctor told me he had scheduled my surgery in just two weeks. My thyroid would be removed, along with any other cancerous tissue in my neck. Powerful radiation therapy would follow a few months after the surgery.

As I left my doctor's office that morning I felt overwhelmed by my diagnosis and by how swiftly my life had changed—literally overnight. I was no stranger to serious illness and to the toll it takes on people's lives. For almost a year, I had been working with a group called 'God's Love We Deliver'. I had been teaching people with AIDS about diet and nutrition and listening to their stories. Now I understood their overwhelming feelings about becoming seriously ill after taking their health for granted.

Had I, too, taken my good health and strong body for granted? Had I assumed I would always remain healthy and that the future was mine for the taking? I had assumed that staying active, avoiding unhealthy habits, and eating mostly healthful foods were enough to keep me strong and well. That might have been enough for some people, but it wasn't for me.

For one thing, I had ignored the toll that stress takes on the body's immune system. My life had been nothing but stressful for several years as I moved from one city to another, started a new career and returned to graduate school. For another thing, my family had a strong history of both thyroid and heart disease, but I had done nothing specific to offset my susceptibility to those illnesses. I was also working very hard and carrying a heavy load at university. In the exciting whirl of all my new activities, I forgot to observe the most famous of caveats among healthcare professionals: 'Physician, heal thyself!'

> *Since the human body tends to move in the direction*
> *of its expectations—plus or minus—it is important to*
> *know that attitudes of confidence and determination*
> *are no less a part of the treatment programme than*
> *medical science and technology.*
>
> —Norman Cousins

As I stood on the pavement outside my doctor's office on a bright autumn day, trying to digest the news of my cancer, I spent a few moments asking myself, 'Why me?' But I didn't linger long with that thought or spend time feeling sorry for myself. Instead, I realized I was lucky in many ways.

First of all, thyroid cancer is one of the most curable cancers, and mine appeared to have been caught early. I had every intention of surviving my disease, and was confident that my strong healthcare background and training would provide me with the tools I needed to speed up and enhance my recovery.

Secondly, I'm an optimist, a doer and a believer in making things happen. (As a youngster, I even came up with a plan to 'feed the world with tofu'.) All my life I've looked for the hidden opportunities in difficult situations, and I'm convinced that any problem can be managed with the right attitude, the right tools and a lot of determination. I saw my cancer as a challenge and a big wake-up call. Not so much a physical wake-up call—I had been fairly healthy up until my diagnosis—but an emotional one. Faced with the possibility of losing my life for health reasons (something I had never imagined before), I suddenly realized how much I valued life. I not only wanted to live, but I wanted to live healthier. I was utterly convinced that I could use it as an opportunity to transform my life for the better.

Maintaining my optimistic beliefs wasn't always easy, because for the next two weeks nothing about my world was normal or routine. I, who had counselled people about how to take control of their health, now felt as if my own was completely beyond my control. My pre-operative days were filled with doctor's visits, surgical consultations, hospital visits, x-rays, CAT scans, MRIs and numerous blood tests after blood tests.

I knew all this activity was part of the process of fighting my disease, but I hated the fact that it felt like I had no control over my own well-being. During this time I made a vow to myself that I would do everything, whatever it took, to stay out of hospitals in the future. I wasn't sure yet what that 'everything' might entail, but I knew it definitely meant taking better and a more conscious control of my health.

> *To exist is to change, to change is to mature,*
> *to mature is to go on creating oneself endlessly.*
> —Henri Bergson

Ironically, it was on the eve of my surgery, in the quiet of my hospital room, that I had the first of many epiphanies about what I would need to do to be truly healthy again. I would have to pursue a new kind of 'active wellness'. When I left the hospital, this new 'active wellness' would encourage me to change some unhealthy behaviours, make conscious, daily choices about my personal health needs and pursue optimal health as a lifelong goal.

I had already begun some client counselling as part of my graduate work, and had witnessed firsthand how even small lifestyle changes can have a profound effect on a person's health. But in the process, I had failed to notice that my own good health had suffered during the past couple of years due to the various, and major, life changes I had experienced.

I also realized, on that evening before surgery, that if I wanted to be truly healthy again—and realize my dream of teaching others about good health—I needed to make my own healing and recovery the number one priority in my life. This new resolve gave me a powerful sense of empowerment as I waited for surgery. It would stand me in good stead down the line, because in less than 24 hours my first wellness project would become obvious.

When I woke up from surgery the next afternoon and tried to talk to my surgeon, I discovered that my voice was almost gone. I soon learned that only half of my voice box was functioning. The nerve to one of my vocal cords had been severely damaged during surgery in an effort to remove all of the cancerous tissue. Now only one vocal cord nerve was working, and I was unable to raise my voice above a mere whisper. According to the surgeon, 'The nerve was damaged pretty badly.' He couldn't make any guarantees that my voice would ever return to normal.

I had no warning, and no expectation, of this development. Needless to say, I was quite upset. Having half a voice is not the worst thing in the world, especially considering the alternatives. But in my new career as a nutritionist and chef, I also planned to work as a healthcare counsellor, teaching others how to make healthy habits a part of their lives. Especially now, with the new insights about changing my approach to good health that I had gained since I had cancer, I believed I had a strong message to share with others. The message about how we all need to take better control of our physical and emotional well-being. And I needed a strong, healthy voice to proclaim that message.

Determined to get my voice back, I put together a recovery plan to regenerate my damaged vocal nerve as soon I left the hospital. With nutrition as the cornerstone of that plan, I started a daily diet of foods that are high in complete proteins and essential fatty acids—both of which are crucial nutrients needed by the body to repair nerve damage.

In addition to my new diet, I also took a good look at the stress in my life and how I could reduce it. I needed to focus most of my energy on my physical healing, but stress is a true energy zapper. So I consciously cut back on my work load to provide myself with some extra and essential recuperation time. I began meditating daily in order to manage stress better and channel my energy into recovery. Finally, I added some generous dollops of commitment, optimism and sheer determination to my personal programme. And it paid off.

After three months of this regimen, and much to the surprise of my surgeon, my damaged vocal nerve regenerated itself and my voice returned to normal. I was thrilled. I had taken personal control of my health, and I had achieved a major goal on my journey to wellness. Though I didn't consciously realize it yet, I had also begun to put together the components of a powerful new wellness programme that would not only serve me well, but would also help others who wanted to make good health their top priority.

Just as my voice returned in January 1992, I was readmitted to the hospital for radiation treatment to destroy any remaining cancer cells in my body. Fortunately, I was feeling newly empowered about regaining my voice—because the radiation treatment proved to be even harder than the surgery.

> *We shall draw from the heart of suffering itself the*
> *means of inspiration and survival.*
> —Sir Winston Churchill

My radiation therapy involved swallowing a 'radioactive cocktail'—two fluid ounces of a vile-tasting liquid that I sipped through a straw from a lead container! It was hard to believe that drinking such a small amount of liquid could kill cancer cells, but I soon learned that this 'drink' was enormously potent.

From the start I was put into isolation, since I became radioactive as soon as I drank the cocktail. This meant that it wasn't safe for others to be exposed to me. I would have to stay in isolation for three days until the radiation levels in my body dropped low enough so that others around me would be safe.

I also had to deal with the warnings about the potential side effects of the treatment. My entire immune system would be weakened, leaving me vulnerable to infections and even serious diseases, such as lupus. I would feel drained and exhausted. I might even lose my sense of taste—a disaster for a chef! All of these possibilities felt almost scarier than my original diagnosis.

By the time I left the hospital, I was physically sick and emotionally drained. The next few weeks were tough. Ironically, I hadn't even felt sick when I was diagnosed with cancer; but now I did. The radiation treatment left me feeling anything but healthy. Instead, my body felt assaulted and polluted. I was also beginning to experience other side effects from both the surgery and the radiation. Because my thyroid had been removed, my body could no longer produce the thyroid hormone that is essential to regulating metabolism. My system had slowed down considerably, and I was gaining weight daily. Both my memory and my thinking became sluggish, and I had problems getting some of the simplest tasks done. I was 28, but I felt more than twice my age. I longed for the days when I had felt positive and full of energy, but I could barely remember them.

What I did remember, however, was the extraordinary sense of optimism and empowerment that I had experienced when I regained my voice just a few weeks earlier. I wanted to experience those feelings again. Faced with another challenge, I dug deep into my personal resources, discovered new reserves of optimism and resolve, and took another leap of faith on the road to recovery.

> *The old woman I shall become will be quite different*
> *from the woman I am now. Another I is beginning.*
> —George Sand

I was newly determined to get healthy—from the inside out—and I was willing to do anything to achieve my goal. Medicine helped me in the short term, but I knew only I could achieve optimal health in the long term. To do that, I needed a powerful personal healthcare regimen that I could easily integrate into my daily life, and then practise for a lifetime. My academic and clinical backgrounds in nutritional healthcare provided the linchpin of my new healthcare programme, but I also investigated other avenues to healing and health. I embarked on my journey to active wellness in earnest.

As I began to put together my personal active wellness programme, the first thing I did was set some reasonable health goals for myself. My long-term goal, of course, was to stay healthy and prevent any more serious illnesses. My short-term goals were to regain my strength, stamina and normal weight; to enhance my immune system; and to detoxify my body of any remaining radiation and cancer. With my long- and short-term goals as the framework, I designed an Active Wellness programme that was unique to my health needs and concerns. I took into consideration my personal lifestyle, my own medical history of cancer and my family's history of thyroid and heart disease. I then identified four key components that were essential to my Active Wellness programme:

⋄ **Optimal Eating:** My eating plan started with eating at least five high-anti-oxidant fruits and vegetables per day, in order to counteract the oxidative effects of the radiation and to enhance my immune system. Whenever possible, I purchased organically grown fruits and vegetables. I ate no meat but had some seafood. I did not consume any caffeine or refined sugars in any form. The goals of my eating plan were to increase and normalize my energy levels (no more 'ups and downs'), strengthen my stamina, and lower my weight.

⋄ **Exercise:** I began my exercise programme slowly and gently by taking 20-minute walks and doing a simple stretching routine every other morning. As I got stronger, I increased my exercise to 30-minute walks along with a stretching routine every other day, plus light weight training on the alternate days. Within a month I was jogging for at least 30 minutes along with the stretching routine every other day, and toning with light weights on the alternate days.

⋄ **Stress Reduction:** To help counteract the stress in my life, I began meditating every morning after my exercise routines, using deep breathing to help focus my mind.

⋄ **Mental and Emotional Growth:** Another key to my personal wellness programme was my decision to embark on a journey of mental and emotional self-discovery and growth. I used therapy, individual and group, as both client and facilitator, to help identify unhealthy patterns that could be creating obstacles in my life. The self-knowledge and self-esteem I gained in therapy were empowering, allowing me to do away with old negative beliefs and behaviours and focus on pursuing happiness and satisfaction in my life, both in work and in love.

I faithfully practised my Active Wellness programme every day and I felt exhilarated about taking control of my well-being and focusing my personal energy on nurturing myself back to health and happiness. By June, I felt better than I had in years. I had achieved each of my short-term goals—stamina, strength and weight loss—and I knew that my long-term goal of lifelong good health was well within my reach.

Moreover, during the first three months of focused self-healing, I gained a new kind of confidence in the mind-body-spirit approach to health. If the components of my personal active wellness programme worked so wonderfully for me, I was convinced they would work just as well for other people who wanted to achieve good health. If I could do it, they could do it. And who better to teach others how to get well and stay well than someone who had made the successful journey herself?

And so, as I finished up my last few weeks of graduate school, I began to think about designing a more encompassing Active Wellness programme. One that people could easily integrate into their daily lives and realistically practise for a lifetime. And one that a variety of people, with a myriad of health concerns, could custom-design to meet their own unique needs. It would take me almost a year to identify and fully integrate all of the various components that are essential to such a wellness programme, but I began that process during the summer after graduate school.

In June 1992, I took a summer job in the nutrition department at Canyon Ranch Spa in the Berkshire Hills in western Massachusetts. Canyon Ranch is a holistically oriented wellness spa that promotes optimal health not only of the body, but also of the mind and the spirit. Guests attend hands-on educational seminars about various aspects of wellness, and are introduced to a variety of health and healing disciplines that treat the 'whole' person—physically, mentally, and spiritually. Canyon Ranch's holistic approach to good health struck a resonant chord in me, and helped broaden the scope of my personal wellness programme.

My personal health programme during the previous spring was grounded primarily in the conventional scientific benefits of nutrition, diet and simple exercise. But at Canyon Ranch I experienced for the first time the power of the holistic approach to good health and the appeal of an environment devoted to healing the whole person. I began to learn in-depth about the health benefits of yoga, meditation, t'ai chi, biofeedback, therapeutic massage, and aromatherapy, among other disciplines. I incorporated many of these alternative approaches into my personal wellness programme. Later, I applied them to my Active Wellness programme as complements to the nutrition and exercise components.

These additions to my Active Wellness programme were, I believe, critical to its later success. My graduate work with clients over the past year had convinced me that people are more likely to stick to a new health programme if they are given a variety of choices within the conventional requirements of good nutrition, low-fat foods, and physical exercise. The various alternative health methods I studied at Canyon Ranch provided exactly the type of variety I sought. Yoga, for example, with its focus on gentle stretching and deep breathing, is an excellent complement to an aerobic exercise plan, a stress management programme, or a combination of the two.

My one concern about the holistic health spa approach was that it reached only a limited audience, one that could afford both the cost and the time away from home and job that the experience demanded. I envisioned my Active Wellness programme as being widely accessible to all people and easily integrated into the daily routine of home and work.

> *Opportunities multiply as they are seized; they*
> *die when neglected. Life is a long line of opportunities.*
> —John Wicker

While continuing my work at Canyon Ranch, I completed my dietetic internship at the Bronx Veterans Administration Medical Center, associated with Mount Sinai Hospital in New York City. Choosing to remain in New York City full time, I began work as a licensed and registered dietitian at Beth Israel Medical Center, as the nutritionist for the Dr. Dean Ornish Lifestyle Programme for Reversing Heart Disease. Dr Ornish is the famed cardiologist and best-selling author of *Dr. Dean Ornish's Programme for Reversing Heart Disease* and *Love & Survival: The Scientific Basis for the Healing Power of Intimacy.* In 1990 he created a sensation in both medicine and the media by publishing research demonstrating that serious heart disease, including blocked arteries, could be reversed non-surgically through a combination of lifestyle changes including a no-fat-added vegetarian diet, exercise, group support and a stress management programme.

While working with Dr Ornish for the next two years, I witnessed firsthand the remarkable changes that occur in people with serious heart disease when they adhere to Dr Ornish's programme of disease reversal. But, like the Canyon Ranch health spa experience, Dr Ornish's programme was also expensive and limited to a select number of people, or those who were covered by their health insurance.

In the early 1990s, health insurance companies would only cover the cost of D. Ornish's programme if the patient had serious heart disease. This policy excluded many individuals who were at increased risk for serious heart disease due to high blood pressure, elevated cholesterol or family medical history—all of whom would have benefited greatly from a preventive programme such as Dr Ornish's. Also excluded—unless they had heart disease—were people with other serious health concerns, such as diabetes and cancer, who wanted and needed to learn the wellness skills that could optimize their health and perhaps prevent future illness.

I saw clearly that these people, and many others outside the hospital arena, needed a less costly but still comprehensive wellness programme to address their unique healthcare needs while also teaching them new, healthy lifestyle skills that would last a lifetime. The programme also had to be flexible and easily integrated into a person's daily routine. My Active Wellness programme met all those requirements.

I formally launched the Active Wellness programme at the National Broadcasting Corporation (NBC) in New York: I led the first classes for their employees in the spring of 1993. After that, I had numerous corporate clients. In cooperation with the New York affiliate of the American Heart Association, I ran Active Wellness programmes at McGraw-Hill, Ogilvy & Mather, Sony and several YWCAs throughout New York. In the spring of 1996, I introduced the Active Wellness Programme at the Beth Israel Medical Center as part of their Wellness Center, alongside the Dean Ornish Programme. It was available to any hospital staff or patient who wanted to try a new kind of wellness weight management programme.

Active Wellness was well received by all its participants as a welcome new approach to long-term success in weight management and healthy living. People appreciated its comprehensive and innovative approach, recognizing that optimal health is a balance of body, mind and spirit. Not only was the programme effective long term, but each person in the programme began to feel healthier and more energetic within a few weeks. As participants achieved their goals, they found themselves feeling younger, stronger, and more attractive than they had in years. A big bonus was that participants didn't feel like they were following a depriving diet, but rather they were on 'a satisfying plan to feel their best and take care of themselves'.

By the summer of 1996, Active Wellness became my full-time career. As a complement to the wellness programme, I also launched the Active Wellness Gourmet in January 1997. Based in New York City, the Active Wellness Gourmet prepares and delivers delicious, nutritious gourmet lunches and dinners to busy but health-conscious individuals who would rather focus their energy and time on fitness and stress management than on cooking meals.

The hallmark of the Active Wellness programme—and the reason for its success—is its recognition that no one diet, exercise regimen, stress management plan or behavioural change can possibly be right for everybody. Individuals have unique healthcare needs, based on their own health history, their family's medical history and their personal lifestyles. Different people also have different healthcare goals within the structure of the same programme. The Active Wellness programme recognizes and honours all healthcare goals and, indeed, celebrates the fact that the path travelled on to optimal health is as unique and multifaceted as the travellers themselves.

> *Dream lofty dreams, and as you dream, so shall you become. Your vision is the promise of what you shall at last unveil.*
>
> —John Ruskin

I am happy to say that seven years after my initial diagnosis of cancer, I have reached my ultimate goal from the outset of my wellness journey: I am happy, healthy and strong. Furthermore, I have so integrated Active Wellness into my daily life that I

now live at my peak level of body-mind-spirit health. Early in my wellness programme, I discovered the health practices that worked for me, that I most enjoyed and
that I could maintain on a long-term basis. They include:

⋄ **An Individualized Eating Plan:** I eat three low-fat meals a day, and I
limit myself to one animal protein meal a day at most. The only animal
protein I eat is seafood and I have recently made soya a bigger part of my
diet. I try to eat at least five servings of fruits and vegetables each day. I do
not drink caffeine. With my meals, I take the vitamins and flaxseed as
recommended in the Active Wellness Guidelines. Occasionally, I have a
dessert that is low in sugar and fat.

⋄ **Running and Weight Training:** I jog every other day for 45 minutes,
accompanied by a 10-minute stretching routine. I may vary my jogging
routine by cycling, rollerblading or taking a cross-training class. On
alternate days, I do weight training and yoga. I also enjoy Latin dancing in
addition to my normal exercise routines.

⋄ **Yoga and Meditation:** I meditate six out of seven mornings a week, after
my workouts and preferably outside. I also do yoga two or three times a
week, on the days when I am not jogging. I use meditation to 'de-stress'
my mind and yoga to 'de-stress' my muscles.

⋄ **A Weekly Support Group:** To keep myself in optimal mental health, I
attend a weekly support group where I continue to work on changing old
behavioural patterns while pursuing self-knowledge, self-esteem and
self-empowerment.

My current wellness schedule takes about one-and-a-half hours each day. This may
seem like a great deal of time, but the benefits greatly outweigh the time invested. I am
able to approach each day with less stress and greater mental focus. I am able to
accomplish more in less time without feeling exhausted at the end of the day. Many
people are amazed at the amount of energy I have. It comes from my genuine excitement about what I'm doing with my life and how good I feel when I'm doing it.

Make no mistake, though, integrating Active Wellness into my life on a daily basis
took concentrated effort and patience. It wasn't always easy to make health my priority, but I learned how to stay focused. What helped me move forward on my journey
was the promise I made to myself at the outset: to make living the Active Wellness
lifestyle a personal priority. Indeed, I felt great as I took control of my health. As I
accomplished each goal, I gained renewed confidence in the fact that I could achieve
anything I set out to do. By focusing on my own goals, I was able to channel my per-

sonal energy into nurturing myself to health, happiness and satisfaction in all aspects of my life.

The Active Wellness programme will help you, too, to focus on your personal health goals and learn to channel your energy into taking care of yourself. It is never too late to achieve your personal level of optimum health. I have had clients embrace the Active Wellness lifestyle at 30, 40, 50, 60, 70 and 80 years of age.

Active Wellness is for anyone at any age, because you can choose a plan that meets your personal taste in food, and your comfort level in exercise and stress management. Your personal goals will help you build the foundation of a programme that works with your lifestyle—at your own pace. You learn how to take care of yourself and your health, regardless of your lifestyle obstacles. If you have children and a job, your Active Wellness programme will work with your schedule, just as it will also work for someone in their sixties looking forward to retirement, or someone in their thirties who may be working long hours and beginning a family. You may identify with some or all of these scenarios. How we feel about ourselves and our health is a concern that is not age dependent. Pursuing optimal health empowers and energizes you to live life at your absolute best, just as hundreds of my programme participants have been doing for years.

Right now you may be saying to yourself, *I've done this before, over and over again, and I never succeed.*

But this time you will, if you follow my lead and each of the 10 steps of the programme. In fact, as your Active Wellness guide, I invite you to make a 'paradigm shift' in your concept of healthy living. Regardless of how many programmes you have tried, you can succeed in meeting your personal health goals and feel satisfied with your healthy lifestyle. I plan to show you how. Whether you're concerned about staying well, managing weight, lowering cholesterol, controlling diabetes, eating a healthy vegetarian diet, or changing unhealthy behaviours, the Active Wellness programme helps guide you through a personal plan of mind-body-spirit wellness that is custom-designed for your unique health needs. And you don't have to pay expensive spa prices or hire a personal trainer.

Active Wellness is designed to fit easily into your daily schedule, so that your wellness programme eventually becomes a natural and lifelong routine. In the process, you will learn how to balance your mental and physical well-being with the demands of your career and family.

The 10 steps of the Active Wellness programme are designed to give you the maximum effect in the shortest period of time—10 weeks. By the end of these 10 weeks, regardless of your lifestyle, health and ageing concerns, you will have acquired all the tools you'll need to maximize your health and pursue optimal wellness for a lifetime.

Together we will develop an owner's manual for your body. We will look at your personal health history, your family's health history and your current lifestyle. Then we will determine the best possible path to wellness for your needs. You will set for yourself some long-term and short-term health goals along that path. Step by step, the Active Wellness programme will provide you with the education, strategies, and tools to reach those goals. Week by week, you will learn new information about nutrition, exercise, stress management, and behavioural change—and you will learn how to integrate these four components of the programme into your daily life. Finally, you will learn how to maintain your new healthy behaviours for the rest of your life.

By the end of the book, you will have the tools you need to maximize any personal health goal—whether it is becoming more fit, more heart healthy or less prone to highs and lows in your energy. By completing the 10 steps of the programme you will, perhaps for the first time in your life, feel in control of your health. You will be well on the road to experiencing Active Wellness for life. May it be as richly rewarding and exhilarating for you as it has been for me.

Gayle Reichler
New York City
Spring 1998

STEP 1

Mentally Preparing Yourself for the Wellness Journey

We are what and where we are because we have first imagined it.
—Donald Curtis

The first step in your Active Wellness journey is to believe you will succeed in achieving your health goals and that you will feel better than you have felt in years. If you have tried other weight-loss or wellness programmes before that have not worked for you, don't despair. You can succeed with Active Wellness!

Participants in the programme have overcome obstacles that frustrated them for years, including craving unhealthy foods and not finding time in their hectic schedule to exercise or relax. The Active Wellness programme works because it's not a diet: it's an energizing, satisfying, healthy way of living, personally designed for you! The Active Wellness programme is founded on several fundamental principles:

⬧ Health should be your top priority.
⬧ Health is available to anyone who is willing to make the commitment.
⬧ Health is an integration of body, mind and spirit.
⬧ Health is best achieved long term if the programme is personalized to fit *your* needs and lifestyle.

With these fundamentals in mind, take a few moments to think about all the things in your life that are most important to you. Is good health near the top of the list? It should be, because living in a state of optimal health makes almost everything else in your life better. If your wellness isn't a priority, you may never be able to live life at your finest. The Active Wellness programme teaches you how to take action to reach your individual health goals, one step at a time. Before you know it, you will see results, whether it be losing weight, lowering high cholesterol, increasing strength, reducing high blood pressure or managing stress.

The Active Wellness programme is a uniquely designed lifetime programme of good health that requires daily practice and commitment. In this programme, wellness isn't simply a goal: It is a way of life and a state of being. The Active Wellness programme doesn't end when you lose those last two stone or complete a 10-kilometre race with energy to spare. Instead, the Active Wellness programme encourages you to practise healthy behaviours throughout your life and, if necessary, to continually reevaluate yourself in order to sustain an optimal level of mind-body-spirit wellness.

Unlike other wellness plans, the Active Wellness programme is custom-designed to fit your unique health and fitness needs based on your current health concerns, your personal medical history, your family's medical history and your individual lifestyle. The early stages of making healthful changes, however good they may be for you, can be challenging.

> *Once begun, a task is easy; half the work is done.*
> —Horace

Taking time to mentally prepare yourself for the Active Wellness journey is a critical step on the road to optimal health. Every successful endeavour first begins in the mind as an idea, a thought, a dream, a conviction. As any great athlete, entrepreneur or performer will tell you, 'You can't do it if your head's not in it.' You also can't do it if you don't know where you're going, or why, or how you're going to get there. Many well-intentioned people have set out to make great changes or accomplish a singular task, only to give up in the early stages because their goals and methods were unfocused, unrealistic or simply impossible. Pursuing wellness is no different than pursuing any goal—except that it may be the most important goal you ever pursue.

As you begin your Active Wellness journey, you need to be crystal clear about what you want to achieve for yourself and how you're going to get it. This chapter is about helping you find that mental clarity and mapping out a strategy for success. Taking this critical step enables the rest of the programme to fall, step by step, spontaneously and logically in place.

As your Active Wellness guide, I can provide you with empowering new knowledge about wellness, basic tools for transforming unhealthy behaviours into healthy ones and abundant encouragement along the way. But only you can do the mental homework that provides the four essential ingredients of any successful endeavour:

- ◇ Vision
- ◇ Planning
- ◇ Time
- ◇ Commitment

These four ingredients form the framework of your Active Wellness journey. They give it purpose, breadth, energy and depth. They provide you with the impetus to begin your journey and the staying power to stick to the path for the long term, despite rough spots and roadblocks. Ultimately, they support your wellness journey for a lifetime. Let's look at each of these ingredients for success and at how they frame and support your Active Wellness programme.

> *First say to yourself what you would be; and then do*
> *what you have to do.*
> —Epictetus

Vision

Take a moment, close your eyes, and conjure up a magnificent vision of yourself in your mind's eye. This vision is not only everything you always wanted to be, but everything you were always meant to be: radiant with health, energy and confidence—on your own unique terms. Guard this vision and hold it close to your heart. It is the reason you picked up this book and have started the Active Wellness journey. It is your motivation behind all the hard effort required to change. It is your impetus for starting down the wellness path as well as your reward for successfully completing the journey. This is a vision of a new, healthful you. Who will that new you be?

Envisioning a New You
A strong mental image of how you want to look and feel at the end of the Active Wellness journey can be a great motivating tool as you progress through each step of your training programme. Clearly you want to be a 'winner'. So for starters, picture yourself at an imaginary finish line, arms raised triumphantly over your head, a broad smile on your face. This triumphant vision is the reward you are working toward.

But who is this 'winner' crossing the finish line? What do you look like? How do you feel? How different are you, inside and outside, from the person who began the race? Asking yourself some pointed questions may help you clarify the vision of yourself you want to see cross the finish line. (Often, the answers reflect what you'd like to change about your current health, appearance and lifestyle.) Other successful Active Wellness participants have asked themselves the following kinds of questions:

- Will I look thinner?
- Will I stop needing my blood pressure medication?
- Will I lower my cholesterol?
- Will I have my blood sugars under control?
- Will I feel less stressed?
- Will I have more energy?
- Will I walk up a flight of stairs without feeling winded?
- Will I wear that suit I bought last year that I can't fit into now?

Ask yourself similar questions or come up with new ones of your own. Then turn those questions into answers—into strong, active and confident statements of belief. Those answers, those beliefs, are part of your Active Wellness vision—the mental images that get you to the starting gate, carry you through the race and send you joyfully across the finish line. The more vivid and clear your images, the more successful you will be in achieving them. Below are some sample Active Wellness images from other individuals who have mastered the programme.

Sample Active Wellness Images
- ◊ I have more energy.
- ◊ I am stronger.
- ◊ I am leaner.
- ◊ I am medication free.
- ◊ I am easily jogging three miles.
- ◊ I am radiating joy and good health.

Now create some Active Wellness images that are uniquely yours. What do you want to achieve from the Active Wellness programme? Think of the above questions that you asked yourself, and turn some of those questions into vivid and positive answers. Write them in the space below or on a card.

Your Active Wellness Images
- ◊ _____
- ◊ _____
- ◊ _____
- ◊ _____

These are the images to carry in your mind's eye throughout the Active Wellness programme—your visual goals. They include various aspects of your vision that you will work towards in each step of your wellness journey. As such, they serve several critical purposes:

- ◊ They inspire you to create attainable long- and short-term health goals.
- ◊ They encourage you to create an eating, fitness and stress-reduction plan that is tailored to your unique needs.
- ◊ They motivate you to find time to follow and practise your Active Wellness programme.
- ◊ They reinforce your commitment to finishing the wellness journey, however bumpy the road may get.

Carry your Active Wellness images in your wallet or purse or post them on your refrigerator door or office bulletin board. Share them with your family and friends and ask them for their support. Taken together, your Active Wellness images are a composite of the new you envisioned at the start of this chapter. You may want to create a self-portrait of that vision—or find a photograph that closely resembles it—and carry that with you as well.

> *Everything's in the mind. That's where it all starts.*
> *Knowing what you want is the first step toward getting it.*
> —Mae West

Having Realistic Expectations

I offer you one warning. Be realistic about your vision of the new you and about the Active Wellness images that you create. You may defeat yourself at the outset of the Active Wellness journey if you have unrealistic expectations about how much you can achieve and how long it will take.

Of course, believing in your new image of yourself is crucial, but make sure that image is also attainable. If you took up playing a new instrument, you wouldn't expect to be performing concert-level sonatas in just 10 weeks. No matter how confident you were and how hard you practised, you would still be a beginner for quite some time until you developed the necessary skills to advance to the next level.

Similarly, you can't remould your body into an entirely new entity without a realistic investment of time and energy. Don't expect to lose a stone in one week on the Active Wellness programme; that would be unhealthy. But you can lose an average of two pounds a week safely, and be well on the way to a leaner and healthier you as you continue to practise your programme. If you're walking for exercise now, expect to increase your strength and stamina in 10 weeks, enabling you to run a mile or more, but not a marathon.

Trust your instincts about how far you need to go to realize the vision of a new you. Most people have an innate sense about what they can achieve for themselves in terms of their health. I have had clients who, over time, returned to their college weight, dramatically lowered their cholesterol, improved their heart health and completely eliminated their need for medication.

Keep your expectations realistic, and you won't be disappointed in the long run. If you try to accomplish too much too soon, you may feel defeated and tempted to give up. Following is a brief self-assessment designed to determine how realistic you are about achieving your vision of a healthier and happier you.

Self-Assessment of Realistic Expectations

◊ I am a unique individual and what works for
other people may not work for me. _____ Yes _____ No

◊ I need to establish my own custom-tailored
plan for Active Wellness. _____ Yes _____ No

◊ I need to make my health goals a top
priority in order to succeed. _____ Yes _____ No

◊ I need to be ready to take action and make
changes or I may not achieve my goals. _____ Yes _____ No

◊ I understand that changing habits takes time. _____ Yes _____ No

◊ If I try to accomplish too many goals at one
time I may not accomplish anything. _____ Yes _____ No

◊ It is healthier to lose weight and start a new
fitness programme slowly rather than quickly. _____ Yes _____ No

◊ It is easier to lose weight, get fit and maintain
a sense of well-being when I combine nutrition,
fitness, and stress management into an
integrated programme. _____ Yes _____ No

◊ Support from close friends and family helps
me achieve my goals. _____ Yes _____ No

The answer to all the above questions is 'Yes'. If you answered 'Yes' to all or most of these questions, you are ready to take the Active Wellness journey, one step at a time, beginning with setting realistic long- and short-term health goals.

> *Reach high, for stars lie hidden in your soul.*
> *Dream deep, for every dream precedes the goal.*
> —Pamela Vaull Starr

Planning

Now that you have a clear mental vision of the person you want to be at the end of your Active Wellness journey, you probably also have an idea of what you need to do to attain your vision. Now is the time to reframe that idea into clear and realistic long-

and short-term goals that you can accomplish one step at a time. You also need to further refine those goals by evaluating your personal health and lifestyle and then your family's health history. Let's start with setting your goals.

Establishing Your Destination: Setting a Long-Term Goal

First, establish a primary, or long-term, health goal that encompasses the vision you are trying to achieve while also becoming your main health objective. Similar to your vision of a new you, your long-term health goal drives your entire Active Wellness programme and urges you onward towards success.

Your long-term goal is also the rationale behind the choices you make about a specific eating plan, fitness regimen, stress-reduction routine and behaviour modification programme. Your long-term goal must be realistic and attainable. Examples of common and realistic long-term goals are:

- Losing weight
- Lowering cholesterol
- Reducing blood pressure
- Normalizing blood sugars
- Increasing strength and flexibility
- Managing stress

You may choose to make your long-term goals more detailed and individualistic, such as fitting into a smaller size or overcoming the need for blood pressure medication. But remember to tackle only one primary goal at a time—you don't want to become overwhelmed or defeat your good intentions before you even have a chance to start your wellness journey. The short-term goals that you establish are designed to counteract that negative effect. They make the process of achieving your primary goal more manageable and enjoyable.

> *I long to accomplish a great and noble task, but it is*
> *my chief duty to accomplish small tasks as if they were*
> *great and noble.*
> —Helen Keller

Getting to Your Destination: Setting Short-Term Goals

You also need to develop some short-term goals, which help you realize your primary goal. The short-term goals you set for yourself serve to both support your long-term goal and provide you with benchmarks along the path to optimal wellness. These checkpoints enable you to measure your success one small step at a time.

For example, if your long-term goal is weight loss, your short-term goals might be:

⋄ Walk half a mile every evening
⋄ Eat two fruits a day instead of dessert
⋄ Eat fish instead of meat at least two nights a week

In this scenario, you are not only losing weight, you are becoming physically fit, lowering your fat intake (and probably your cholesterol at the same time), and taking preventive measures against heart disease and cancer. You are well on your way to realizing optimal wellness and achieving your primary goal at the same time.

Effectively Wording Your Short-Term Goals

While your long-term goal may be generalized and broad in scope, your short-term goals need to be concrete, specific, and include parameters of achievements, since they are meant to give you direction and to serve as benchmarks when checking your progress. Choosing the right words for your short-term goals markedly increases your chances for success. Notice that each effectively phrased goal includes an action followed by a measurable time, quantity, or distance. Below are some examples of effective words and phrases for framing your short-term goals.

Effective Words for Framing Your Goals
⋄ I will *increase* my stamina/strength/energy.
⋄ I will *lower* my blood pressure/cholesterol.
⋄ I will *reduce* my weight/my fat intake.
⋄ I will *eliminate* junk food/sugary desserts.
⋄ I will *limit* my meat intake.
⋄ I will *add* more fruits and vegetables to my diet.

Effectively Phrased Goals
⋄ I will reduce my weight by two stone.
⋄ I will develop a new eating plan to lower my cholesterol in six months.
⋄ I will add two fruits to my diet each day.
⋄ I will walk two miles a day.

Ineffectively Phrased Goals
⋄ I want to be thin.
⋄ I have to control my cholesterol and blood pressure.
⋄ I must become less stressed.

Take a moment now to fill in the Goal Chart below. This is an important step because when you write down your goals you acknowledge them concretely and underscore your desire to achieve them.

No doubt you have a clear long-term goal in mind. Write that down now. You may also have a good idea of the short-term goals you would like to achieve. If so, write those down as well. If you're not sure at this point about all of the short-term goals you want to pursue, leave that section blank until later in your Active Wellness programme. After assessing your personal health and your family's health history, or after starting your eating plan or fitness regimen, you may have a better idea of some practical short-term goals.

As you begin to practise short-term health goals, consider keeping a wellness journal to chart your successes. The more you recognize your achievements, the better you will feel about the programme and, more importantly, about yourself.

Goal Chart

Long-Term Goal:

◇ _____

Short-Term Goals:

◇ _____

◇ _____

◇ _____

◇ _____

Our plans miscarry because they have no aim. When a man does not know what harbour he is making for, no wind is the right wind.
—Seneca

Assessing Your Personal Health History and Lifestyle

As mentioned earlier, you may want to modify your short-term health goals after assessing your personal health, your lifestyle, and your family's health history. The Personal Health History and the Lifestyle Assessment and the Family Medical History Chart all include illness and nutrition assessments that significantly affect your personalized wellness plan, and therefore your long- and short-term goals.

Please take the time to answer the questions on pages 34-36. Write your answers in the spaces provided, so you will have a record of your health history and lifestyle at the beginning of your Active Wellness programme. As you answer each question, record the points that correspond to your answers on a separate piece of paper. At the end of the Personal Health History and the Lifestyle Assessment, tally your points to determine your needs for the Active Wellness programme.

A Note on Cholesterol and Triglycerides

If you haven't had your cholesterol and triglycerides checked, or if you don't know the breakdown of the types of cholesterol, I recommend that you contact your doctor. Ask him or her to check your cholesterol and triglycerides, and to thoroughly explain the numbers to you. Compare the numbers with the acceptable ranges listed in the chart below. Please note whether your numbers are high, low or normal. Then fill in your results to categories 1 and 2 under Personal Health History.

Recommended Cholesterol and Triglyceride Levels

Cholesterol	In mg/dl	Risk Level
Low-Density Lipoprotein (LDL Cholesterol):	<100	Desirable (with heart disease)
	<130	Desirable (if no heart disease)
	130 to 159	Borderline High
	>160	High
High-Density Lipoprotein (HDL Cholesterol):	<35	High Risk
	36 to 59	Desirable
	>60	Most Desirable
Total Cholesterol:	150-200	**Desirable**
	200-220	**Borderline High**
	>220	**High**
Total Cholesterol/HDL Ratio:	<3.0	Desirable
	3.0-4.0	Borderline High
	>4.0	High
Triglycerides:	<200	Normal
	200 to 400	Borderline High
	400 to 1,000	High
	>1,000	Very High

(These numbers are based on fasting plasma triglyceride levels.)

Personal Health History

1. Please record your current cholesterol levels:
   a. Total cholesterol____ (If >200 mg/dl, give yourself 0 points; if your levels are <200 give yourself 5 points.)
   b. Your HDL cholesterol____ (If <35 mg/dl, give yourself 0 points; if your levels are >35 give yourself 5 points.)
   c. Your LDL cholesterol____ (If >130 mg/dl, give yourself 0 points; if your levels are <130 give yourself 5 points.)

2. Please record your triglycerides____ (If >200 mg/dl, give yourself 0 points; if your levels are normal give yourself 5 points.)

3. Alcohol intake:____ drinks per day
   (Use the following point scale for alcohol: 0-1 drink/day = 5 points; 2 or 3 drinks/day = 2 points; 3 to 5 drinks/day = 0 points.)

4. Tobacco intake:____ nonsmoker (5 points)
   ____ quit smoking (3 points)
   ____ smoker (0 points)

5. Exercise:
   If your exercise routine includes:
   a.____ Aerobic exercise

0 times/week	(0 points)
1 or 2 times/week	(3 points)
3 or 4 times/week	(5 points)

   b.____ Strength training

0 times/week	(0 points)
1 time/week	(2 points)
2 times/week	(4 points)
3 or more times/week	(5 points)

   c.____ Stretching exercise

0 times/week	(0 points)
1 or 2 times/week	(2 points)
3 or 4 times/week	(4 points)
every day	(5 points)

PERSONAL HEALTH HISTORY SUBTOTAL: _____

Lifestyle Assessment

1. Over the course of a week, how would you describe your overall energy level? Rate your energy level, based on the scale listed below. At one end of the spectrum is 'Full of Energy' (5 points), and at the other is 'Exhausted (1 point). Indicate how you feel most of the time:

Full of Energy   5   4   3   2   1   **Exhausted**

2. Over the course of a week, how would you describe your overall stress level? Rate your stress level based on the scale listed below. At one end of the spectrum you are 'Stress Free' (such as relaxing on holiday with no worries). At the other extreme is 'Highly Stressed' (at the end of your rope and about to blow a fuse). Three is neutral. Pick the place on the continuum from 1 to 5 that describes how you most often feel during the course of a week:

Stress Free   5   4   3   2   1   **Highly Stressed**

3. How well do you sleep? (tick the one that applies to you)
   _____ I almost always get the amount of sleep I need; I rarely feel tired. (5 points)
   _____ I feel tired because I usually get a few hours too little sleep each night. (2 points)
   _____ I never get the amount of sleep I need and I am always tired. (0 points)

4. When you eat, are you:
   a. Eating on the run?
      _____ Yes (0 points)
      _____ No (5 points)
      _____ Sometimes (2 points)
   b. Eating when you're not hungry?
      _____ Yes (0 points)
      _____ No (5 points)
      _____ Sometimes (2 points)

5. When you eat, do you:
   a. Eat quickly (finish your meal within 10 to 15 minutes)?
      _____ Yes (0 points)
      _____ No (5 points)
      _____ Sometimes (2 points)

b. Skip meals?
____ Yes (0 points)
____ No (5 points)
____ Sometimes (2 points)
c. Eat late (after 9.00 p.m.)?
____ Yes (0 points)
____ No (5 points)
____ Sometimes (2 points)

LIFESTYLE ASSESSMENT SUBTOTAL: ____

PERSONAL HEALTH HISTORY AND LIFESTYLE ASSESSMENT TOTAL: ____

When you tally the total points in your Personal Health History and Lifestyle Assessment, you get a good picture of how well you are living an Active Wellness lifestyle. For example:

⬥ If your score is **85**, you are doing an excellent job at maintaining Active Wellness and can use the programme to achieve an even better level of optimal mind-body-spirit health.

⬥ If your score is **60-84**, you are doing fairly well at living an Active Wellness lifestyle, but you have some room for improvement. Use the programme as your guide to incorporate the changes you need in order to achieve your optimal level of mind-body-spirit health.

⬥ If your score is **41-59**, you are not doing very well at living an Active Wellness lifestyle, and you are putting yourself at risk for further health complications. You stand to gain greatly from your Active Wellness programme.

⬥ If your score is **2-40**, you are leading a lifestyle of high health risk. You will feel healthier as you progress in your Active Wellness programme. By following the programme you can improve your chances of reducing disease risks. The lower the numbers in the categories above, the greater your health risks.

Your Family's Health History: Charting Your Susceptibility to Disease

The personal assessment you've just completed gives you a clear indication of where you are vulnerable or at high risk because of your current medical conditions and lifestyle choices. But another critical component of the planning stage of your Active Wellness programme is assessing your genetic predisposition to certain diseases and medical conditions. This predisposition is linked to your family's history of illness.

Like our fingerprints, each of us is unique, based on our genetic makeup. Diseases that appear in our adult years can occur when genes we inherited from our family members are triggered by a variety of environmental factors—some within our control, such as diet and unhealthy behaviour, and some beyond our control, such as environmental pollution. Such diseases are considered *multifactorial* because, in addition to your genetic predisposition, diet, physical activity, healthy or unhealthy lifestyle choices and environmental exposures also play a part.

The multifactorial diseases that arise most frequently in adulthood include most forms of heart disease, cancer, non-insulin-dependent diabetes, obesity, and hypertension. The sooner you become aware of your genetic predisposition to specific diseases, the sooner you are able to put together a preventive healthcare programme. That programme should minimize your health risk factors for those diseases and maximize your resistance to them.

In order to determine any diseases and medical conditions that you are genetically predisposed to, chart your family's medical history. Using the chart on page 43, start with yourself and your first-degree relatives (parents and siblings). Then go down the list of medical conditions and diseases and place an 'F' for each condition or disease that has occurred. Do this first for yourself, then your father, your mother, and/or your siblings. Go through the same procedure for your second-degree relatives (grandparents, aunts, uncles and/or cousins), placing an 'S' in the appropriate boxes.

Check to see whether you have two first-degree relatives with the same condition or disease, or three or more first- and second-degree relatives with the same condition or disease. If you do, you may have an increased predisposition to that illness yourself. Use this information in Step 2 when you are choosing the Active Wellness Eating Plan that is best suited for you.

The medical histories on the more senior members of your family, even if they are deceased, are especially important. Many individuals display their most critical genetic health-risk traits at an older age. Knowing about these can help you discover health-risk traits in yourself before they become obvious.

On my family health chart, I had thyroid cancer, my cousin had hyperthyroidism and my younger sister was diagnosed with Hashimoto's thyroiditis hypothyroid. Clearly, our family's thyroid gene is undergoing a type of genetic alteration.

If you discover a medical trait that appears three times or more on your family's chart, don't panic. Simply be aware of the situation and inform your doctor of your discovery. Diseases run along a continuum, so you may exhibit tendencies toward a disease, but never have the full-blown symptoms. For example, you may have parents who are diabetic, while you are sensitive to sugar highs and lows.

In some cases, full-blown symptoms of a disease may not appear unless your body undergoes prolonged or severe stress and your resistance to disease decreases. Whether or not you get a disease also depends on the impact of a variety of factors. The air and pollutants you breathe and ingest, the foods you eat, the toxins you're exposed to, the unhealthy behaviours you indulge in, and the medicines you do or don't take all take their toll.

As you begin to build your Active Wellness programme, you can continually use your family health history chart as a reference. If you find some common disease traits among your family members, your Active Wellness programme will be custom-designed to help you reduce your risk for that trait through a conscious preventive wellness programme of appropriate diet, exercise and stress management.

As you've been mentally preparing yourself for the Active Wellness journey, you may have noticed that the first two ingredients of a successful journey—vision and planning—are fairly easy to grasp. We all have a pretty good idea of how we want to look and feel, and we certainly believe that the pursuit of wellness is a worthy aim. When we trust our instincts and create realistic expectations, we get a good sense of the specific health goals we need to set in order to achieve Active Wellness.

But the last two ingredients of a successful journey—time and commitment—are tougher hurdles to clear. First, take a look at time.

Time

Linda started the programme because she wanted to lose weight. She was a nurse working 46 hours a week, commuting to and from work three hours a day, five days a week, and had a husband and two children at home. Linda had difficulty figuring out when she was going to find time for herself and her programme. The answer was her lunch hour. Once she identified that island of time for herself, Linda savoured it every day, using it to practise various components of her programme. When she finished her Active Wellness programme, she had achieved all the goals she had set for herself—at her own pace.

A common concern among new Active Wellness participants is that they never seem to have enough time for the little things in life, let alone a comprehensive wellness programme. But if Linda can do it, so can you! And the enormous benefits to your physical, mental, emotional and spiritual health far outweigh the initial time you invest.

Still, one of the first and greatest challenges of most Active Wellness participants is carving out a block of time in their schedule for practising their programmes every day. Why is this?

Why Finding Time for Yourself Is Difficult

Most of us work harder and longer hours than our parents and grandparents did. We manage homes and careers in a results-oriented world that pushes us to perform and produce faster and faster each day. In addition to that, many of us are taking care of our children and our parents, and juggling home, job and community commitments. Without a doubt, we don't have much time to ourselves. But in many cases, we have only ourselves to blame. We've traded on time in the name of success and security. Worse, when we sacrifice our bodies and souls on the altar of time and success, we often ignore the price we're paying in diminished health.

The Price You Pay for Trading on Time

We are dying for lack of time in our lives. We are exhausted, but we ignore the signals our bodies send us. Feeling tired, having headaches and heartburn, and experiencing tension and anxiety have become normal states. We drink coffee to stay awake, order fast food because we worked too late, drink alcohol to relax and smoke cigarettes to soothe our nerves. Ironically, we seem to have no problem developing time-consuming bad habits that put even more stress on our exhausted bodies and souls. In the process, we increase our risk for heart disease, diabetes, cancer, stroke and other illnesses.

We must make time for ourselves! We can start by getting our priorities straight.

Setting Your Priorities

When we don't find time for Active Wellness in our lives, the trade-off in bad health is enormous. We need to find that time—and find it fast!

Incredibly, many of us think nothing of investing hours in research and then days and weeks in shopping for a new car or a refrigerator. But we baulk at the idea of carving out 30 minutes a day to do something healthful for ourselves.

Yet you have the power to choose your priorities. Family, work, and friends are important—perhaps the most important in your life. But they all will be seriously threatened, if not entirely lost, if your health is irreparably damaged because you didn't find time to practise wellness in your life. By all means, keep family and work, partner and children, lovers and friends your top priorities. But make good health and Active Wellness an unshakable top priority.

Things which matter most must never be at the mercy
of things which matter least.
　　　　　　　　　　　　—Johann Wolfgang von Goethe

Making Time for Yourself

The Active Wellness programme requires that you practise some component of the programme every day for the next 10 weeks. Whether reading this book, restocking your pantry with healthy foods, creating a meal plan, walking a mile, doing a stretching routine, lifting light weights or exploring stress-reduction techniques, you will need at least 30 to 45 minutes a day to practise your programme. The sooner you devote that time, the sooner you will see results; and the sooner you see results, the more encouraged you will be to stick with your programme. The participants who achieve the best results in the Active Wellness programme are those who work toward their wellness goals every day throughout the 10 weeks.

Here are some of the ways successful participants have found extra time to practise Active Wellness:

- Getting up 30 to 45 minutes earlier each day and using the time for walking, stretching, meditation, yoga or planning meals

- Using the 30 to 45 minutes before bedtime for practising stress reduction, doing stretching routines or writing in one's progress journal

- Using lunch hours for aerobic workouts, light weightlifting, jogging, walking or meditation (and eating a light lunch afterwards)

- Using weekend mornings or afternoons for extended fitness workouts and cross-training routines

- Giving up a favourite evening television programme and using that time to meditate, do yoga, practise stress reduction or lift light weights

If you have your diary handy, block out some Active Wellness time right now. Writing it down helps reinforce your commitment to practise your programme at a specific time every day. But be flexible with yourself. If a time you've chosen doesn't work on a particular day, try to grab some makeup time that evening, the next day or on the weekend. I prefer to use the morning, before my day begins, because I have fewer distractions and the day gets off to a wonderful start.

Once you have chosen a time to practise your programme every day, you are almost ready to begin your Active Wellness training. But first you need to take a brief look at the final ingredient of your successful wellness journey—the hard-to-define 'glue' that binds the other ingredients together: commitment.

If you wish in this world to advance,
Your merits you're bound to enhance;
You must stir it and stump it,
And blow your own trumpet,
Or trust me, you haven't a chance.
—W. S. Gilbert

Commitment

Rose, an Active Wellness winner, recommends thinking back to an accomplishment that you never imagined you would be able to do. For her it was learning how to play the recorder—a lifelong dream. At the age of 60, Rose finally began taking recorder lessons. She didn't think she was ever going to get it when she first started, but she was determined to keep on trying. So Rose stayed focused on her goal and practised, practised, practised. Now, three years later, she is playing classical music with a group of professional recorder musicians.

When Rose began the Active Wellness programme to lose weight and lower her cholesterol, she applied the same tenacity and determination to her health goals as she had to her music goals. She said to herself, "If I learned how to play the recorder at age 60, I can certainly do this." And she did. After losing 1 stone 4 pounds, reducing her cholesterol, and strengthening her heart, Rose is now helping others get started in the programme.

You can't teach commitment. In many ways, it's both elusive and undefinable. It is equal parts desire (the need to achieve something), opportunity (the time and ability to do it) and character (the capacity to stick with it). And it is more than that. It is the 'thing' that some people have that gets them out of bed on a dreary morning to do their daily run. And it's the 'thing' that other people don't have when they turn over and go back to sleep on that same dreary day.

If you have taken the time to read this far and do all the exercises and suggestions in this chapter, you are no doubt committed to beginning your Active Wellness journey. Look at some of the things you have already accomplished:

- ◇ Envisioned a new healthful you
- ◇ Set long- and short-term health goals
- ◇ Evaluated your current health and lifestyle
- ◇ Charted your family's genetic history of disease
- ◇ Found time to practise your programme every day

Whether you finish the Active Wellness journey depends very much on keeping your level of commitment strong and steady. With each new step, you will be encouraged to stay on the path and you'll receive suggestions about how to work the programme more effectively. As your Active Wellness guide, I will teach you new and innovative ways to eat healthfully. I will show you how to balance your meals for optimum nutrition, how to incorporate a variety of physical fitness routines into your life, how to practise stress-reduction techniques, and how to change unhealthy behaviours into healthy, lifetime habits.

But only you can bring the critically important ingredient of 'commitment' to each and every one of the 10 steps. One of the ways you can keep up your level of commitment is to incorporate the 'Three Ps'—practice, pacing, and patience—into your programme.

Practice. Practising your programme—each step, each new behaviour, each new routine—every day is the key not only to mastering the step, behaviour or routine, but to mastering the art of living a life of Active Wellness. By practising new skills every day, they eventually become second nature to you and empower you to master more new steps, routines and behaviours.

Pacing. Every movement towards a healthy change or healthy habit is progress. But some changes come slowly, with more difficulty. That's why following the Active Wellness programme one step at a time is important. It enables you to garner new knowledge and confidence about your wellness journey as you move through each of the steps. The steps are meant to be both incremental and cumulative: You begin with small changes and short-term, attainable goals. As you progress through the programme, you add larger changes and more complex goals. Eventually your reach the point where Active Wellness has permeated every part of your life.

Patience. Above all, be patient with yourself. However slowly and steadily you are moving, remember that you are probably confronting a lifetime of unhealthy behaviours. Don't despair. Forgive yourself and just move on. Sooner than you think, you will be enjoying one small success after another. By the end of your Active Wellness programme, your string of small successes will have become the basis for a lifetime of wellness.

Keep in mind what Ralph Waldo Emerson said: 'We find in life exactly what we put into it.' If you remain focused on reaching your goals, you will get there.

During your Active Wellness journey, you will be introduced to new foods, new behaviours and new lifestyles. You will be encouraged to be adventurous and to try new activities, such as yoga, t'ai chi or power walking. You will begin to view your life with an Active Wellness perspective, and you will feel better and happier in body, mind, and spirit. I guarantee it. So—let's get started!

FAMILY MEDICAL HISTORY CHART

	FIRST-DEGREE RELATIVES			SECOND-DEGREE RELATIVES					
	You	Mother	Father	Siblings	Grandmother	Grandfather	Aunts	Uncles	Cousins
High Total Cholesterol									
High LDL Cholesterol									
High Triglycerides									
High Blood Pressure									
Cancer (indicate type)									
Breast									
Bowel									
Lung									
Other									
Diabetes (non-insulin)									
Diabetes (insulin-dependent)									
Stroke									
Osteoporosis									

STEP 2

Part I

Getting Started with Your Personal Eating Plan: Rethinking Food, Fat and Calories

Never eat anything at one sitting that you can't lift.
—Miss Piggy

In Step 1 you identified your long-term and short-term wellness goals, created a family medical history chart to spotlight illnesses to which you might be susceptible, and took a long, hard look at your personal health history and lifestyle. Now that you have a good sense of your health needs and your personal wellness goals, it's time to take the next step to Active Wellness by initiating your personal eating plan.

Your eating plan is the cornerstone of your Active Wellness programme. Therefore, designing and following an eating plan that is personalized to fit your specific nutritional needs and wellness requirements is one of the most important factors in achieving your goals. Optimal nutrition strengthens and nourishes you physically, mentally, and emotionally. It prepares you to practise and enjoy the other components of the programme—physical exercise, stress management and behaviour modification.

Whatever your long-term and short-term goals are, this chapter will show you the types of foods, combinations of foods and amounts of foods you need to eat every day in order to achieve any one of a variety of wellness goals, including:

- ◇ Losing weight
- ◇ Increasing energy and stamina
- ◇ Living a healthier lifestyle
- ◇ Managing your food cravings
- ◇ Lowering cholesterol and blood pressure
- ◇ Controlling diabetes
- ◇ Preventing osteoporosis
- ◇ Minimizing risk factors for heart disease, stroke or cancer

Before you can begin to create your personalized eating plan, you need to throw out some of your old ideas about food, fat and calories and reframe your notion of what good nutrition is and isn't.

Food As Energy

Your body is a magnificent machine that performs a myriad of tasks every moment of every day: breathing, thinking, running, walking and lifting, to name just a few. The body's heart, brain, lungs, liver, kidneys, bones, muscles, skin and tissues—all synergistically linked by a complex system of biochemical messengers that travel through the body via the bloodstream—strive to work together harmoniously and efficiently to keep the body-machine running at peak capacity. To do that, the body needs to be fuelled regularly with energy to build and maintain its systems. And the source of this energy is the nutrients found in the food you eat.

> Start thinking of food as fuel for your body and *not* as calories that make you fat!

The Six Basic Nutrients

Different bodies have various nutritional requirements, but all bodies need the same six basic nutrient groups, which are considered essential to life:

- Water
- Vitamins
- Minerals
- Proteins
- Carbohydrates
- Fats

Of these six essential nutrient groups, only proteins, carbohydrates and fats can be transformed into fuel for your body. In addition to providing you with energy, each of these nutrient groups plays its own distinct role in your body. Proteins drive the vital reactions that run our bodies, including growth and tissue repair. Carbohydrates turn into quality fuel to run the body. Fats help form our cells and hormones, and transport nutrients that are used by the body. In the case of essential fatty acids, these 'good' fats help protect the body by promoting immune function, rebuilding cell membranes and lowering blood levels of total cholesterol.

The energy released from food is measured in units called calories, which may explain the long-time fixation among dieters and weight watchers on 'counting calories' as a way of measuring the energy consumed. By balancing the energy you consume with the energy you use, you will maintain your weight. However, if you create a surplus of energy by consuming more than your body expends, you will gain weight. And if you create a deficit by eating less than you use, you will lose weight.

> Energy In > Energy Used (weight gain)
> Energy In = Energy Used (weight maintenance)
> Energy In < Energy Used (weight loss)

However, it is not just the number of calories consumed that creates weight and nutritional problems, it is also the kinds of calories consumed. In fact, focusing only on counting calories omits an important consideration—the nutritional quality of the foods you are eating.

Why We Are Overweight—and Undernourished

Your body's energy requirements are unique to you. They depend on many factors, including your height, weight, age, gender, activity level and general health. Therefore, the number of calories you need to consume as energy every day to feel good and perform well is also unique to you. If you eat more calories than your body can convert into energy, the excess energy left over in your body turns into fat and remains in your body as 'storage fuel'. Fat is an efficient way to store calorie reserves because it contains more than twice the energy (9 calories per gram) than either protein (4 calories per gram) or carbohydrate (4 calories per gram). This is also true of the nutrients in the food we eat.

Storing fat as fuel for some future emergency is a leftover survival mechanism from our ancient ancestors, who faced famine on a regular basis and needed to utilize their bodies' reserves of fat simply to live. The average Westerner rarely faces famine, yet regularly packs away more storage fat than our ancestors ever dreamed of having. And stored fat is a culprit in obesity, as well as a contributing factor to heart disease, cancer and diabetes.

Sadly, and despite the fitness craze that has swept the West in the last two decades, we are getting fatter every year and jeopardizing our physical health and emotional well-being in the process. A 1996 survey revealed that 60 per cent of British men and 50 per cent of women were overweight or obese, and the figures are rising. Three simple reasons can help explain why this is happening:

- We regularly consume *more calories* than we need daily.
- We consume a higher percentage of calories as *fats*, which contribute excess energy that our bodies cannot use.
- We expend *less physical energy* due to increasingly sedentary habits in our everyday lives.

Our sedentary lifestyles and poor diets are wreaking havoc with our bodies, so it comes as no surprise that most Active Wellness participants want, and need, to change their eating habits and lose weight. Though they often have other health concerns or medical problems, their overriding concern is usually excess weight. And along with that extra weight comes low energy, fatigue, and limited stamina.

The first thing most of my Active Wellness clients request is help in rethinking their approach to food, nutrition, and dieting. What they develop—and what you will create for yourself here—is a personalized eating plan that accomplishes the following objectives:

- Provides a full complement of healthful nutrient groups to satisfy each individual's unique energy requirements.
- Helps each individual lose weight (or maintain weight) and regain physical energy and stamina.
- Guides each individual to eat the specific foods and food combinations that help her or him stay well and prevent or control certain illnesses and medical conditions.
- Promotes personal preferences of foods so you can create an eating plan you find satisfying and enjoyable.

The first step in creating such an eating plan is determining how much energy your body needs every day.

How Much Energy Does Your Body Need?

Energy, in the form of food calories, is needed for digestion, physical activity, and healing the body. The amount of calories that your body needs varies with your age, gender and height. To determine how much energy your body needs, you should know about how many calories your body burns as fuel on a daily basis. The Daily Calorie Intake charts *(pages 52 and 53)* will help you determine what your ideal daily calorie (energy) intake should be—whether for weight loss or weight maintenance.

Your body is smart. If you don't give it enough calories to function, it conserves energy by slowing down your metabolism. And a slow metabolism can be a problem, particularly when you are trying to lose weight. Your body does not burn food calories as efficiently as it should, and weight loss slows or stops altogether. Further, when your body is not getting enough calories, especially the right kinds of calories, you are more susceptible to illness and disease. Even if you're not trying to lose weight or don't have any particular health concerns, a slow metabolism affects how you look and feel, and how energetically and effectively you perform your daily tasks.

Designing Your Personal Eating Plan

Whether you are choosing to maintain or lose weight, your Active Wellness personal eating plan is designed to meet your metabolic needs so you can increase your energy, burn calories more efficiently and feel your best. Just as important, it helps you learn which foods are ideally suited for your overall wellness goals and health concerns.

Designing your personal eating plan involves four key steps:

⬦ Choosing a reasonable weight-loss goal for your gender and height
⬦ Choosing a daily calorie level
⬦ Choosing the most appropriate Active Wellness Eating Plan for your specific health concerns
⬦ Choosing your favourite healthy foods to correspond to your eating plan

Following the four steps to personalizing your eating plan is easy. As we take a closer look at each step, we will use Rose as our example. Rose is a 60-year-old, 5-foot-4-inch (1.63 m) woman weighing 154 lb (70 kg) who wants to lose weight and control her elevated cholesterol.

Choosing a Reasonable Weight-Loss Goal

Most Active Wellness participants want to lose weight, and are often reasonable about setting a healthy weight goal, but not realistic about the time frame in which they can lose their excess weight. At first everyone looks for the 'quick fix'—10 lb (4.5 kg) in one to two weeks. But it soon becomes apparent that a steady weight-loss goal of an average of 1–2 lb (0.45–0.90 kg) per week is a comfortable effective rate for long-lasting results. Some weeks you may notice larger drops in weight, but keep in mind that you can be losing weight and not detect it on the scale for several weeks. So be patient, because if you are following your eating and exercising plans, your weight will come off. If the scale discourages you, check your weight only once every two weeks.

Knowing your healthy weight level and choosing a reasonable weight-loss goal are the first requirements for setting up a personal eating plan that promotes both good health and weight loss. Once you have decided on your desirable weight goal, use the Weight for Height Charts (*opposite and page 50*), to confirm that your weight goal is reasonable.

If you generally have not been overweight during the last 10 years but weight gain has become a fairly recent problem, use the Weight for Height Chart I (*opposite*). According to this chart, a reasonable weight range for a 5-foot-8-inch (1.72 m) woman is 140–150 lb (63.5–68 kg).

If you have been very heavy or overweight for most of your life, use the Weight for Height Chart II (*page 50*). According to this chart, a reasonable weight range for a 5-foot-8-inch (1.72 m) woman is 175–187 lb (79–85 kg).

If the weight ranges from either chart seem too high or too low for you, ask yourself the following questions:

1. *Have I always been on the thin side or on the heavy side?*
   If you have always been on the thin side or are small boned, the lower end of the weight range for your height may not be low enough. If this is the case, you should subtract 5–10 lb (2.2–4.5 kg) from the lower weight and

confirm your healthy weight range by checking your body mass index (BMI) on page 51. Conversely, if you are large boned or on the heavy side, the higher weight may be too low. If this is the case, add 5–10 lb (2.2–4.5 kg) to the higher weight, and check your BMI in order to confirm your healthy weight.

2. *Have I been this weight during the last 10 years and have I been able to maintain it, plus or minus 2 lb (0.90 kg)?*

If the weight you choose for yourself is one you have maintained for a year or more sometime during the last 10 years, it is probably a reasonable goal.

Weight for Height Chart I*							
Use this chart if you are at a good weight or if you have put on weight during the last 10 years.							
Women				Men			
Height		Weight		Height		Weight	
ft/in	*m*	*lb*	*kg*	*ft/in*	*m*	*lb*	*kg*
5 ft	1.5 m	90-110	41-50	5 ft	1.5 m	96-116	44-53
5 ft 1 in	1.55 m	95-115	43-52	5 ft 1 in	1.55 m	102-122	46-55
5 ft 2 in	1.57 m	100-120	45-54	5 ft 2 in	1.57 m	108-128	49-58
5 ft 3 in	1.6 m	105-125	48-57	5 ft 3 in	1.6 m	114-134	52-61
5 ft 4 in	1.63 m	110-130	50-60	5 ft 4 in	1.63 m	120-140	54-64
5 ft 5 in	1.65 m	115-135	52-61	5 ft 5 in	1.65 m	126-146	57-66
5 ft 6 in	1.68 m	120-140	54-64	5 ft 6 in	1.68 m	132-152	60-69
5 ft 7 in	1.7 m	125-145	57-66	5 ft 7 in	1.7 m	138-158	63-72
5 ft 8 in	1.73 m	130-150	60-68	5 ft 8 in	1.73 m	144-164	65-74
5 ft 9 in	1.75 m	135-155	61-70	5 ft 9 in	1.75 m	150-170	68-77
5 ft 10 in	1.78 m	140-160	64-73	5 ft 10 in	1.78 m	156-176	71-80
5 ft 11 in	1.8 m	145-165	66-75	5 ft 11 in	1.8 m	162-182	73-83
6 ft	1.83 m	150-170	68-77	6 ft	1.83 m	168-188	76-85
6 ft 1 in	1.85 m	155-175	61-79	6 ft 1 in	1.85 m	174-194	79-88
6 ft 2 in	1.88 m	160-180	73-82	6 ft 2 in	1.88 m	180-200	82-91
6 ft 3 in	1.9 m	165-185	66-84	6 ft 3 in	1.9 m	186-206	84-93
6 ft 4 in	1.93 m	170-190	68-86	6 ft 4 in	1.93 m	192-212	87-96

* Based on the Hamwai Method for Determining Ideal Body Weight, a standard equation used to estimate weight for height.

Weight for Height Chart II*
Use this chart to determine your weight if you have been overweight or very heavy for most of your life.

Women				Men			
Height		Weight		Height		Weight	
ft/in	m	lb	kg	ft/in	m	lb	kg
5 ft	1.5 m	125-138	57-63	5 ft	1.5 m	133-145	60-66
5 ft 1 in	1.55 m	131-144	59-65	5 ft 1 in	1.55 m	140-152	64-69
5 ft 2 in	1.57 m	138-150	63-68	5 ft 2 in	1.57 m	148-160	67-73
5 ft 3 in	1.6 m	144-156	65-71	5 ft 3 in	1.6 m	155-168	61-76
5 ft 4 in	1.63 m	150-162	68-73	5 ft 4 in	1.63 m	162-175	73-79
5 ft 5 in	1.65 m	156-168	71-76	5 ft 5 in	1.65 m	170-182	68-83
5 ft 6 in	1.68 m	163-175	74-79	5 ft 6 in	1.68 m	178-190	81-86
5 ft 7 in	1.7 m	169-181	77-82	5 ft 7 in	1.7 m	185-197	84-89
5 ft 8 in	1.73 m	175-187	79-85	5 ft 8 in	1.73 m	193-205	88-93
5 ft 9 in	1.75 m	181-193	82-88	5 ft 9 in	1.75 m	200-212	91-96
5 ft 10 in	1.78 m	188-200	85-91	5 ft 10 in	1.78 m	208-220	94-100
5 ft 11 in	1.8 m	194-206	88-93	5 ft 11 in	1.8 m	215-227	98-103
6 ft	1.83 m	200-212	91-96	6 ft	1.83 m	223-235	101-107
6 ft 1 in	1.85 m	206-218	93-99	6 ft 1 in	1.85 m	230-242	104-110
6 ft 2 in	1.88 m	212-224	96-102	6 ft 2 in	1.88 m	238-250	108-113
6 ft 3 in	1.9 m	219-231	99-105	6 ft 3 in	1.9 m	245-269	111-122
6 ft 4 in	1.93 m	225-237	102-108	6 ft 4 in	1.93 m	253-265	115-120

* Based on the Hamwai Method for Determining Ideal Body Weight, a standard equation used to estimate weight for height.

❖ Rose ❖

Rose's desired weight goal is 120 lb (54.4 kg). She gained 34 lb (15.4 kg) during the last 10 years, so she referred to Weight for Height Chart I. After checking her weight level, a weight goal of 120 lb (54.4 kg) appears to be reasonable for her, especially since she used to be that weight 10 years ago; but to make sure it is not too low a weight, she will check her Body Mass Index level as well.

Don't weigh yourself every day! Weight fluctuates from day to day, depending on a variety of factors. Seeing a gain of 2–3 lb (0.9–1.3 kg) when you've been sticking to your diet can be discouraging. If you feel you *must* weigh yourself, do it only once every two weeks. Your progress will be abundantly clear and your commitment will be renewed.

Body Mass Index (BMI)

One of the best ways to identify if your weight goal is reasonable is to determine your body mass index (BMI). The BMI is a unique weight-to-height mathematical ratio that indicates excess body fat (measured as weight in kilograms/height in metres squared). First use the Body Mass Index equation below to determine your current BMI, then assess your weight goal.

The healthiest BMI is one that is below 25, and ideally as low as 20—this is the desirable range. A BMI below 20 is considered underweight. A person with a BMI of 30 or more is considered obese, and a BMI greater than 40 is extremely obese. Anyone who has a BMI greater than 25 is considered at higher health risk for diseases associated with excess weight.

Now determine your BMI level using your weight goal. If the resulting BMI falls within the desirable range, you have chosen a reasonable weight goal.

CAUTION: A BMI should not be used to predict body fat in children, pregnant or breast-feeding women, the frail, the elderly, or serious bodybuilders.

You can use this BMI equation, which also has equivalents in pounds and inches for easy use:

$$\text{Body Mass Index} = \frac{\text{Weight in kilograms}}{\text{Height in metres}^2} \quad \text{or} \quad \frac{\text{Weight in lb} \times 704}{\text{Height in inches}^2}$$

❥ Rose ❧

Rose's current BMI puts her at a level of increased health risk. Since her weight goal of 120 lb (54.4 kg) is not on the chart, she calculated her BMI using the equation above. Rose's BMI = 20. When Rose loses her excess weight, it will put her at a desirable BMI and reduce her health risks.

Once you confirm your desirable weight goal, enter it below.

Record Your Weight Goal Here: _____

Once you have established a reasonable weight goal for yourself, you are ready to choose your maximum daily calorie level: one that promotes weight loss (or maintains your current weight) and also targets specific health conditions.

Choosing Your Daily Calorie Level

For starters, use the Daily Calorie (Energy) Intake Charts *(below and page 53)*. If you want to lose weight, find your height in the first column and the corresponding daily calorie level in the second ("Weight Loss") column. Following this daily calorie level ensures a slow but steady weight loss of about 1–2 lb (0.45–0.90 kg) a week.

Women's Daily Calorie (Energy) Intake Chart for Weight Loss and Weight Maintenance			
Height		Calorie (Energy) Intake for Weight Loss	*Calorie (Energy) Intake for Weight Maintenance
5 ft	1.5 m	1,200	1,400
5 ft 1 in	1.55 m	1,200	1,400
5 ft 2 in	1.57 m	1,300	1,500
5 ft 3 in	1.6 m	1,300	1,500
5 ft 4 in	1.63 m	1,400	1,600
5 ft 5 in	1.65 m	1,500	1,700
5 ft 6 in	1.68 m	1,500	1,700
5 ft 7 in	1.7 m	1,600	1,800
5 ft 8 in	1.73 m	1,600	1,800
5 ft 9 in	1.75 m	1,700	1,900
5 ft 10 in	1.78 m	1,800	2,000
5 ft 11 in	1.8 m	1,800	2,000
6 ft	1.83 m	1,900	2,100
6 ft 1 in	1.85 m	1,900	2,100
6 ft 2 in	1.88 m	2,000	2,200
6 ft 3 in	1.9 m	2,000	2,200
6 ft 4 in	1.93 m	2,100	2,300

* Calorie levels for weight maintenance take into consideration that you have incorporated an exercise plan into your routine—three or four times a week, for a minimum of 30 minutes per session. If you do not meet this minimum level of exercise, follow the calorie level indicated for weight loss.

> ## ❖ Rose ❖
> At 5 ft 4 in (1.63 m) Rose's daily calorie level for weight loss is 1,400.

Men's Daily Calorie (Energy) Intake Chart for Weight Loss and Weight Maintenance

Height		Calorie (Energy) Intake for Weight Loss	*Calorie (Energy) Intake for Weight Maintenance
5 ft	1.5 m	1,200	1,400
5 ft 1 in	1.55 m	1,300	1,500
5 ft 2 in	1.57 m	1,300	1,500
5 ft 3 in	1.6 m	1,400	1,600
5 ft 4 in	1.63 m	1,500	1,700
5 ft 5 in	1.65 m	1,500	1,700
5 ft 6 in	1.68 m	1,600	1,800
5 ft 7 in	1.7 m	1,700	1,900
5 ft 8 in	1.73 m	1,700	1,900
5 ft 9 in	1.75 m	1,800	2,000
5 ft 10 in	1.78 m	1,900	2,100
5 ft 11 in	1.8 m	1,900	2,100
6 ft	1.83 m	2,000	2,200
6 ft 1 in	1.85 m	2,000	2,200
6 ft 2 in	1.88 m	2,200	2,400
6 ft 3 in	1.9 m	2,200	2,400
6 ft 4 in	1.93 m	2,400	2,600

* Calorie levels for weight maintenance take into consideration that you have incorporated an exercise plan into your routine—three or four times a week, for a minimum of 30 minutes per session. If you do not meet this minimum level of exercise, follow the calorie level indicated for weight loss.

If you want to maintain your current weight, find your height in the first column and the corresponding daily calorie level in the third ('Weight Maintenance') column.

When choosing your personalized eating plan, you will use your daily calorie level to determine the most appropriate foods and servings of foods to encourage weight loss, promote optimal health and help control or prevent specific health concerns.

Record Your Daily Calorie Level Here: _____

Choosing Your Active Wellness Eating Plan

When you choose your personalized eating plan, it should be consistent with the health goals you established in Step 1. Refer to the charts entitled Choosing an Eating Plan to help determine the best eating plan for your needs.

If you want to choose an eating plan for overall health, vegetarian eating or one primary health concern, use the chart for Choosing an Eating Plan I *(page 57)*. If you want to choose an eating plan that targets multiple health concerns, use the chart for Choosing an Eating Plan II *(page 58)*.

Once you determine the type of plan you will be using, you can locate the more detailed individualized eating plans, complete with their general nutritional guidelines, beginning on page 85 later in this chapter.

Record the Name of Your Active Wellness Eating Plan: _____

Choosing the Right Foods for Your Eating Plan

Now that you've identified your reasonable weight goal, determined your daily calorie level, and chosen your Active Wellness Eating Plan, you're ready to translate your energy (calorie) needs into delicious and nutritious foods to eat. Part II of this chapter focuses on choosing the right foods for your customized eating plan.

You'll find general eating guidelines that apply to all the eating plans. They also include recommendations for taking vitamin and mineral supplements and explanations of the difference between 'good' and 'bad' fats. And you'll see a substantial list of foods, together with appropriate serving sizes, that fulfill all your unique nutritional needs.

The Active Wellness Eating Plans are specifically designed to help you focus on nutritious foods, not calories. You won't be counting the calories in the foods you eat on this plan. Instead, you'll be keeping track of the types and serving sizes of foods you eat and making smart choices about those foods. Making smart food choices—not counting calories—is the key to eating healthfully, getting optimal nutrition and preventing disease. Counting calories has an inherent danger, because it inadvertently encourages cheating. Those 260 calories you allotted for breakfast can include a banana and bowl of cereal with low-fat milk—or be used to scoff down one plain chocolate bar!

Now that you've laid the groundwork for designing a customized eating plan that's unique to your needs, let's begin putting it all together. Believe me, it's easier than you think—and the rewards are great!

Special Lifestyle and Health Needs

Age: If you are 50 and over, your calorie level drops by 10 per cent per decade, because your metabolism naturally decreases. Therefore, if you are 60 years of age, you should adjust your calorie requirements by following the equation below:

Chosen calorie level x .90 = _____ = calorie level to use with
food portion charts.

Athlete: Use the Active Wellness Basic Eating Plan 1 *(page 85)*. If you are an athlete who exercises 5 to 7 times a week for approximately one hour of high-intensity exercise, you will need to take into consideration the energy expenditure from exercise. You will need to increase the amount of calories listed by following the equation below:

Calorie level for maintenance x 1.6 = _____ = calorie level needed
to maintain weight.

Choose the lower number if your number is between two calorie levels. If you are exercising more than an hour a day, you will need to consume extra calories. The best snacks are carbohydrate foods, such as fruits and starchy foods, and grains such as cereals, breads, potatoes and pasta. Dairy is a good third choice; good low-fat snacks are low-fat or fat-free yoghurts and smoothie shakes with fruit and low-fat cheese.

Check the calorie level chart with your new calorie level. Use the portions of food associated with this calorie level to determine your daily food intake.

Vitamin Supplementation: Excessive vitamin supplementation does not improve performance and can be dangerous. If you eat a balanced diet, you should not need more vitamins than those recommended in the Active Wellness Guidelines.

Prior to an event, you will want to consider your nutrient needs before, during, and after the competition. For more information on eating for optimal performance, you can contact the Active Wellness website or contact a registered dietitian.

Pregnant or Breast-Feeding: If you are pregnant, you will need to consume 300 more calories a day during pregnancy. Use the following equation to calculate your estimated needs:

Calorie level for maintenance _____+ 300 calories = _____ = calorie
level for pregnancy or maintaining weight while breast-feeding.

If you are breast-feeding you will need an additional 300 calories per day to compensate for the energy used during breast-feeding. If you are not trying to lose post-pregnancy weight, you can follow the equation on page 55. If you are trying to lose weight, follow the equation for weight loss and add 300 calories to your total. Also, if you are pregnant or breast-feeding:

⋄ Ask your doctor about your vitamin supplements.
⋄ Avoid caffeine and alcohol.

Concerns that Alter Types of Foods and How You Eat

Digestive Problems: If you have any of the following digestive difficulties—hietal hernia, peptic ulcers, diverticulitis, irritable colon—it is important to eat small meals and eat more often. If you have flare-ups of your symptoms, contact your doctor.

Hypoglycaemia (low blood sugar): If your blood sugar drops after a meal, do not eat sugary foods or refined carbohydrates, such as white bread, pasta, pizza dough, fruit juice or sweets. Avoid any foods that cause large swings in your blood sugar level. Eliminate caffeine and decaffeinated beverages, and avoid alcohol. It is usually helpful to eat smaller meals more often, about every three hours, to prevent large swings in your energy level and blood sugar. You may use the diabetic meal plan as a guide.

Intolerance to Foods

Lactose Intolerance: This is an intolerance to lactose, a sugar in milk products. Generally, most people have some degree of tolerance at small doses. Fermented dairy products such as yoghurt and buttermilk are usually easier to digest.

Gluten Intolerance (Coeliac Sprue): This is an intolerance to the protein gliadin found in wheat, oat, barley and rye products or products made with these ingredients. If you have this condition, substitute maize, rice, buckwheat, soya bean or potato.

Gout: Avoid or reduce purine-rich foods to prevent pain. High-purine foods include: organ meats, meat extracts, meat broth/stock, anchovies, scallops, mussels and mackerel. Loss of excess weight also helps relieve symptoms.

Allergies: Food allergies can cause a range of reactions including nausea, itching, rashes, asthma and anaphylactic shock. Some of the most common food allergies are to peanuts, tree nuts, eggs and shellfish. In general, if you have a reaction to a food that makes you uncomfortable, isolate the food item and avoid it altogether.

Renal (Kidney) Disease: For detailed instructions, contact your doctor and have a consultation with a dietitian to understand your restrictions. Your restrictions will depend on the severity of your disease.

If you want to follow an overall healthy eating plan or a vegetarian eating plan, and you have only one primary health concern, use this chart to choose your Active Wellness Eating Plan.

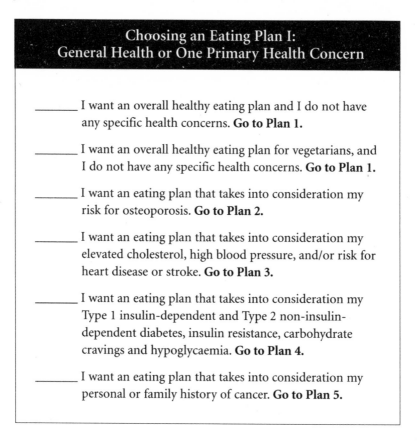

Choosing an Eating Plan I: General Health or One Primary Health Concern

_____ I want an overall healthy eating plan and I do not have any specific health concerns. **Go to Plan 1.**

_____ I want an overall healthy eating plan for vegetarians, and I do not have any specific health concerns. **Go to Plan 1.**

_____ I want an eating plan that takes into consideration my risk for osteoporosis. **Go to Plan 2.**

_____ I want an eating plan that takes into consideration my elevated cholesterol, high blood pressure, and/or risk for heart disease or stroke. **Go to Plan 3.**

_____ I want an eating plan that takes into consideration my Type 1 insulin-dependent and Type 2 non-insulin-dependent diabetes, insulin resistance, carbohydrate cravings and hypoglycaemia. **Go to Plan 4.**

_____ I want an eating plan that takes into consideration my personal or family history of cancer. **Go to Plan 5.**

If you have multiple health concerns, use this chart to choose your Active Wellness Eating Plan. Note that certain health conditions and illnesses may override other health concerns.

Choosing an Eating Plan II: Multiple Health Concerns

If you have:

_____ Type 1 insulin-dependent and Type 2 non-insulin-dependent diabetes, insulin resistance, carbohydrate cravings and hypoglycaemia plus any other health concerns. **Go to Plan 4.**

_____ Heart disease, including elevated total cholesterol or LDL cholesterol, and/or high blood pressure plus diabetes, insulin resistance or carbohydrate cravings. **Go to Plan 4.**

_____ Heart disease, including elevated total cholesterol or LDL cholesterol, and/or high blood pressure plus any other health concern other than diabetes. **Go to Plan 3.**

_____ Cancer plus any other health concern. **Go to the plan for the other health concern; also read the additional information about cancer on page 95.**

_____ Osteoporosis plus any other health concern. **Go to the plan for the other health concern; also read the additional information about osteoporosis on page 86.**

Putting It All Together

Tell me what you eat and I will tell you who you are.
—Anthelme Brillat-Savarin

When you look at the charts for the Active Wellness Eating Plans *(pages 85-96)*, you will see that the seven food groups plus alcohol—across the top of each chart—are included in each plan. They are illustrated below on the Active Wellness Plate.

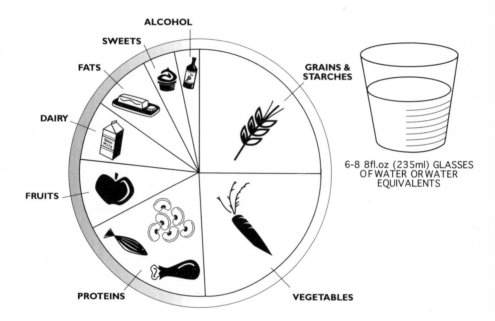

6-8 8fl.oz (235ml) GLASSES OF WATER OR WATER EQUIVALENTS

The seven food groups plus alcohol and your daily water requirement are included to emphasize the importance of variety and nutritional balance in any good eating plan. The food groups, each designated by its own distinctive symbol, include:

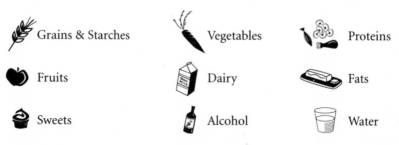

Grains & Starches   Vegetables   Proteins

Fruits   Dairy   Fats

Sweets   Alcohol   Water

In the first column of your eating plan chart is a series of daily calorie levels. Locate the daily calorie level you chose for yourself earlier in this chapter. Across from your calorie level, you will find the number of servings from each food group that you may eat every day to meet your nutritional needs.

For example, if you have chosen Plan 1, the Active Wellness Basic Eating Plan for Good Health, and a daily calorie level of 1,600 calories, you may eat the following each day:

- Seven servings of grains and starches
- Four servings of vegetables
- Five servings of protein
- Three servings of fruit
- Two servings of dairy
- Four servings of fat
- One serving of sweets
- One optional serving of alcohol
- Six to eight 8 fl. oz (235 ml) glasses of water

You don't even have to worry about calculating how much food belongs in a 'serving'. All of that is done for you in the Active Wellness Guide to Foods and Serving Sizes, which begins on page 63. It lists a variety of foods from each food group, together with their appropriate serving sizes.

For the first week or two, until you feel confident about choosing foods and designing meal plans, you may want to follow one of the starter eating plans provided in the Appendix. The starter plans provide a menu of foods and servings that can serve as a guide while you are getting established in your new eating routine. I encourage you to start expanding on the starter plan by including other foods within each of your food groups as soon as possible. Aim for a variety of tastes, textures and colours in your foods.

Everyone who has been successful in the Active Wellness programme used the Daily Allowance Cards to help keep track of the amount of foods they were eating each day. A blank sample card is illustrated at the top of page 61. You may photocopy this sample card or make up your own allowance cards. As you will see, it lists each of the seven food groups that comprise your plan, plus water (a must!) and the distinctive symbols for each of the food groups.

In the column next to the food group name, fill in the number of daily servings your eating plan allows. For example, if you are following Plan 1, the Active Wellness Basic Eating Plan, your filled in Daily Allowance Card might look like the one illustrated at the bottom of page 61. As you finish your meals, cross off the servings of each food group you've eaten. At the end of the day, you can review your eating patterns and see where you may have 'overspent' your food budget or scrimped on nutrition.

DAILY ALLOWANCE CARD												DATE: / /	
	NO.												
WATER													
GRAINS & STARCH													
VEGGIE													
PROTEIN													
FRUITS													
DAIRY													
FATS													
SWEETS													
ALCOHOL													

Even if you are following one of the starter plans in the Appendix, use your allowance cards to reinforce your new eating behaviours. Think of your daily allotment of foods as your 'nutrition bank account'—the card helps you to keep track of how you 'spend' your food portions. It is up to you to decide when you would like to eat them.

Use your Daily Allowance Cards until you are comfortable with the amount of food

DAILY ALLOWANCE CARD		Plan 1									DATE:	11/7/99	
	NO.												
WATER	6												
GRAINS & STARCH	7												
VEGGIE	4												
PROTEIN	5												
FRUITS	3												
DAIRY	2												
FATS	4												
SWEETS	1												
ALCOHOL	1												

that meets your daily nutritional requirements. At a minimum the Daily Allowance Cards should be used for the first two weeks that you are on the Active Wellness eating plan. From the time you wake up until the time you go to bed, check off everything you eat on your card. If you 'underspend' and have servings left over at the end of the day, don't worry. It is more important to be concerned if you find yourself 'overspending' by eating more food than your daily allowance. If this is the case, just make a note of it and start anew the next day. Take your new eating plan one day at a time: Don't focus on how much weight you're losing, but on how good you're feeling! You'll reach your optimal wellness goal and lose the weight faster than you ever expected.

Now you are ready to start choosing the foods you will eat on your new Active Wellness eating plan. On the following pages the Active Wellness Guide to Foods and Serving Sizes offers a multitude of delicious and nutritious food choices in every food group. Best of all, it takes the guesswork out of how much food equals 'one serving' on your Daily Allowance Card.

Quick and Easy Ways to Estimate Serving Sizes

One quick and easy way to estimate food portions is to use your hands.

- One handful equals about 4 fl. oz (120 ml); two hands together equals about 8 fl. oz (235 ml).
- The amount of animal protein you need each day is usually equal to the size of the palm of your hand, which does not include your fingers.
- 1 oz (30 g) of cheese is about equal to the length and width of your thumb.
- You can use a soup spoon to approximate 1 tablespoon (15 ml), and a common teaspoon as 1 tsp (5 ml).

To make estimating serving sizes easier, many of the portions in the lists that follow and in the recipes in this book are expressed as volumes rather than weights.

These simple guidelines can help you master portion control and keep you from overeating. If you are trying to lose weight, simply cutting back on your portions makes a big difference in your rate of weight loss.

Active Wellness Guide to Foods and Serving Sizes

The Grains/Starches Group

(Bread and Bread Alternatives, Cereals, Starchy Vegetables, Pasta, Rice and Other Grains, and Beans, Crackers and Snacks)

Each Grain/Starch Serving contains approximately 80 Calories, 15 grams Carbohydrate, 3 grams Protein, 0 to 1 gram Fat, 2 grams Fibre

Bread and Bread Alternatives

Food	Equivalent of One Active Wellness Serving
Bagel, large	¼ bagel = 1 oz (30 g)
Bagel, small (mini)	½ bagel = 1 oz (30 g)
Bread, reduced calorie	2 slices = 1 oz (30 g)
Bread (wholemeal, whole grain)	1 slice = 1 oz (30 g)
Breadcrumbs	1 oz/30 g = 4 tbsp (60 ml)
Breadstick, crisp	1 oz/30 g = 4 tbsp (60 ml)
Dinner roll	1 small roll
Egg-roll wrapper (not fried)	1 wrapper
English muffin	½ muffin
Hamburger bun (wholemeal, whole grain)	1 bun
Hard roll (wholemeal, whole grain) ½ roll	
Low-fat muffin (blueberry, banana, etc.)	
3 oz (85 g) muffin (small)	½ muffin
6 oz (170 g) muffin	¼ muffin
Pancakes (4 in/10 cm across)	2
Pitta bread (wholemeal, oat, whole grain)	
Mini	5 pittas
Medium	1 pitta = 1 oz (30 g)
Large	½ pitta
Tortilla (corn or wholemeal)	
6 in/15 cm tortilla	1 tortilla
8 in/20 cm tortilla	1 tortilla
10–12 in/25–30 cm tortilla	½ tortilla

Waffles	1
Wonton wrapper	4

Cereals

Food	Equivalent of One Active Wellness Serving
Cereal, dry (whole grain, without nuts)	8 fl. oz (225 ml) or serving equivalent listed on box
Cereal (dry puffed)	12 fl. oz (340 ml)
Cereal, hot	1 pack of instant or 8 fl. oz (225 ml) cooked
Unprocessed bran	2.5 fl. oz (70 ml)
Wheat germ	3 tablespoons (45 ml)

Starchy Vegetables

Food	Equivalent of One Active Wellness Serving
Corn/maize	1 6-in (15 cm) corn on the cob or 4 fl. oz (115 ml) cooked
Peas	4 fl. oz (115 ml) cooked
Plantains	4 fl. oz (115 ml) cooked
Potatoes (white, sweet)	½ medium potato or 4 fl. oz (115 ml) cooked
Squash (butternut, acorn, etc.)	4 fl. oz (115 ml) cooked

Pasta, Rice and Other Grains and Beans

(Cooked and Uncooked)

Food	Equivalent of One Active Wellness Serving
All pasta, rice and other grains, and beans (cooked in water or stock)	4 fl. oz (115 ml) cooked*
Bean soup	8 fl. oz (225 ml)
Miso (soya product)	3 tablespoons (45 ml)

* Refer to cooking charts in Step 10 for dry equivalents of cooked grains and beans.

Crackers and Snacks

Food	Equivalent of One Active Wellness Serving
Pretzel	1 large
Digestive biscuits	2
Other crackers	Refer to serving equivalent listed on package.
Popcorn, plain (air popped or low fat)	24 fl. oz (680 ml)
Popcorn, lite (packaged)	1 oz = 8 fl. oz (225 ml)
Potato or tortilla chips (fat free)	1 oz = 8 fl. oz (225 ml)
Rice cakes	2 large or 6 mini
All other low-fat snacks	Use serving equivalent listed on package.

Vegetables

**Each Vegetable Serving contains approximately 25 Calories,
5 grams Carbohydrate, 2 grams Protein, 0 grams Fat, 2 grams Fibre**

You may eat an unlimited number of vegetable servings (except for the starchy vegetables listed under Grains/Starches). You may use fresh or frozen vegetables, as long as they are prepared without added fat. However, vegetable juice and tomato sauce should be limited to two servings per day. For purposes of keeping track of the number of units you eat, one serving of vegetables is equivalent to the following:

Food	Equivalent of One Active Wellness Serving
Cooked vegetables	4 fl. oz (115 ml)
Raw vegetables	8 fl. oz (225 ml)
Tomato sauce	4 fl. oz (115 ml)
Vegetable juice	8 fl. oz (225 ml)

Proteins

Try to eat mostly protein foods from the lean category. If you are a vegetarian this rule does not apply.

Lean

**Each oz/gram of lean protein contains approximately 55 Calories,
0 grams Carbohydrate, 7 grams Protein, 1 to 3 grams Fat, 0 grams Fibre**

Food	Equivalent of One Active Wellness Serving
Beans, dried or split peas	2 fl. oz (55 ml) cooked
Beans, puréed (e.g. hummus)	1 fl. oz (30 ml)
Bean soup	4 fl. oz (115 ml)
Egg substitute	2 fl. oz (55 ml)
Egg whites	2
Fish	1 oz (30 g) cooked
Game duck, pheasant (no skin), goose, rabbit (venison, buffalo, ostrich)	1 oz (30 g) cooked
Lean beef (sirloin, top loin) tenderloin, roast (rib, rump) steak (cubed, T-bone), trimmed of all visible fat	1 oz (30 g) cooked
Lean ham, Canadian bacon	1 oz (30 g) cooked
Meat analogs (fat free)	See Nutrition Facts label on package.
Pork, fresh ham, trimmed of , all visible fat	1 oz (30 g) cooked
Poultry, chicken or turkey (skinless)	1 oz (30 g) cooked
Shellfish	1½ oz (45 g) cooked
Textured vegetable protein	1 oz (30 g) cooked
Veal, trimmed of all visible fat	1 oz (30 g) cooked
Vegetarian burgers, hot dogs (fat free, low fat)	1 burger cooked

Medium Fat

Use these foods for vegetarian protein sources.

Each ounce of medium-fat protein contains approximately 75 Calories, 0 grams Carbohydrate, 7 grams Protein, 5 grams Fat, 0 grams Fibre

Food	Equivalent of One Active Wellness Serving
Baked tofu (soya product), tempeh	2 oz (55 g)
Meat analogs (low fat)	See Nutrition Facts label.
Tofu, tempeh	4 oz (115 g)
Whole egg	1

Fruits

(Fresh and Frozen Fruits, Unsweetened Fruits Canned in Water,
Fruit Juices and Dried Fruits)

Each Fruit Serving contains approximately 60 Calories,
15 grams Carbohydrate, 0 grams Protein, 0 grams Fat, 2 to 3 grams Fibre

Fresh or Frozen Fruit

Food	Equivalent of One Active Wellness Serving
Bananas	½ large or 1 small
Cherries	10 (1 handful)
Fresh berries	8 fl. oz (225 ml)
Fresh fruit	1 piece (the size you can hold in your hand, except for below)
Grapefruit	½
Grapes	15 (1 handful)
Honey dew	2-in (5 cm) slice
Melon, cantaloupe	⅓ melon
Pineapple	6 fl. oz (170 ml) cubed
Watermelon	1 slice (1 in/2.5 cm thick), 10 fl. oz (285 ml) cubed

Fruit Juices

4 fl. oz (115 ml)

Dried Fruits

Food	Equivalent of One Active Wellness Serving
Apple halves	4 slices
Apricot halves	8 halves
Dates	3
Figs	1
Prunes	3 medium
Raisins, cherries, cranberries	2 tablespoons (30 ml)

Dairy

(May be exchanged for soya-based or rice-based dairy alternatives)

**Each Dairy Serving contains approximately 100 Calories,
12 grams Carbohydrate, 8 grams Protein, 0 to 3 grams Fat, 0 grams Fibre**

Milk

Food	Equivalent of One Active Wellness Serving
Buttermilk, low fat	8 fl. oz (225 ml)
Evaporated, skimmed	4 fl. oz (115 ml)
Milk, skimmed (non-fat—can be protein fortified) or low fat (1%)	8 fl. oz (225 ml)
Non-fat dry milk powder	2.5 fl. oz (70 ml)
Non-fat or low-fat yoghurt	8 fl. oz (225 ml)
Rice milk, non-fat or low fat	8 fl. oz (225 ml)
Soya bean milk, non-fat or low fat	8 fl. oz (225 ml)

Cheeses and Soured Cream

Food	Equivalent of One Active Wellness Serving
Cottage cheese	4 fl. oz (115 ml)
Hard cheese (less than 3 grams of fat per serving)	2 oz (55 g)
Parmesan cheese, grated or shredded	2 tablespoons (30 ml)
Ricotta, low fat or fat free	4 fl. oz (115 ml)

Fats

A certain amount of fat is necessary in everyone's diet. The 'trick' is to choose your fat servings carefully, so that you use it where you will most enjoy it. Here are suggestions for doing just that. On the next page are servings for foods high in unsaturated fats ('good fats'). Nuts can also be good sources of vitamins and minerals and contribute a small amount of protein to your diet.

**Each Fat Serving contains approximately 45 Calories,
0 grams Carbohydrate, 0 grams Protein, 5 grams Fat, 0 grams Fibre**

Food	Equivalent of One Active Wellness Serving
Oils	
Monounsaturated:	
Olive oil, peanut oil	1 teaspoon (5 ml)
Polyunsaturated:	
Corn, safflower, sesame, soya, sunflower, walnut	1 teaspoon (5 ml)
Nuts and Seeds	
Almond butter	1 teaspoon (5 ml)
Almonds	6
Cashews	6
Chestnuts	6
Chestnuts, water	6
Hazelnuts	1 tablespoon (15 ml)
Macadamia nuts	1 tablespoon (15 ml)
Peanut butter, natural	2 teaspoons (10 ml)
Peanuts, small	20
Pecans	4 halves
Pine nuts	15
Pistachios	15
Pumpkin seeds	1 tablespoon (15 ml)
Sesame seeds	1 tablespoon (15 ml)
Sunflower seeds	1 tablespoon (15 ml)
Tahini (sesame paste)	1 teaspoon (5 ml)
Walnuts	4 halves
Most other nuts	1 tablespoon (15 ml)
Most other nut butters	1 teaspoon (5 ml)
Dressings, Condiments, and Miscellaneous	
Avocado pears	2 tsp = ⅛ fruit (1oz/30 g)
Bacon, back	1 slice
Cream cheese, fat free	2 tablespoons (30 ml)
Cream cheese, low fat	1 tablespoon (15 ml)
Creamers, powder or liquid	1 tablespoon (15 ml)
Horseradish	1 tablespoon (15 ml)
Mayonnaise, fat free, low fat	1 tablespoon (15 ml)
Olives, black (large)	8
Olives, green (small)	10

| Salad dressing, low fat | 2 tablespoons |
| Soured cream, low fat | ¼ cup = 4 tablespoons |

Sweets/Desserts

Enjoy your sweets, but be aware that they provide very little nutritional value. Sweets may also promote sweet cravings.

**Each Sweets Serving contains approximately 100 Calories,
18 grams Carbohydrate, 0 grams Protein, 0 to 3 grams Fat, 0 to 2 grams Fibre**

Food	Equivalent of One Active Wellness Serving
Cake (less than 3 grams of fat per serving)	one ½-in/1-cm-wide slice
Biscuits (less than 3 grams of fat per serving)	2
Low-fat ice cream	4 fl. oz (115 ml) = small serving
Non-fat frozen yoghurt	4 fl. oz (115 ml) = small serving
Whole grain bars, fruit bars	½ bar
Other low-fat or fat-free desserts	See serving size on package.

Alcohol

Alcohol can be enjoyable, but limit yourself to one serving a day. More can be harmful to your health.

**Each Alcohol Serving contains approximately 100 Calories,
0 to 12 grams Carbohydrate, 0 grams Protein, 0 grams Fat, 0 grams Fibre**

Beverage	Equivalent of One Active Wellness Serving
Beer, light	12 fl. oz (340 ml)
Distilled spirits (80 proof)	1½ fl. oz (45 ml)
Wine	5 fl. oz (140 ml)

Water or Water Equivalents

Everyone should try to replenish their body with 6–8 8 fl. oz (225 ml) glasses of water per day.

Beverage	Equivalent of One Active Wellness Serving
Club soda	8 fl. oz (225 ml)
'Fizzy water', flavoured but unsweetened	8 fl. oz (225 ml)
Herbal teas, hot or cold	8 fl. oz (225 ml)
Mineral water	8 fl. oz (225 ml)
Stock, broth, consommé	8 fl. oz (225 ml)
Tonic water, sugar free	8 fl. oz (225 ml)
Water	8 fl. oz (225 ml)

Foods to Use Sparingly

The foods listed below *do not* have to be tallied on your Daily Allowance Card. Use them sparingly throughout the day, up to 3 times per day.

Food	Active Wellness Suggested Servings
Sweeteners	
Honey	1 tablespoon (15 ml)
Maple syrup	1 tablespoon (15 ml)
Sugars	1 teaspoon (5 ml)
Treacle	1 tablespoon (15 ml)
Condiments and Spreads	
Cocoa	1 tablespoon (15 ml)
Cream cheese, fat free	1½ tablespoons (20 ml)
Fruit jam, naturally sweetened	1 tablespoon (15 ml)
Ketchup	1 tablespoon (15 ml)
Mayonnaise, fat free	1 tablespoon (15 ml)
Mustard	1 tablespoon (15 ml)
Oil spray	2 to 3 sprays
Soured cream, fat free	2 tablespoons (30 ml)

Foods to Use Anytime

Flavouring extracts
Herbs, seasonings and spices
Salad dressing, fat free
Sauces, fat free (i.e. Tabasco, Worcestershire)*
Stock or broth
Tea, herbal
Unflavoured or sugar-free gelatine

* Food items that can be high in sodium.

Combination Foods

There are many foods that are combinations of several food groups, such as pizza, lasagne or stew. If the meal is made with low-fat ingredients, you can determine how to check it off on your Daily Allowance Card by considering all the servings of food groups that were combined to create the meal.

> *For example:* 1 Slice of Low-Fat Fresh Cheese Pizza (thin crust) is made of the following ingredients: The crust (approximately 1½ Servings Grains/Starches Group) + Tomato Sauce (Vegetable Group) + Part Skimmed Mozzarella (1½ Servings Dairy Group).

Please Note: If you do not see a food item you desire on the list, determine the food category in which it belongs and compare its nutrition information with the requirements for calories, carbohydrate, protein and fat listed in the Active Wellness food list. If the food item is comparable in energy nutrients and calories, feel free to use it in your eating plan. Servings are adapted from the American Diabetes Association and the American Dietetic Association Exchange Lists for Meal Planning.

The Active Wellness Basic Food and Nutrition Guidelines

❦ **Eat low-fat, whole foods as the mainstay of your daily eating plan.** Purchase individual food items that have 3 grams or less of total fat per serving* or prepared meals that have 30 per cent or less of total calories from fat. *Soya products and fish high in omega-3 fatty acids are an exception to this guideline.

❦ **Greatly reduce or eliminate decaffeinated beverages and caffeine from your diet.** This includes the caffeine in coffee, tea, colas, cocoa and chocolate.

❦ **Vegetables are unlimited.** Try to eat a minimum of five different dark green, orange, red and yellow fruits and vegetables a day.

❦ **Supplement your diet with the following vitamins and minerals, unless you are consuming more than five servings of fruits and vegetables a day.** Food is the best source for any nutrient. It is difficult, however, to eat adequate amounts of a variety of foods daily, especially if you are trying to lose weight. The supplements listed below will provide you with nutrients to meet your needs and protect you against cell damage and diseases. Keep in mind that vitamins should be taken on a full stomach for best absorption.

❦ **Vitamin C** (500 mg per day), taken in two 250 mg doses with breakfast and dinner. (The body cannot absorb the full 500 mg dose at one time.)

❦ **Vitamin E** (100 IU per day) (If you have high blood pressure, check with your doctor before taking a vitamin E supplement.)

❦ **Selenium** (50 mcg per day)

❦ **Folic acid** (200 mcg per day)

❦ **Multivitamin** (One multivitamin per day.) It is best to take a multivitamin that contains 100 per cent of the daily value for most vitamins and minerals. See below and the next page for specific guidelines for calcium, vitamin D, vitamin B_{12} and iron.

For every serving of calcium-rich dairy and soya foods you do not eat, make sure your supplement contains 300 mg of calcium. (Refer to the Calcium Food Chart on page 88.) If necessary, take an added calcium supplement that contains vitamin D, for optimal absorption.

If you are younger than 50 years of age and you follow the Active Wellness guidelines, you will be meeting your daily requirement of 200 IU of vitamin D. If you are over 50 years of age, a 400 IU of vitamin D is recommended daily, especially if it is not included in your daily supplement and you do not spend much time outdoors. If you are over 60 years of age, make sure your supplement contains 25 mcg of vitamin B_{12}—if not, consider taking a supplement. If you are 70 years of age or older, take 600 IU of vitamin D daily.

CAUTION: If you currently have or are at risk of heart disease, or if you are a male, make sure that your multivitamin does not contain iron. Recent research indicates that iron, an oxidizing agent, may increase your risk for heart attack. If you are a female, who is a vegetarian or premenopausal, supplemental iron is usually not a problem.

☀ **Eat low-fat and fat-free sweets sparingly, and eliminate high-fat desserts from your diet.** Most sweets and desserts are sources of 'empty' calories, because they do not contain many nutrients.

☀ **Eat polyunsaturated and monounsaturated fats. Avoid saturated fats. Eliminate hydrogenated fats and fried foods.** To help provide the proper balance of essential fatty acids (omega-6 and omega-3) take daily: 1½ tablespoons (20 ml) of flax- seed or 1½ teaspoons (7.5 ml) of flax oil.

Make sure you eat at least two to three servings per week of a food or fish that is high in omega-3 essential fatty acids.

☀ **Drink 6–8 8 fl. oz (225 ml) glasses of water or water equivalents every day.**

☀ **Eat mainly whole-grain products. Limit foods made with refined carbohydrates and processed white flours.** Whole-grain products are higher in fibre and help prevent carbohydrate cravings. Refined and processed carbohydrates to limit include foods made with white flour, most pastas, white rice, sugars and syrups.

☀ **Avoid alcohol or drink in moderation.** Alcohol, like sugar, provides calories with little nutritional value. Excessive drinking of alcoholic beverages can cause health problems.

A Closer Look at the Basic Food and Nutrition Guidelines

Reducing the Fat in Your Diet

Almost all packaged foods are now marked with Nutrition Information labels like the one at right. They show fat, sugars and calories per serving, among other details.

A good rule of thumb to follow when choosing low-fat foods is to check the nutrition label on the packages. Only purchase foods that contain either 3 grams or less of total fat per serving for individual items or 30 per

NUTRITION		
TYPICAL	A 200g	100g
COMPOSITION	serving provides	provides
Energy	730kj/172kcal	360kj/86kcal
Protein	3.0g	1.5g
Carbohyrdate	22.4g	11.2g
of which sugars	3.0g	1.5g
Fat	7.8g	3.9g
of which saturates	3.0g	1.5g
Fibre	3.0g	1.5g
Sodium	0.8g	0.4g
This pack contains 2 servings		
INFORMATION		

cent or less of total calories from fat for meals. By following this guideline, you will also be limiting your saturated fat intake, since most low-fat foods are also low in saturated fat.

Cutting Out Caffeine

Caffeine is a member of a group of drugs called methylxanthines that can stimulate your appetite, act as a diuretic and indirectly contribute to elevated blood cholesterol. Also, caffeine can actually make you feel like you have less energy by inducing a stress response. The graph over on the next page helps to show you how caffeine works on your system.

Within five minutes after you drink your morning coffee, the caffeine begins to stimulate your central nervous system, triggering the release of stress hormones in your body, causing a stress ('fight or flight') response. The stress hormones are useful if you need to prepare yourself to fight or flee a dangerous situation, but if you are simply sitting at your desk you may feel a short charge of alertness, quickly followed by feelings of agitation. Within the next hour or so, after the stress response dissipates, you will probably feel more tired and hungry. At these low-energy times, many people reach for another cup of coffee, or eat a snack that is often high in sugar to 'pep' themselves up and stay alert. However, both caffeine and sugar only give you temporary feelings of increased energy, which quickly dissipate. For some people, this cycle of low energy followed by an infusion of caffeine or food continues the entire day—leaving them feeling exhausted and unable to focus by 3.00 p.m. because they are drained from the ups and downs in energy their body endured throughout the day. By eliminating caffeine, you will feel like you have more energy, because your energy level stays at an even level throughout the day.

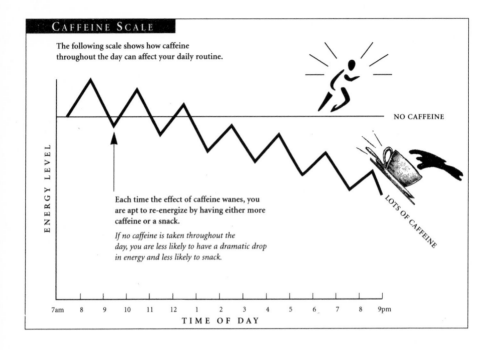

CAFFEINE SCALE

The following scale shows how caffeine throughout the day can affect your daily routine.

NO CAFFEINE

ENERGY LEVEL

Each time the effect of caffeine wanes, you are apt to re-energize by having either more caffeine or a snack.

If no caffeine is taken throughout the day, you are less likely to have a dramatic drop in energy and less likely to snack.

LOTS OF CAFFEINE

7am   8   9   10   11   12   1   2   3   4   5   6   7   8   9pm

TIME OF DAY

Caffeine also affects the body in many other unhealthy ways, including changing blood sugar and triglyceride levels, increasing blood pressure and heart rate, constricting blood vessels, inducing anxiety, disrupting sleep patterns, and inhibiting the body's absorption of iron, zinc, calcium, potassium, magnesium and sodium. In addition, caffeine has been linked to fibrous breast tissue, cancer and cardiovascular disease.

I strongly recommend that you eliminate the caffeine in your diet, particularly if you have heart disease, high blood pressure or osteoporosis, or if you want to increase your energy and lower your stress level.

Participants of the Active Wellness programme have been amazed at how energetic and calm they feel when they stop consuming caffeine. You can either eliminate all the caffeine in your diet right away, or slowly reduce the caffeine you consume over the course of several weeks. After two weeks of caffeine reduction you can decide whether you feel like you have more energy and/or fewer cravings for sweets and refined carbohydrates.

To reduce the caffeine in your diet, start by determining where your caffeine is coming from. The chart on the next page lists the levels of caffeine in a variety of foods. You can see that different beverages have different amounts of caffeine. Even decaf coffee has some caffeine, but far less than regular coffee.

Caffeine Content of Common Foods and Beverages		
Source	**Caffeine Content in Milligrams (mg)***	
	Range	Average
Coffee (5 fl. oz/140 ml)		
Drip	60-180	115
Espresso	50-120	85
Percolator	40-170	80
Instant	30-120	65
Decaffeinated, brewed	2-5	3
Decaffeinated, instant	1-5	2
Tea (5 fl. oz/140 ml)		
Brewed	25-110	65
Instant (1 tsp/5 ml powder)	25-50	35
Iced (12-oz. glass)	67-76	70
Soft Drinks (12 fl. oz/340 ml)		
Colas and diet colas	30-60	40
Cocoa and Chocolate Beverages		
Chocolate Milk (8 fl. oz/225 ml)	2-7	5
Cocoa beverages (5 fl. oz/140 ml)	2-20	4
Solid Chocolate and Syrup		
Plain chocolate (1 oz/30 g)	5-35	20
Milk chocolate (1 oz/30 g)	1-15	5
Bakers chocolate (1 oz/30 g)	26	26
Chocolate syrup (1 oz/30 g)	4	4
Coffee-flavoured low-fat yoghurt	45	45

* Source: U.S. Food and Drug Administration and M. L. Bunker & M. McWilliams, 'Caffeine Content of Common Beverages',*Journal of the American Dietetic Association*, Vol. 74, pages 28-32, January 1979.

When you eliminate or greatly reduce the caffeine in your diet, you may experience mild withdrawal symptoms, such as headaches, because caffeine is a mild drug. Aspirin can help with the headaches, and you will invariably feel better within three to four days. If you have been drinking large amounts of coffee or tea (five or more cups per day), decrease your caffeine gradually by switching to a mix of half-regular and half-decaf coffee or tea.

> Don't eat on the run! Sit down to eat every meal. Chew slowly and savour the scent, flavour and texture of your food.

Eating Five or More Fruits and Vegetables Daily

You can get most of your essential vitamins and minerals from fresh fruits and vegetables, which are more readily absorbed by the body. Vitamins and minerals are essential to the many biochemical functions that keep the body strong, healthy and disease free. One research study after another reports that people whose diets are rich in fruits and vegetables have lower incidences of heart disease, stroke and cancer. Additionally, the dark green, orange, yellow and red fruits and vegetables are high in antioxidant vitamins, which can prevent cell damage from oxidants. Oxidants include substances that can cause cell damage such as environmental pollutants, food additives, pesticides, trans fatty acids and over-supplementation of certain vitamins and minerals. (See the Foods Rich in Antioxidants and Other Vitamins chart on page 79.)

Many fruits and vegetables also contain phytochemicals, plant compounds that appear to have the ability to enhance the immune system and protect against cancer and heart disease. The most common fruits and vegetables that contain phytochemicals include citrus, garlic, onions, tomatoes, broccoli, cabbage, Brussels sprouts, kale and carrots.

Fruits and vegetables are also naturally low in fat and high in fibre. The additional fibre adds bulk to your diet, which is good for intestinal health and helps lower cholesterol levels. Fibre also helps you feel fuller for a longer period after meals, which discourages overeating.

Taking Vitamin and Mineral Supplements

I recommend taking supplements when you cannot eat a variety of foods every day, including five servings or more of different fruits and vegetables each day, and at least three servings of calcium-rich foods each day. All supplements should be taken on a full stomach or with meals.

It is often difficult to consume enough of the right foods to get adequate amounts of the essential vitamins and minerals that we need for optimal health.

Antioxidants found in fruits and vegetables, including vitamins C and E, carotenoids, and the mineral selenium are important for maintaining good health. Not only do they act as oxidants, but these vitamins and minerals also help inhibit the development of certain diseases by fighting off the damaging 'free radicals' in the body.

Free radicals are highly reactive molecules produced by environmental influences, including stress, radiation, air pollution, smoking and excessive oxygen in the body (caused by overexercising or by certain vitamins and minerals, such as iron). Free radicals can damage the cells of the body, which may result in wrinkled skin, cataracts, premature ageing, arterial plaque and, according to some researchers, certain cancers.

If you do not consume at least five fruits and vegetables listed in the Foods Rich in Antioxidants and Other Vitamins chart, make sure you obtain these nutrients in supplemental form.

An important fact to understand when taking supplements is that more is not necessarily better. Actually, too much of any one vitamin or mineral can inhibit the absorption of other essential nutrients. In addition, large doses of some vitamins and minerals are actually harmful. The guidelines provided by Active Wellness are safe levels of supplementation. Please see a registered dietitian before deciding to take other supplements that provide more than 100 per cent of the recommended dietary allowances (RDA).

Foods Rich in Antioxidants and Other Vitamins

Food Group	Carotenoids	Vitamin C	Vitamin E	Folic acid
V E G E T A B L E S	Asparagus Carrots Dark green, leafy vegetables (Dandelion Greens, Kale, Spinach, Mustard Greens, Chicory) Pumpkin Tomatoes Broccoli	Broccoli Cabbage Cauliflower Dark green, leafy vegetables (Kale, Collard, Mustard and Turnip Greens) Peppers (green and red) Brussels Sprouts Radishes Chili Peppers	Dark green, leafy vegetables (Spinach, Kale, Collard Greens Swiss Chard) Asparagus Broccoli	Asparagus Broccoli Beetroot Cauliflower Dark green, leafy vegetables (Spinach, Kale, Collard Greens) Seaweed Onions Artichoke
F R U I T S	Papaya Melon Apricot Mango Nectarine	Papaya Strawberries Orange Grapefruit Kiwi	Avocado pear Olives Papaya Mango Blueberries	Avocado pear Mango Papaya Banana Blackberries

> When purchasing supplements, make sure that you examine the expiration date so that you buy only active ingredients.

Eating Sweets Sparingly

Refined sugar acts on the body in a way similar to caffeine—it produces a cycle of unnatural energy highs and energy lows. Additionally, it stimulates the body into a 'false' sense of hunger and cravings, usually for sugary and fat-laden snacks, and it can elevate your triglyceride levels.

When you eat sugary foods, the body releases insulin that absorbs the sugar into your cells where it is used for energy. As your blood sugar level rises, you may feel like you have more energy. But that energy is short lived. When blood sugar levels inevitably decrease—because the sugar in your blood has all been absorbed—you tend to feel tired and low in energy. And at this low end of the sugar cycle, people often crave another sugary snack to give them another energy boost, thus starting the (vicious!) cycle again.

> A spoonful of sugar makes your energy go down...!

Avoiding 'Bad' Fats and Eating 'Good' Fats

Not all fats are bad for you. In fact, some fats are essential to good health. These 'good' fats help to build and maintain cellular tissue, transport vitamins and manufacture hormones. The five major types of fats found in food are:

- Saturated fats
- Hydrogenated fats—trans fatty acids
- Polyunsaturated fats
- Monounsaturated fats
- Essential fatty acids—omega-6 (alpha-linoleic acid) and omega-3 (linolenic acid) fatty acids

Saturated Fats and Hydrogenated Fats. These are the 'bad' fats that have a detrimental effect on your health and should be avoided. Saturated fat is the most prevalent fat in the diet and is a leading contributor to high cholesterol levels, fatty plaque deposits in the coronary arteries and cardiovascular disease in general. Foods such as lard, butter, full-fat dairy products, meats, palm oil and coconut oil contain saturated fats, which are solid at room temperature.

Hydrogenated fats are liquid oils made solid by the addition of hydrogen, as in margarine. They typically appear in baked goods, cereals, snack foods and fast foods. Once presumed 'healthier' than saturated fats, current research indicates that hydrogenated fats raise total blood cholesterol levels and LDL cholesterol. In terms of your health, hydrogenated fats (margarines) are just as bad as saturated fats (butter).

Additionally, when fats are hydrogenated they produce a very damaging form of fats called trans fatty acids, which have recently been the subject of much cardiovascular research. Trans fatty acids create damaging free radicals that cause damage to our cells and arteries. Free radical damage also caused by oxidants have been linked to cancer, heart disease and premature ageing.

Polyunsaturated and Monounsaturated Fats. These are the good 'fats' that have a positive effect on your health. Both types of fat are liquid at room temperature and have beneficial effects on blood cholesterol levels.

Polyunsaturated fats are found mainly in plant foods, such as nuts, seeds, corn (maize) and corn, safflower and sunflower oil. They lower total cholesterol levels and 'bad' LDL cholesterol levels. Our LDL (low-density lipoproteins) is the 'least desirable' to have at high levels, because it is the carrier that is responsible for depositing cholesterol on our arterial walls, creating plaque that can lead to a heart attack or stroke.

Monounsaturated fats are found in peanuts, avocado pears, olive oil and peanut oil. Monounsaturated fats not only lower total and LDL cholesterol levels, but they also appear to raise the 'good' HDL cholesterol levels that are associated with a decreased risk of heart disease. HDL (high-density lipoproteins) are highly desirable because they are responsible for picking up cholesterol to be re-used by the body. I like to think of them as 'recyclers' that pick up waste (excess cholesterol) and carry it back to the liver to be re-used. The more HDL you have, the better, because it will help clear the excess cholesterol from your system and reduce the problems that can be caused by your LDL cholesterol.

Bad Fats	Good Fats	
Saturated Fats	Polyunsaturated Fats	Monounsaturated Fats
Coconut oil	Safflower oil	Olive oil
Butter	Sunflower oil	Peanut oil
Beef fat	Corn oil	
Lard		
Full-fat dairy foods		
Palm oil		

Essential Fatty Acids—Omega-6 (alpha-linoleic acid) and Omega-3 (linolenic acid). Essential fatty acids, also called omega-6 and omega-3 fatty acids, are part of the polyunsaturated fat family and are members of the 'good' fats group. They are called essential, because the body cannot make them and must obtain them from foods.

Omega-3 fatty acids in particular have multiple beneficial effects on the body and should be eaten on a daily basis, since most diets are deficient in them. Flaxseed is an excellent source of omega-3 fatty acids; 1 tablespoon (15 ml) contains 2,000 milligrams of omega-3. Among the many health benefits of omega-3 fatty acids, the major ones include:

⬧ Lowering triglycerides
⬧ Decreasing inflammation (and pain) in connective tissues diseases such as arthritis

◇ Inhibiting the blood-clotting mechanism that causes heart attacks and strokes
◇ Thinning the blood and increasing the availability of oxygen to the body's tissues
◇ Lowering blood pressure

Fish Rich in Omega-3 Fatty Acids	
Based on a 3½-oz (100 g) serving: Contains 500 to 1,000 or more milligrams of omega-3 fatty acids.	
Anchovies	Squid (Calamari)
Carp	Striped Sea Bass
Halibut	Swordfish
Herring	Trout, Rainbow
Mackerel	Tuna, Albacore, Bluefin
Salmon	Turbot
Sardines	Whitefish
Shark	

Omega-3 fatty acids can be found in many 'fatty' fish, the most common of which are illustrated in the chart above. Try to add two to three servings of these fish foods to your diet each week. You can also get your omega-3 fatty acids from plant sources including flaxseed, green leafy vegetables, nuts and especially soya products (soya beans, tofu, tempeh).

Omega-6 fatty acids, which in the diet are derived primarily from vegetable oils, are also essential to good health. Currently, they make up the greater percentage of essential fats in the diet. Over the course of time, and with the development of technology for manufacturing oils, the diet has become disproportionately high in omega-6 fatty acids, creating an imbalance.

The general population does not consume enough omega-3 fatty acids. Currently, the ratio of omega-6 to omega-3 in the diet is about 10:1, but a healthful diet has a ratio around 2:1—only two times the amount of omega-6 instead of 10 times the amount. In order to create a healthful balance, it is important to make sure you are eating a greater amount of foods that are rich in omega-3 fats. You can do this by following the Active Wellness recommendation to increase omega-3-rich fish in your diet and to incorporate 1½ tablespoons (20 ml) of flaxseed per day, or 1½ teaspoons (7.5 ml) of flax oil into your diet. If you are a vegetarian, the flaxseed will help you meet recommended levels of omega-3 fats. The best supplement is the seed itself, which can be sprinkled on salads, on cereals or on yoghurt. Capsules often go rancid, and for this reason they are not recommended.

Plant Sources Rich in Omega-3 Fatty Acids
(Not including nuts)

Based on the servings below, these plant sources contain 500 to 100 milligrams of omega-3 fatty acids.

Berries—Strawberry, Raspberry, Blueberry (8 fl. oz /225 ml)	Tempeh ('4 fl. oz/115 ml)
	Tofu (4 fl. oz/115 ml)
Dried Beans (8 fl. oz./225 ml)	Soyabeans, young green (4 fl. oz/115 ml)
Dark Green Leafy Vegetables (i.e. spinach) (8 fl. oz/225 ml)	Soyabeans, roasted (1 oz/30 g)

Drinking 6–8 8 fl. oz (225 ml) Glasses of Water or Water Equivalents Daily
Over 60 per cent of your body is water. For your body to function efficiently, it must be well hydrated. If you are trying to lose weight, drinking water also helps curb your appetite.

Using Alcohol in Moderation
A little alcohol goes a long way. Recent research from the University of Milan and the Georgetown University Medical Center reaffirms that moderate intakes of alcohol from wine, beer and spirits can help protect against heart disease by reducing the stickiness of the blood and interfering with blood clots.

However, drinking moderate amounts of alcohol also has several downsides. Studies associating cancer with alcohol consumption found that alcohol consumption may increase the risk of several cancers, including breast cancer, lung cancer, and cancer of the mouth, larynx, oesophagus and liver.

Alcohol also stimulates the appetite and can alter your perception of how hungry you really are. So if you are trying to lose weight, consider avoiding alcohol as a good strategy. Furthermore, alcohol contains many calories and very little nutrition.

If you are a non-drinker you should not start drinking to benefit your health. If you do drink and are concerned about its effects, weigh your personal risks and benefits. You should definitely avoid alcohol if you have very high triglycerides, uncontrolled hypertension, liver disease, breast cancer or risk of breast cancer, abnormal heart rhythms, peptic ulcers, or sleep apnoea.

All the Active Wellness eating plans recommend you limit yourself to one drink a day, equivalent to 5 fl. oz (140 ml) of wine, 12 fl. oz (340 ml) of beer, or 1½ fl. oz (45 ml) of distilled spirits (80 proof).

Eating Mainly Whole-Grain Products
The amount of refined carbohydrates (white bread, pasta and crackers) that you should eat does reach a limit. Consuming a lot of bread products that are not whole

grain can raise your triglycerides, particularly if they're already elevated. By including more whole-grain products and fewer refined bread products in your diet, you can help decrease your triglycerides. Whole grains are also high in fibre, which adds bulk to your diet helping you to feel full and prevent overeating. Fibre can also help reduce your cholesterol and prevent bowel cancer.

> Remember to use your Daily Allowance Cards to reinforce your new, healthier eating behaviours.

STEP 2

Part II

The Active Wellness Eating Plans

Plan 1
Active Wellness Basic Eating Plan
for Good Health

General Nutrition Guidelines for Plan 1

Plan 1 is a general eating plan designed to promote optimal health and well-being. It is based on a breakdown in energy nutrients of 60 per cent carbohydrates, 20 per cent proteins and 20 per cent fats. Combine your eating plan with The Active Wellness Basic Food and Nutrition Guidelines on pages 73-74.

This plan is suitable for the various types of vegetarians: vegans, who eat no meat, fish, poultry, eggs or dairy products; ovo-vegetarians, who eat eggs; ovo-lacto-vegetarians, who eat eggs and milk; and semi-vegetarians, who eat some fish and chicken, but no beef. Vegans tend to have the lowest levels of body fat, blood pressure and cholesterol.

If you wish to start following a vegetarian diet you can use this plan to help you incorporate more vegetarian eating into your life. Begin by eating a vegetarian meal one or two nights per week. In order to make your vegetarian or non-vegetarian meals more appetizing, fill your plate with vegetables, grains, and proteins that have a variety of colours, textures, and tastes. To expand your choices of foods, experiment with eating new foods, such as different beans, fruits, fish, vegetables and the many new soy products on the market.

> Family and friends are there for you! Ask them for support as you make these positive changes in your life.

Plan 1 Chart
Active Wellness Basic Eating Plan
for Good Health

Calorie level	Grains/ Starches	Veggie	Protein	Fruit	Dairy	Fat	Sweets	Alcohol
1,200	4	4	3	2	2	3	1	1
1,300	5	4	4	2	2	3	1	1
1,400	6	4	4	2	2	3	1	1
1,500	6	4	4	2	3	4	1	1
1,600	7	4	5	3	2	4	1	1
1,700	8	5	5	3	2	4	1	1
1,800	9	4	5	3	2	5	1	1
1,900	10	4	5	3	2	5½	1	1
2,000	11	3	5	2	3	6	1	1
2,100	12	4	5	2	3	6	1	1
2,200	12	4	6	3	3	6	1	1
2,300	13	5	6	3	3	6	1	1
2,400	13	5	7	4	3	6	1	1
2,500	14	5	8	3	3	6½	1	1
2,600	15	6	8	3	3	6½	1	1

Plan 2
Active Wellness Eating Plan for Preventing Osteoporosis

General Nutrition Guidelines for Plan 2

One in three women and one in twelve men in the UK will develop osteoporosis in their lifetime. The disease costs the NHS and the British government over £940 million every year. Worryingly, the incidence of osteoporosis is increasing by 10% a year.

Plan 2 is based on a breakdown in energy nutrients of 60 per cent carbohydrates, 20 per cent proteins and 20 per cent fats. This plan emphasizes servings of high-calcium foods to meet elevated demands for those who are concerned with consuming adequate amounts of calcium to maintain bone mass and bone density. Combine Plan 2 with The Active Wellness Basic Food and Nutrition Guidelines, for a well-balanced plan that will help prevent osteoporosis and promote optimum health. After the body reaches the age of 30 the majority of bone is formed. From that point on, if calcium levels drop in the blood, your body extracts the calcium it needs from your bones. This depletes bone density and mass, particularly after menopause, and significantly increases the risk for serious bone fractures. Therefore, you need to consume optimal levels of calcium every day, via foods and supplements, to maintain an adequate calcium balance in your body.

You need to do four things to maximize calcium levels in your blood:

⋄ Take enough calcium to meet your daily needs. Calcium is best absorbed from foods. Intake goals, based on the report of the Panel on Dietary Reference Values of the Committee on Medical Aspects of Food Policy, for calcium are as follows: adolescents should consume 800 to 1,000 mg per day, 25- to 50-year-old adults should consume 700 mg per day, and females over 51 (or on oestrogen replacement) and men over 65 should consume 700 mg per day. If you cannot meet your needs with the foods you eat (see the Calcium-Rich Foods chart opposite), a supplement is recommended. However, do not take a calcium supplement with 2,500 mg (or more) per day, because it can raise the risk of kidney stones and interfere with the absorption of other essential minerals, such as iron, zinc and magnesium.

⋄ Consume ample quantities of foods or vitamin and mineral supplements that enhance the absorption of calcium, including soya-based foods, vitamin D and vitamin C. Soya-based foods contain phyto-oestrogens, which may inhibit the loss of calcium from your bones. Vitamin D is essential for the absorption and utilization of calcium. It is a nutrient naturally made by our bodies upon exposure to 10 to 15 minutes of sunlight; however, this ability declines with age. If you do not spend time outdoors or are over 50 years of age, you should consider taking a daily vitamin D supplement of 400 IUs to 800 IUs, which can be part of your calcium supplement. Low- fat or skimmed milk is fortified with approximately 100 IUs of vitamin D per 8 fl. oz (225 ml). Vitamin C also helps enhance the absorption of calcium. The amounts of vitamin C in the Active Wellness eating plans will adequately meet your requirement, but it is also a good idea to eat calcium-rich foods (yoghurt, cottage cheese, milk) with fruits or vegetables that are high in vitamin C. (See the lists of fruits and vegetables in the Foods Rich in Antioxidants and Other Vitamins chart on page 79.)

⋄ Avoid foods and minerals that inhibit the absorption of calcium, including excess protein, salt, iron, beetroot greens, and spinach. Beetroot greens and spinach are high in calcium, but are also high in substances called oxalates, which inhibit calcium absorption. Substitute soya-based food products (soya milk, tofu and soya beans) for some of the protein in your diet. And limit salt intake to 2,300 mg (1 teaspoon/5 ml) or less per day.

◇ Weight-bearing exercises are important to maintaining bone mass. Choose an exercise that you enjoy and try to do it for at least 30 minutes each day.

If you do take calcium supplements, for best absorption, take them with food in 500 mg dosages or less, spaced throughout the day. According to recent research from Tuft University's Human Nutrition Research Center on Aging, if you are taking 1,500 mg of calcium daily you should complement this with 10 mg of zinc, because high levels of calcium inhibit zinc absorption. Check your multivitamin levels of zinc before you take an additional supplement. Another mineral that contributes to the formation of strong bones is magnesium. Magnesium is found in whole grains, nuts, beans, tofu and dark green leafy vegetables. Your multivitamin will help ensure that you are taking in adequate levels of magnesium each day.

CAUTION: Too Much of a Good Thing
Please be aware that the US National Academy of Sciences has set tolerable upper intake levels (UL) for calcium at 2,500 mg per day and vitamin D at 2,000 IU (50 mcg) per day. Health problems can occur when your daily intake is at the UL levels or above.

Calcium-Rich Foods		
Food	Serving	Calcium (mg)
Yoghurt, non-fat, plain	8 fl. oz/225 ml	452
Yoghurt, low- fat, plain	8 fl. oz/225 ml	415
Yoghurt, low- fat, vanilla	8 fl. oz/225 ml	389
Evaporated milk, skimmed	4 fl. oz/115 ml	371
Collard greens, cooked	8 fl. oz/225 ml	357
Ricotta cheese, part skimmed	4 fl. oz/115 ml	337
Parmesan cheese, hard	1 oz/30 g	336
Orange juice, calcium fortified	8 fl. oz/225 ml	333
Milk, skimmed	8 fl. oz/225 ml	302
Milk, 1% fat	8 fl. oz/225 ml	300
Soya milk, fortified	8 fl. oz/225 ml	200 to 300
Soya beans, dry roasted	4 fl. oz/115 ml	232
Tofu, firm	4 fl. oz/115 ml	100 to 200

Plan 2 Chart
Active Wellness Eating Plan for Preventing Osteoporosis

Calorie level	Grains/ Starches	Veg	Protein	Fruit	Dairy	Fat	Sweets	Alcohol
1,200	4	3	2	2	3	3½	1	1
1,300	4	3	2	2	4	4	1	1
1,400	4½	4	3	2	4	4	1	1
1,500	5	4	3	3	4	4	1	1
1,600	5	2	4	4	4	4½	1	1
1,700	6	2	5	4	4	4½	1	1
1,800	7	4	5	3	4	5½	1	1
1,900	7	4	4	3	5	6	1	1
2,000	7	5	5	5	4	6	1	1
2,100	8	5	5½	5	4	6½	1	1
2,200	9	5	6	5	4	6½	1	1
2,300	10	5	6	5	4	6½	1	1
2,400	11	6	6	5	4	6½	1	1
2,500	11	6	6	5	5	7	1	1
2,600	12	6	6	5	5	7½	1	1

Plan 3
Active Wellness Eating Plan for Prevention of Heart Disease, Stroke, Elevated Cholesterol and High Blood Pressure

General Nutrition Guidelines for Plan 3

Plan 3 is based on a breakdown in nutrients of 65 per cent carbohydrates, 20 per cent proteins and 15 per cent fats. This plan includes 5 per cent more carbohydrates and 5 per cent less fat than in the Active Wellness Basic Eating Plan, in order to help prevent diet risks associated with heart disease.

In conjunction with the general Active Wellness guidelines, which are beneficial for preventing heart disease, Plan 3 also emphasizes potassium-rich foods and foods rich in vitamins B_6 and B_{12} and folic acid. Other lifestyle risk factors associated with heart disease include smoking, sedentary lifestyle and obesity.

Preventing Heart Disease, Stroke and Elevated Cholesterol

Reducing your risks for heart disease and stroke and lowering your cholesterol levels requires that you watch your total intake of fat, trans fatty acids and saturated fat. Fats and elevated cholesterol can clog arteries, decreasing blood flow to the heart, causing heart disease and possible heart attacks. You can refer to the guidelines in Step 1 to reassess your risk based on your current cholesterol levels.

Aim to keep your triglyceride level below 100, since recent research from the University of Maryland's Center for Preventive Cardiology links readings above 100 with more than twice the risk of heart disease. Triglycerides can be elevated by refined sugars, processed flours, bread products, sweets, alcohol and fat—so try to avoid those foods.

A number of recent cardiovascular research studies around the world indicate that a fourth substance in the blood, an amino acid called homocysteine, significantly increases the risk for heart attack when found in high levels. Elevated levels occur when homocysteine is not broken down properly in the body, due to a genetic or environmental defect. Vitamins B_6 and B_{12} together with folic acid can break down homocysteine to safe levels, which is why Plan 3 specifically recommends them. Foods rich in vitamins B_6 and B_{12} include poultry, fish, pork, beans, whole grains, fortified soya foods, lean meats and milk. Folic acid can be found in leafy vegetables, pulses and fortified cereals. It is a good idea to take the recommended folic acid supplement listed in the guidelines. Also check your multivitamin to see if it has at least 4 mg of vitamin B_6 and 8 micrograms of vitamin B_{12}.

Omega-3 essential fatty acids can help lower cholesterol and reduce the risk for heart disease, as discussed in the Active Wellness Basic Food and Nutrition Guidelines. Although omega-3 supplements and vitamin E can help you, the wrong dosage may increase your risk for stroke. Therefore, be sure to consult your doctor before taking fish-oil or vitamin E supplements.

It is also beneficial to consider moving toward a more vegetarian diet, because plant foods are naturally low in fat, high in protective antioxidants and phytochemicals, and higher in fibre, all of which can help you reduce your risks for heart disease.

Preventing High Blood Pressure

High blood pressure is defined as anything at or above 140/90 ml of mercury. An optimal blood pressure is equal to or less than 120/80 ml of mercury. High blood pressure may be the result of several factors: excess weight, lack of exercise, excessive sodium intake (if you are salt-sensitive), excessive fat consumption, lack of fruits and vegetables in your diet, smoking or high levels of stress.

Too much salt in the diet is commonly believed to be a major cause of high blood pressure associated with heart disease, but in fact only half the people who have elevated blood pressure are sensitive to salt. A doctor can determine if you are salt-sensitive by finding out if you have low levels of the enzyme renin, which helps regulate blood pressure. If your renin levels are low, you are probably salt-sensitive and should reduce your intake of salt (sodium) to 1 teaspoon (5 ml) a day or less.

However, salt intake does appear related to stroke risk. Keeping your blood pressure at normal levels is particularly important for preventing strokes. In a project conducted by the US National Institutes of Health, both men and women aged 60 to 80, who reduced their excess weight and sodium intake were 50 per cent more likely to maintain normal blood pressure levels without medication.

Recent research from Johns Hopkins University indicates that the mineral potassium plays a significant role in regulating blood pressure. Supplementing your diet with 2,300 mg of potassium can significantly lower blood pressure if you also get at least 2,500 mg of potassium in your food daily. While many people do take potassium in supplemental tablet form, getting your potassium through foods is the optimal way to reduce your blood pressure. The chart below lists the most potassium-rich foods by serving size. Try to incorporate as many of these foods as possible into your eating plan.

Potassium-Rich Foods

Food	Serving	Potassium (mg)
Banana	1 large size	451
Melon	8 fl. oz/225 ml	494
Dried prunes	5	313
Figs	5	666
Kidney beans	4 fl. oz/115 ml	357
Potatoes	1 large size	844
Raisins	2 fl. oz/60 ml	563
Spinach	4 fl. oz/115 ml	419
Swiss chard	4 fl. oz/115 ml	483

CAUTION: Please consult your doctor before taking potassium supplements. If you take prescription medications called angiotensin-converting enzyme (ACE) inhibitors to lower your blood pressure, or if you have impaired kidney function, heart disease, or diabetes, taking extra potassium can be dangerous.

Plan 3 Chart
Active Wellness Eating Plan for Prevention of Heart Disease, Stroke, Elevated Cholesterol and High Blood Pressure

Calorie level	Grains/ Starches	Veg	Protein	Fruit	Dairy	Fat	Sweets	Alcohol
1,200	5	4	3	2	2	2	1	1
1,300	5	5	3	3	2	2	1	1
1,400	6	5	3½	3	2	2	1	1
1,500	7	5	4	3	2	2	1	1
1,600	8	5	4½	3	2	2	1	1
1,700	9	5	4½	3	2	3	1	1
1,800	9	5	5	4	2	3	1	1
1,900	9	6	5½	5	2	3	1	1
2,000	10	6	5½	5	2	3	1	1
2,100	10	6	5½	5½	3	3	1	1
2,200	10	6	6	6½	3	3	1	1
2,300	10	6	7	7	3	3½	1	1
2,400	11	6	7	7½	3	3½	1	1
2,500	11	6	8	8½	3	3½	1	1
2,600	12	7	8	8½	3	3½	1	1

Plan 4
Active Wellness Eating Plan for Type 1 Insulin-Dependent and Type 2 Non-Insulin Dependent Diabetes, Insulin Resistance, Carbohydrate Craving and Hypoglycaemia

General Nutrition Guidelines for Plan 4

The eating plan for insulin-dependent and non-insulin dependent diabetes is designed to keep blood sugar levels down and also reduce triglyceride and cholesterol levels. Current research from Stanford University indicates that diabetics can reduce their blood sugar levels and triglycerides by eating a diet that is slightly higher in monounsaturated fats than what is recommended in the Active Wellness Basic Eating Plan. Plan 4, therefore, is comprised of 50 per cent carbohydrates, 20 per cent proteins and

STEP 2, PART II

30 per cent fats, with the additional fats in the form of monounsaturated fats. This eating plan applies to diabetics as well as to the other conditions: insulin resistance, carbohydrate craving and hypoglycaemia (low blood sugar).

In general, the key to keeping your blood sugar levels under control is to use food to your advantage by carefully planning mealtimes and food portions. Three main components of every meal affect the elevation of blood sugar: the types of food you eat; the amount of food you eat; and the amount of fibre in the food you eat.

Types of Food You Eat

Carbohydrates are metabolized into sugar in the bloodstream, and therefore you must monitor carbohydrate intake closely, including the carbohydrates in grains, starchy vegetables, sugary foods and fruits. In particular refined (processed) carbohydrate foods should be avoided, including sugar, fruit juice, white bread, pre-cooked rice, pasta and most refined cereals. A good rule of thumb is to limit yourself to a total of three servings of the high-carbohydrate food groups at any one meal, the grains/starches group, which includes starchy vegetables (corn/maize, peas, mashed potatoes) and the fruit group. Vegetables are unlimited, but one can eat sweet vegetables such as carrots and beets in moderation. If you want a sweet, sugar-free sweets are good choices, or sweets that are low in sugar (made with unsweetened fruits). It is best to eat sweets after a meal and limit yourself to one serving a day or less. Proteins and fats do not elevate your blood sugar unless they are prepared with a sweet sauce.

Eat a Variety of Nutrient Groups at One Meal

Each nutrient group—proteins, carbohydrates, and fats—are digested at different rates. Both proteins and fats are slower than carbohydrates, and when combined with carbohydrates can slow down the absorption of sugar into your body. Eating a variety of foods at a set number of meals slows down your rate of digestion while also slowing down the absorption of carbohydrates. In turn, slowing down the rate at which carbohydrates are absorbed helps keep blood sugar levels normal.

Amount of Fibre in the Food You Eat

High fibre foods, such as whole grains, brown rice and beans, add bulk to the diet and slow down digestion. As noted above, slowing down digestion also slows down the absorption of carbohydrates (which are metabolized into sugar) and thus helps keep blood sugar levels stable.

Checking your blood sugar levels regularly is also important in order to determine what specific foods may cause unnecessary elevations in your blood sugar. Artificial sweeteners are acceptable to use. Alcohol is not recommended, but if you want to drink, limit yourself to one drink a day.

A Note for Insulin-Dependent Diabetics

Timing meals with insulin injections is the most important dietary aspect of managing insulin-dependent diabetes. The goal is to avoid wide swings in blood glucose levels. Many people eat breakfast, lunch and dinner and at least one evening snack. A good rule of thumb is to avoid eating more than 3 units of grains or starchy vegetables at any one meal: this alleviates wide swings in your blood sugar. Desserts are best eaten following a meal. Fruit, which is high in sugar, can be eaten after a meal or as part of a snack. (See the Appendix for meal plan ideas.)

Plan 4 Chart
Active Wellness Eating Plan for Type 1 Insulin-Dependent and Type 2 Non-Insulin Dependent Diabetes, Insulin Resistance, Carbohydrate Craving and Hypoglycaemia

Calorie level	Grains/ Starches	Veg	Protein	Fruit	Dairy	Fat	Sweets	Alcohol
1,200	3	3	3	2	2	5½	1	1
1,300	3	3	3	2	3	6	1	1
1,400	3	4	4	2	3	6½	1	1
1,500	4	4	4	2	3	7	1	1
1,600	4	4	5	3	3	7	1	1
1,700	5	4	5	3	3	7½	1	1
1,800	6	3	6	3	3	7½	1	1
1,900	7	3	6	3	3	8	1	1
2,000	6	5	6	3	4	9	1	1
2,100	7	5	6	3	4	9½	1	1
2,200	7	6	6	4	4	10	1	1
2,300	7½	6	7	4	4	10	1	1
2,400	8½	5	8	4	4	10	1	1
2,500	9	6	8	4	4	10½	1	1
2,600	9	6	8	5	4	11½	1	1

Plan 5
Active Wellness Eating Plan for Individuals
with a Personal or Family History of Cancer

General Nutrition Guidelines for Plan 5

The Active Wellness Basic Food and Nutritional Guidelines on pages 73-74 are consistent with recommendations for prevention of cancer. Plan 5 follows those guidelines and is comprised of 60 per cent carbohydrates, 20 per cent proteins and 20 per cent fats. Plan 5 enhances the general plan by recommending a higher intake of fruits and vegetables that contain protective phytochemicals and antioxidants to fight the damaging free radicals linked to cancer and other diseases. Fat intake is somewhat limited in Plan 5 because of the link between excess fat and several cancers, particularly breast cancer. Plan 5 foods are also high in fibre, which has been shown to reduce the risks for both colon and breast cancers.

Avoid foods that have been barbecued, smoked, or pickled, since those foods have been linked with some stomach and oesophagus cancers. Also avoid alcohol if you are concerned about cancer of the liver, head or neck (including the larynx, pharynx, mouth and oesophagus). Excessive alcohol intake also weakens the immune system.

If you or someone you know is undergoing radiation or chemotherapy for cancer, bear in mind the importance of consuming enough calories to keep the body strong and help promote healing. In particular, the appetite may be reduced or the taste buds impaired while undergoing chemotherapy, so finding appetizing and tasty foods is a worthy challenge. If chewing is a problem, liquid shakes made with fruit and skimmed milk or non-dairy milk are excellent nutritional supplements.

> Eating excessive amounts of refined sugar also inhibits your body's absorption of vitamin C from fruits and vegetables.

Plan 5 Chart
Active Wellness Eating Plan for Individuals
with a Personal or Family History of Cancer

Calorie level	Grains/ Starches	Veg	Protein	Fruit	Dairy	Fat	Sweets	Alcohol
1,200	2	4	4	4	2	3	1	1
1,300	3	4	5	4	2	3	1	1
1,400	4	4	5	4	2	3	1	1
1,500	4	4	5	4	3	4	1	1
1,600	5	4	6	5	2	4	1	1
1,700	6	5	6	5	2	4	1	1
1,800	7	4	6	5	2	5	1	1
1,900	7	5	5	5	3	6	1	1
2,000	9	3	6	4	3	6	1	1
2,100	10	4	6	4	3	6	1	1
2,200	10	4	7	5	3	6	1	1
2,300	12	5	7	5	3	6	1	1
2,400	12	5	8	6	3	6	1	1
2,500	13	7	8	4	3	6½	1	1
2,600	14	8	8	4	3	6½	1	1

Congratulations! You have taken a monumental leap toward optimal Active Wellness with all the work you've done in Steps 1 and 2. You've taken a look at your own health and lifestyle, reviewed your family's medical history and set yourself some reasonable but challenging long- and short-term health goals. You decided what you wanted and needed from a nutritional programme and designed your own customized eating plan for maximum health and well-being. Now all you need to start eating right is a larder full of healthy and appetizing foods. Throw out those hot dogs, soft drinks and cakes! It's time to go shopping and set up your own Active Wellness kitchen!

STEP 3

Setting Up Your Active Wellness Kitchen

One should eat to live, not live to eat.
—Molière

One of the best ways to stay on your personal eating plan is to be prepared. Stocking your kitchen with the right foods makes healthy eating much easier and more enjoyable. Start setting up your Active Wellness kitchen by getting rid of all those high-fat, high-sugar and low-nutrition foods that may tempt you away from your path of healthy eating!

Cleaning Out the Kitchen

Your first plan of action is to discard all the high-fat items from your kitchen shelves and to restock them with new and appetizing foods. If you are the only one in your family who is following the Active Wellness eating plan, you may want to set up a shelf in one of your cupboards and in your refrigerator with foods that are just for you. That way, you won't be as tempted by the rest of the family's 'goodies'.

> *The 3 Grams Fat Rule:* Discard any food product that contains more than 3 grams of fat per serving or that derives more than 30 per cent of its total calories from fat.

Go through your cupboard, refrigerator and freezer shelves and remove all of the high-fat items, except actual fats such as oil and butter. Use as your guide the nutrition label on each product and discard any food that contains more than 3 grams of fat per serving. Any food product with 3 grams of fat or less per serving is considered a low-fat food; most of these are also low in saturated fats.

Now go through your freezer shelves and remove any prepackaged, frozen meals or side dishes that derive more than 3 grams of fat per serving. The nutrition label on prepackaged foods often lists the weight of fat in 100 g of the product. This will give your the percentage of fat contained in the product. For example, 3.9 g total fat in

100 g of a product is 3.9 per cent . . . and should be discarded.

Also discard any foods that contain hydrogenated vegetable oil. Hydrogenated fats (the fats that contain damaging trans fatty acids) will be listed in the ingredients information on the package. Many prepared rice and pasta dinners come with flavouring packets that contain hydrogenated fats. These flavouring packets are often high in sodium as well. You can discard the packets and keep the rice and pasta.

If you're also cutting down on or eliminating caffeine, now is the time to rethink how many high-caffeine items you want to discard or give away, including espresso, dark roast coffee, decaf coffee, tea and colas.

Restocking the Kitchen:
Shopping the Active Wellness Way

When you begin the Active Wellness way of life, food shopping becomes fun, instead of a chore. Eventually you'll learn how to work your way around the supermarket in record time because you'll be avoiding some food aisles completely.

Do plan to spend some extra time when you take your first Active Wellness shopping trip. You'll be reading the Nutrition Information labels on all the items you purchase—checking for fat, sodium and sugar contents. And you'll be looking for new food products that satisfy your plan's nutritional requirements.

One of the key facts to know about supermarkets, which will streamline your shopping time, is that all of the fresh food items, including fruits, vegetables, fruit juices, meat, poultry, seafood, dairy and sometimes even frozen food and bread products, are usually located around the perimeter of the store. Packaged and canned items are located in the center aisles of the store. Knowing this helps make healthy shopping easy and quick, since the majority of foods you will buy on a regular basis are fresh foods that are found on the outside aisles. A good place to begin your Active Wellness shopping trip is in the produce section.

Vegetables and Fruits

Fresh Produce

Vegetables, fruits and the starchy vegetables, which are members of the grains/starches group on your eating plan, are found primarily in the fresh produce section of supermarkets. Vegetables and fruits are essential to good health and your daily eating plan. Pound for pound, they are the best supermarket buy. They add flavour, colour, vitamins, minerals and fibre to your meals and are invariably low in fat, sugar and sodium. The most flavourful vegetables and fruits are those that are fresh and in season. Out of season produce is usually picked before it has ripened, and the ripening then takes place during shipping. Reducing the plant's natural ageing process in this way also reduces both flavour and nutritional value.

Farmers' markets are often good sources for fresh, ripe produce. If you have a weekly market in your area, try to take advantage of it. You may also find fresh produce stands and stores that are open year round. It is usually worth the trip to these specialty produce markets, because you benefit by finding freshly picked produce. Keep in mind that the vegetable portions in your plan are minimum guidelines—fresh vegetables should be considered unlimited foods in your eating plan.

Antioxidant Shopping Tip: An easy way to spot antioxidant-rich vegetables and fruits is to shop by colour. Vegetables and fruits that are yellow, orange, red and dark green generally pack the most nutrition per bite. Orange produce such as carrots, tomatoes and melon, as well as dark green leafy vegetables, are high in carotenoids. Strawberries, broccoli, red pepper and oranges are good sources of vitamin C, and vitamin E can be found in corn/maize, kale, spinach and sweet potatoes.

As you shop in the produce section, be adventurous and try some of the many unique varieties of fruits and vegetables that are now available. Fresh and loose produce is best, but if you are short on cooking time, you can buy prepackaged fruits and vegetables from the produce section or precut produce from the salad bar. This will save you preparation time at home. The special bags used for premixed salads and other fruits and vegetables help retain their freshness, but they usually aren't as flavourful or as nutritious as loose produce. Both light and heat can enhance the loss of vitamins and minerals in foods.

The produce section may also be where you will find excellent vegetable protein sources, such as tofu and tempeh, low-fat salad dressings and fresh vegetable and fruit juices.

Buying Organic—Is It Better?

Although it's difficult to determine whether organic produce is more nutritious, produce labelled 'organic' should contain less pesticide residue. The effects of long-term ingestion of pesticide residue is inconclusive, but it is always advisable to minimize your exposure to it when you can. You can identify organic produce by the label, which should show the name of the Soil Association or a related organisation, which verifies that the product was grown without pesticides. Keep in mind, however, that organically grown products may not necessarily be pesticide-free, since airborne pesticides may drift onto organic produce from neighbouring fields. Also keep in mind that even if organic produce isn't available, the benefits of eating fresh fruits and vegetables certainly outweigh any risk from pesticide residues.

> *Fibre Shopping Tip:* When looking for fibre-rich fruits, a good rule of thumb is to buy those that have edible skins and seeds, such as apples and strawberries. Dried fruits are also high in fibre because they are dehydrated, and therefore more concentrated. But eat them sparingly if you are watching your weight, because they are also high in calories.
>
> Since most vegetables are high in fibre, refer to the antioxidant shopping tip *(opposite)* to find the vegetables that are good sources of vitamins and minerals. For best nutrition, avoid vegetables that are pale green, such as iceberg lettuce and peeled cucumber. Fibre-rich vegetables and fruits include broccoli, carrots, Brussels sprouts, berries, potatoes with skin, apples and corn/maize.

Frozen and Canned Produce
You can also find produce in the frozen and canned food sections of the supermarket. Flash-freezing helps retain most of the nutritional quality of frozen produce, so frozen fruits and vegetables—without added sauces and sugars—are the best substitute for fresh produce. Frozen produce may be more nutritious than fresh, depending upon how the fresh produce has been handled and ripened.

Canned fruits and vegetables, packed in water, are available in low-sodium and low-sugar varieties. They are good alternatives to fresh produce. Look for canned fruits that are packed in water, not sugar syrup. Canned fruits retain most of their vitamin content, but canned vegetables may lose some vitamins during the canning process, particularly vitamins B and C. Since these vitamins are often found in the liquid in which the foods are canned, use that liquid when you're cooking canned vegetables.

Vegetable and Fruit Juices
Vegetable and fruit juices can help fulfill your eating plan's vegetable and fruit requirements. One vegetable and one fruit serving are equivalent to 8 fl. oz (225 ml) vegetable juice and 4 fl. oz (115 ml) fruit juice, respectively.

Vegetable juice makes a great snack. Check the labels on canned and bottled vegetable juices because some are high in sodium. V-8® juice, as well as several other brands, now produce low-sodium vegetable juices. A wide variety of fruit juices are available, but check the nutrition labels carefully: many contain as little as 10 per cent real fruit juice. If the juice isn't labeled 100 per cent fruit juice, or is called a 'fruit drink', it probably contains a high percentage of water and sugar. Avoid these fruit juices if you're trying to lose weight. Look for calcium-fortified orange juice, to help meet your daily calcium requirement. Remember that fruit juice doesn't contain the fibre that fresh fruit does, so it won't fill you up as much as fresh fruit.

Remaining on the perimeter of the supermarket, move on from produce to the dairy section, and then on to fresh seafood and the deli.

Dairy

At the dairy section, the simple rule of thumb to follow with all the products is this: Every dairy purchase you make should be low fat or fat free.

Milk
Buy skimmed (non-fat) milk or 1 per cent low-fat milk.

Yoghurt
Fat-free and low-fat yoghurts are great snack foods, particularly if you are trying to boost your calcium intake. The best yoghurts are those that have live bacteria cultures, which is marked right on the container. Both organic and non-organic yoghurts, with or without fruit, are good choices. Many are also made with natural sweeteners, such as fruit juice, rather than refined sugars. If you are avoiding sweets, avoid the highly sweetened yoghurts.

Soured Cream, Cheeses and Spreads
Soured cream now comes in low-fat forms, some of which taste just as good as their full-fat counterparts. Good low-fat cheeses are hard to find, no doubt about it. But finding them is not impossible. There are a number of excellent tasting brands of low-fat goat cheese and farmers' cheese. Several low-fat versions of processed cheese are on the market. Although highly processed, they still make good substitutes for their high-fat counterparts. Kraft® makes low-fat ('lite') Philadelphia cream cheese.

If you do not eat dairy products or want to try a new type of low-fat cheese substitute that melts well, try low-fat or fat-free soya cheeses. These taste quite good and have no dairy fat, so you may want to give them a try. You can find soya cheeses in health food shops and in some supermarkets.

Eggs

Whole eggs are fine to purchase, but if you are watching your fat and cholesterol, you should remove the yolk before cooking or use egg substitutes. Try egg substitutes that contain only egg whites with added vitamins and food colouring if you want to reduce both the fat and cholesterol in your diet. Experiment with the different brands, since each has a distinctive taste.

Seafood

Try the many distinct varieties of fresh and seasonal seafood that are now available in supermarkets. If you would like to increase your intake of omega-3 essential fatty acids, refer to the listing of fish that are rich in these fatty acids on page 82 in Step 2. You'll also find a variety of seafood marinades in the fish section of the store. Many of these are delicious and low fat or fat free. If you are watching your sodium intake, check the nutrition labels on the marinades, as some are high in salt.

Frozen seafood is a good alternative to fresh, unless it is fried, breaded or preserved in an oily dressing.

Poultry and Meat

The leanest forms of poultry are chicken and turkey—both without the skin. The leanest cuts of beef are topside, rump, top rump and silverside. The leanest cut of pork is pork loin. If you want lean mince, ask the butcher to grind the meat from the rump or purchase 95 per cent lean beef mince.

When you shop for beef, remember that the more white marbling in the beef, the higher its fat content.

The Deli

Unfortunately, the deli section is limited in low-fat choices. Most of the deli meats are high in fat. The leanest choices of meat at the deli are turkey breast, roast beef with the fat removed, and ham. Roast chicken is a good choice, but remove the skin before you eat it, since that's where most of the fat is. Look for low-fat, pre-packaged sandwich meats in the meat section.

The prepared meat and fish salads in the deli section are usually high in fat because they are mixed with mayonnaise or oil. Avoid these items, or ask the shop staff about the ingredients in any particular salad.

You should also look out for interesting specialty breads, biscuits and crackers, including pitta breads and flatbreads. Check their labels for fat content. Remember to buy products made from whole grains, such as five-seed bread, whole-grain rye and wholemeal. (See the Breads section on page 106 for more information.)

Now that you've toured the perimeter of the supermarket, it is time to begin tackling each of the centre aisles. When reading the labels on the prepared foods, please be aware that ingredients are listed on a package by weight, from highest to lowest. For example, if you look at the ingredients list below you will see that there is more sugar in this product than oil.

Ingredients List: wholemeal flour, oats, skimmed milk, sugar, bicarbonate of soda, vanilla, raisins, salt, oil.

If you're watching your salt intake, make sure salt is one of the last ingredients listed on the package. Before you check the ingredients list, you can also refer to the Nutrition Information label as a guide. As a rule of thumb, when watching your salt content, use only products that contain 350 mg or less of sodium per serving (unless you are further restricted for medical reasons). If the package is labelled low sodium, it is a sure sign that it is acceptable. Since sodium is found in both natural and packaged foods, try to limit yourself to about 1,500 mg per day of sodium from packaged foods.

Continue your tour of the packaged-food aisles starting with beverages.

Beverages

Water
Bottled sparkling and non-sparkling water can help you meet your Active Wellness daily water allotment. There are regulations for bottled water. Bottled water must meet the same standards as tap water; water labelled 'spring water' must come from a natural spring source; and mineral water that contains a significant amount of calcium, iron and sodium must list the nutrition contents on the label. Some mineral waters can help you meet your daily requirement for calcium and iron.

Don't be fooled by the many 'imitation water' products, which are clear in colour but high in sugar or syrups. Many have the same amount of calories as a piece of fruit, but none of the nutritional value. Check the Nutrition Information labels on these products carefully.

Caffeinated Beverages
If you're not restricting your caffeine intake, here is where you'll find many caffeinated beverages, including diet colas and iced teas. Be cautious when buying any of the herbal bottled drinks that are now available: Many are heavily sweetened with honey and thus are high in sugar—so high, in some cases, that they count as a 'sweets' serving.

Bottled Juices
Bottled juices and other natural drinks are better choices than caffeinated beverages. However, they are often flavoured with a good deal of sugar, fruit juice concentrate, honey or syrup, which makes them high in sugar. Check the nutrition label: if the fruit drink is not mostly juice, you should consider it a 'sweets' serving, not a fruit serving.

Cereals

Look for hot and cold whole-grain cereals. Cereals are a terrific way to meet your daily servings of whole grains. But read the cereal labels carefully. Many are high in fat, sodium and sugar—exactly what you should avoid. Instead, look for cereal labels that list the grain (*not* the sugar) first. Try to find cereals that list sugar as the fourth or fifth ingredient. A good rule is to look for cereals that contain no more than 1 gram of sugar for every 5 grams of total carbohydrates. Also look for cereals that are high in fibre: If the label says the cereal contains 7 or more grams of fibre per serving, it is a high-fibre food. Cereals containing 3 to 6 grams of fibre per serving are a moderate-fibre food.

Avoid cereals that contain hydrogenated or partially hydrogenated oil, palm oil, cottonseed oil and coconut oil. These are all considered 'bad' fats.

If you are trying to restrict your sodium intake, check the cereal label to make sure it contains 300 mg or less of sodium per serving.

If you are confused about how much of your favourite cereal is equal to one Active Wellness serving, you can identify the amount of a serving by using the serving size listed on the cereal's Nutrition Information label.

Breads, Baked Snacks and Biscuits

Make a point of looking for whole-grain breads. Don't be fooled by breads that look brown, but aren't whole grain. Check the nutrition label. If the first ingredient listed is *not* white flour, but whole-wheat flour, oat flour, rice flour or rye flour, then the bread is probably a whole-grain product. Check the fibre content as well. Bread with 2 grams or more of fibre per serving is an excellent choice.

If you are trying to lose weight, avoid breads that contain dried fruit, which is often high in calories. Remember to follow the low-fat rule to determine which bread products qualify: 3 grams or less of fat per serving. A slice of bread (1 oz/30 g) equals one grain unit on your Active Wellness eating plan.

Baked Snacks

I am often asked how baked snacks (including cream crackers and the like) equal one grains serving. With the wide variety of crackers and baked snacks available, the serving size on the nutrition label is a reliable guide to how much of an item equals one serving. Also check the nutrition label for fat and sodium content, particularly if you are trying to lose weight or restrict your salt intake. Check the fibre content as well. Crackers and snacks with 1 gram or more of fibre per serving are considered high-fibre options. If they are high fibre, they are probably also whole-grain products, the preferable choice for the Active Wellness eating plan.

Biscuits

As a population, we eat tons of sweet biscuits and cookies every year, and most of those are high in fat and sugar. But there are some exceptions. Look for biscuits that have 3 grams or less of total fat per serving, such as digestive and ginger biscuits. Many low-fat and fat-free cookies make a guilt-free treat. However, keep in mind that fat free does not mean calorie free. Many fat-free biscuits are high in sugar. Two biscuits or cookies usually count as one sweets serving on your Active Wellness eating plan. Always confirm an Active Wellness serving with the Nutrition Information label serving if you are unsure of how much to eat.

Beans

Beans make great soups and stews. They are also terrific additions to salads, adding colour, texture and fibre. Beans—which are also referred to as pulses—are an excellent source of both low-fat and high-fibre protein. Experiment with the many types of beans in both dried and canned forms. Canned beans are just as good as dried. If sodium intake is a concern for you, check the can for the sodium content. It can be quite high. Since most of the sodium is in the canning liquid, just rinse the beans well before using them.

Lentils and split peas, especially good in soups, are often available only in dried form, but they cook quickly (in about 20 minutes). If you are new to dried beans, follow the cooking directions on the package or those offered in Step 10.

To reduce the wind produced by beans, cover them with cold water and soak them overnight. Drain them well under running water, then place them in a pot and cover them with fresh water. Boil the beans until they are tender.

On your Active Wellness eating plan, beans can satisfy either your protein or grains/starches requirements. Main-course bean dishes are excellent substitutes for animal protein—4 fl. oz (115 ml) of beans equals about 1 oz (30 g) of animal protein.

Grains, Pasta, and Rice

Almost all grains, pasta, and rice make good choices for your eating plan. But be cautious when buying pre-packaged frozen and boxed blends of grains, pasta and rice that contain flavour packets. Many of these flavourings contain ingredients that are high in butter solids and hydrogenated oils. It is helpful to look for preboxed grains when you are trying out new varieties. The box will guide you with cooking and serving directions. You can also use Step 10 to guide you with grain cookery, particularly if you are buying your grains in bulk.

Try the many different types of grain and rice from the Middle East, Africa and Spain now available at most supermarkets. Each one has its own distinct texture and taste. Whole grains are best if used within a month, otherwise their natural oils may go rancid. On your Active Wellness eating plan, grains, rice and pasta all fall into the whole grains/starches group.

Soups

Choose from a wide variety of canned, frozen and dried soups. All are good choices for your eating plan, since soups are quick and delicious ways to satisfy hunger and fill you up. Soups also offer a tasty way to start eating beans. If you are watching your sodium intake, you may need to avoid many of the dried soups and some of the canned soups, both of which tend to be high in salt.

Soup can fall into one of three areas in your diet. One cup of vegetable soup or stock is a 'free' food. If it is bean soup, it is either a serving from the whole grains/starches group or proteins group—depending on how you choose to spend your 'food servings'. If it contains mostly meat and vegetables (for example, stew), do your best to estimate how much meat is in the soup and count it in the proteins group. The rest of the ingredients are free.

Spreads, Dips, Sauces, Salad Dressings and Marinades

Spreads and Dips

While most people use mayonnaise as a spread, it is truly a fat and a saturated one at that. Avoid it whenever possible. The best alternative is fat-free mayonnaise.

Other sandwich spreads, such as mustard and ketchup, are usually fine to use because they are low fat or fat free. But if you are watching your sodium intake or trying to lose weight, check the sugar and sodium content on the nutrition labels of mustards and ketchups.

Vegetable and bean spreads are increasingly popular items. They make a wonderful snack when you spread them on low-fat crackers or use them as dips for raw vegetables. You can find them ready-made in most supermarket delis or produce sections or in health food shops. Gourmet vegetable spreads sold in supermarkets and specialty shops include pumpkin spread, aubergine spread and roasted red pepper spread. Again, if necessary, check the salt, fat, and sodium content on the label.

Sauces, Salad Dressings, and Marinades

Check all sauces, salad dressings, and marinades for fat, sodium, and sugar content. A wide variety of these products are available, and their ingredients vary considerably. Follow these rules when buying any of these items:

◇ Total fat per serving should be 3 grams or less
◇ Sodium per serving should be 350 mg or less

Tomato sauces and other pasta sauces—except the creamed sauces—are generally healthy alternatives as toppings for pasta, chicken, fish and even beans. If you like salad dressings, look for those that are low fat and fat free.

Fats and Oils

Avoid saturated fats, including butter, lard, and hydrogenated vegetable oils such as margarine. If you must use margarine, choose one of the liquid varieties. When buying oils, choose olive oil, or peanut oil. Oil sprays also offer good choices.

Frozen Entrées

Excellent low-fat and vegetarian frozen entrées are available in most supermarkets. Always check their nutrition labels for fat, sodium and sugar content. Look for low-calorie dinners that derive less than 30 per cent of their calories from fat. Frozen dinners are good in a pinch, but shouldn't be relied on every day. They are often low in vitamin A, vitamin C, fibre and calcium. If you eat a lot of frozen dinners, supplement them with fruits, vegetables and low-fat dairy products to get extra nutrition.

To translate frozen dinner entrées into Active Wellness serving units that satisfy your eating plan requirements, make a best-guess estimate based on how much of the meal, in ounces/grams, is grain, beef, chicken or fish.

Also check out the frozen food section for vegetable burgers—low-fat, nutritious, and delicious alternatives to meat for lunch or dinner. You can also find low-fat specialty foods, such as burritos, and a vast array of other international cuisines, including Indian, French, Spanish and Chinese foods, in the frozen food section. Be adventurous, but remember to check all of the nutrition labels for fat, sodium and sugar content.

Frozen Desserts, Cakes and Pies

Many frozen desserts, including frozen yoghurt and ice cream, sorbet, fresh fruit lollies and ice-cream sandwiches, come in low-fat or no-fat versions. They make great treats and have the additional advantages of helping curb your appetite and satisfying your sweet tooth.

Low-fat and fat-free cakes are available in frozen and fresh versions. Be cautious when buying these, since many are high in sugar and calories. Check the nutrition label and make sure that low-fat cakes fall within these guidelines:

◇ 3 grams or less of fat per serving
◇ 125 calories or less per serving
◇ sugar is not the first ingredient listed

Pies are also available in the frozen food section, but very few of them offer nutritious choices. Making a good pie is almost impossible without adding a lot of butter to the crust. Even if the filling is sugar free, the crust is probably high in fat. Pie is simply not the best dessert choice for your Active Wellness eating plan.

If you must have a piece of pie, fruit pies are the best choice. Have a very small piece, so that you can stay within the guidelines of 3 grams or less of fat per serving and 125 calories or less per serving.

Snacks

Snacking is almost everyone's favourite pastime. But finding nutritious snacks can be difficult, and determining what makes a healthy portion can be even more difficult. Fortunately, snack foods such as popcorn, tortilla crisps and potato crisps now come in low-fat varieties. Pretzels are almost always low fat. However, they are also made with processed flours. If you can find wholemeal pretzels, try to purchase them instead. For snack foods and pretzels, count the serving size listed on the package as equal to one serving of whole grains/starches on your Active Wellness eating plan.

Nuts, in small quantities, may be eaten as snacks. Be cautious about how many you eat, however, since they are high in fat. Indeed, nuts fall into the 'fats' category on your eating plan. See Step 2 for specific serving sizes for different varieties of nuts.

Muesli bars and energy bars have become increasingly popular as snack foods, but they invariably are high in sugar and often high in calories. Therefore, they qualify as 'sweets' on your eating plan. Look for muesli and energy bars that are 150 calories or less per serving.

Soya Products and Non-dairy Alternatives

Soya and non-dairy alternative food products are easily found in health food shops and are increasingly found in supermarkets. They are worth hunting down.

Soya Products

Soya products, made from the soya bean, are a great source of nutrients that also provide essential fatty acids. Soya products include tofu, tempeh (fermented soya), baked tofu, soya custard, soya protein, soya cheese, soya burgers and soya nuts, a terrific snack-food item. (One serving of dry roasted soya nuts is equivalent to one grains/starches or proteins Active Wellness serving on your eating plan.) If you want to incorporate more soya in your diet, I encourage you to try dry roasted soya nuts. Many soya products also come in low-fat versions. All the soya products are nutritious alternatives to meat, poultry and fish. They also help cut down on the saturated animal fats in your diet.

Non-dairy Alternatives

If you cannot tolerate cow's milk, try soya bean milk or rice milk. They both come in a variety of flavours. Several rice milk desserts are available as well.

Setting up your Active Wellness kitchen and restocking your pantry takes time, but the dividends are worth it. With delicious, nutritious and healthy foods close at hand, you're more likely to follow your eating plan and to enjoy the process of eating well!

Now that you've laid a solid nutritional foundation for yourself, it's time to move on to Step 4. We'll look at the triggers that first set off your thoughts and feelings and at concrete examples of how you can handle those triggers more effectively.

Changing Old Patterns
and Forming New Healthy Habits

Change your thoughts and you change your world.
—Norman Vincent Peale

As you settle into your Active Wellness lifestyle, you may start each day with the best of intentions only to be sidetracked by some old, unhealthy habits that get in the way of your success.

Habits are acquired behaviour patterns that are regularly repeated over time until they become nearly involuntary or unconscious actions in our everyday lives. Many habits are constructive and good for our health. Exercising regularly, eating right, practising relaxation and brushing one's teeth are just a few examples.

Unfortunately, many other habits are bad for our health and are destructive. Often, these are habits that we develop as coping mechanisms for negative or uncomfortable feelings and events. These 'coping' habits too often work against our goals for good health, including smoking when we are stressed, overdrinking when we are upset or overeating when we are depressed. Even seemingly innocuous behaviours can become obstacles to our success—always having coffee with breakfast or a sugary treat in the late afternoon, never sitting down to savour a meal or constantly working until no time is left for exercise.

Long-established habitual routines may seem like natural patterns in your life, but are they helping you or hurting you? If some of your habitual behaviours are preventing you from living a healthy life or enjoying a healthy self-image, they are definitely hurting you. Now is the time to develop strategies for changing old behaviours into new and healthy habits. This chapter will teach you how to do that, beginning with a look at how habits are formed, followed by a discussion of the tools you can use to help change them.

The Anatomy of a Habit

A habit is the end result of a chain reaction that begins with a triggering *event*. That initial event is translated into a *thought* or thought pattern that soon produces emotional or physical *feelings*. Those feelings are then 'coped with' by a particular action. The action taken may become a habit if it is repeated. The diagram below illustrates this chain reaction. Let's take a closer look at each of the links in the chain.

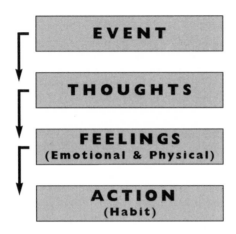

Event

The triggering event that starts the chain reaction that leads to a particular habit may be significant or insignificant: a sudden shock or a well-known circumstance. It can be a serious emotional trigger, such as an argument with a loved one, or a banal event, such as walking past a bakery.

Depending on your circumstances and your emotional and physical states, such triggers can set off a series of thoughts and unconscious behaviours that ultimately sabotage whatever good intentions you had before the event occurred. Below is a list of common triggers that many Active Wellness participants have identified as obstacles on their own wellness journeys. As they tried to make healthy changes in their lives, such as improving their diets, losing weight, reducing stress and exercising more, they faced these familiar temptations. See if any of these ring true for you.

Common Triggers

- ◇ Celebrating a special occasion
- ◇ Watching television
- ◇ Success at a job
- ◇ Having a disagreement with the boss
- ◇ Having to work late
- ◇ Sitting in mother's kitchen
- ◇ Being late for an appointment
- ◇ Feeling lonely
- ◇ Argument with a loved one

Thoughts

Once a trigger or circumstance occurs that ignites our thoughts, we begin a dialogue with ourselves that stress experts and psychologists call 'self-talk'.

For example, reading this book may be triggering self-talk in your own head. Perhaps you are thinking, 'I don't believe this programme will work for me. It may work for other people, but not for me.' This is the typical kind of negative self-talk that almost always leads to defeat when you are trying to change specific behaviours and habits. The talk is not even rooted in fact, but is merely an assumption, probably based on past 'failures'. The truth is, you don't know what works for you, unless you give it a try. And any attempt to change—no matter how small—is never a failure, but always a positive step forward. A more empowering type of self-talk when facing the challenge of changing unhealthy habits is, 'This just might work for me. I can certainly give it my best effort.'

Self-Talk

It is critical at this juncture in your Active Wellness journey to 'listen' to your self-talk as you try to make healthy changes in your life. Changing your self-talk can help you take more positive actions—because new thoughts generate new feelings, which in turn can translate into different, healthier responses (actions/habits). As you learn to change your self-talk, you'll need to acknowledge the original negative thought and change it to a positive thought. You'll soon create a cascade of changes that will follow sequentially down your habit chain—ultimately helping you change your old habit!

The ability to listen to your self-talk is a fundamental first step in acquiring the skills to transform unhealthy habits into healthy ones. As you develop new healthy-habit skills, you can apply your new self-talk phrases to each of the steps in the Active Wellness programme. Whether you are embarking on a new eating plan, learning to incorporate exercise into your daily life, or practising stress management, listening to your self-talk will enable you to transform negative thoughts into positive ones, defeatist behaviours into successes and triumphs. Eventually, you can apply self-talk skills to any area of your life that you want to change—work, relationships, parenting, or self-esteem.

We talk to ourselves hundreds of times a day, but do we recognize the self-talk that leads to undesired actions or bad habits? What kinds of things do you say to yourself? Are they invariably negative or positive? What emotional feelings and physical sensations accompany those thoughts? Try to keep a daily list of your repetitive and negative self-talk in a personal journal or The Habit Diary shown at the end of this chapter. Words that can help you identify negative self-talk include can't, won't, shouldn't, never and not. Positive, proactive and transformational words include can, will, want, should, always and I am.

Many Active Wellness participants find it extremely helpful to fill out their own Habit Chain as practice in observing their self-talk. Take a moment to fill out the diagram below. Think about an action you took recently that you wish you could have prevented and write it on the line beside 'Action (Habit)'. Then work your way backward through the Habit Chain to see what initial event triggered your action. Working backwards is an easier approach when you are reflecting on a past action. Try to remember how you felt (emotionally and physically) before and after the triggering event and the thoughts that accompanied those feelings. Now write down the event that triggered the feelings and thoughts. If identifying one particular event is difficult, just focus on the feelings you had before your action or habit took place.

After you have recorded the feelings that resulted from the event, try to come up with new self-talk. Your new 'self-talk' phrase can be a thought that is more positive and empowering, or that focuses on what you need to do for yourself. Notice if your new thought leads to more positive feelings, and then ask yourself, 'Would I have taken the same action if I had changed my thoughts and had different feelings?' On page 117 is a completed Habit Chain, using Tom's scenario as an example. The diagram shows where Tom could change his thoughts and ignite a change in feelings—transforming an old action into a healthier action response (habit).

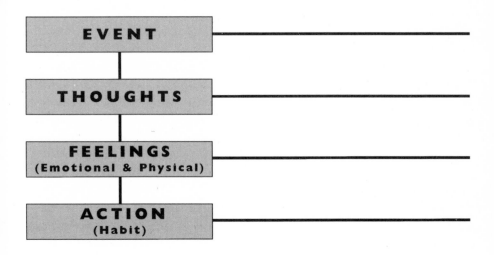

✦ Tom's Story ✦

Let's use the 'having to work late' trigger to describe the chain of events that led to Tom's habit of eating unhealthy and fattening foods. An Active Wellness participant who was trying to lose weight, Tom frequently had to put in extra hours at the office. When this happened, his thoughts were: 'I hate that I have to work late. They are not paying me enough for all the hours I put in, I'm not appreciated.' The event (having to work late) triggered negative thoughts and self-talk. Those thoughts, in turn, triggered negative feelings, both emotional and physical, which led Tom to engage in a self-destructive habit.

In this case, Tom's thoughts caused him to feel both angry about working late and stressed because he didn't believe his work was being recognized or rewarded. The stress resulted in physical tension, which he felt throughout his neck and back. Tom turned to a compensating habit. He purchased several bars of chocolate that he would eat all at once, even though he was trying to lose weight.

Soon, eating the sweets became more than just Tom's unhealthy habit, it became a new triggering event. Now Tom felt guilty about eating the sweets because he was trying to lose weight. In turn, this made him feel ugly and fat. Feeling defeated, Tom's negative feelings led him to eat even more, and feel bad about himself, which further discouraged him from restarting his healthy eating plan the next day.

This seemingly self-perpetuating chain of unhealthy behaviours may feel defeating, but you can break the chain by changing the old thoughts that are triggered by an event. Tom broke his own habit chain by changing his thoughts about work. When the old thoughts surfaced, he acknowledged them and changed them to his new self-talk: 'I have been given this work because they think I do a good job. But I cannot let my work get in the way of my health.' With this new thought, Tom was able to change his feelings over time from anger and stress to positive feelings of pride in his work and a sense of control over his life. Feeling empowered to make the healthy changes he needed, Tom no longer needs sweets to get through the day. Instead, he focuses more on his needs than on the feelings of anger that get in his way. When these feelings occur he manages them by taking a walk outside the office for a few minutes as a 'breather'.

Tom's Habit Chain

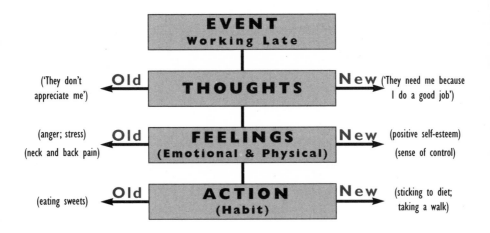

Feelings aren't facts!
—Unknown

Feelings

Recognizing or acknowledging our feelings is not always easy, especially if we have never stopped to think about them before, and many of us don't. With old habits in particular, we often move directly from a triggering event to the action or habit we use as a coping mechanism, without stopping to observe the feelings we experience between the two. In many ways, we form our unhealthy habits in an effort to ignore or bypass our unwanted or uncomfortable feelings.

According to Dr Susan Jakubowicz, a psychoanalyst who works with the Active Wellness programme, the only way to stop an unhealthy habit is to 'digest' or 'own' the feelings that trigger and propel the habit. Dr Jakubowicz also emphasizes that before you can give up your old habit, it is crucial to understand how that behaviour serves you. This means you need to 'feel' the feelings you are avoiding, not smother them with an unhealthy habit. When you acknowledge your feelings—instead of jumping over them to a compensating habit—you may no longer need the old behaviour. But first you need to acknowledge and name the feelings you are experiencing, so you can feel in control and respond rather than react. Keep in mind that the emotional system functions like the digestive system. Feelings, like food, need to be digested and eliminated. We can't get rid of a feeling by not wanting to have it—a feeling will linger in our system and affect us as destructive actions or behaviours until it is digested.

Recognizing Your Feelings

We all experience hundreds and hundreds of feelings of varying intensity. As you observe yourself in different situations, you will begin to recognize your own unique way of feeling. Essentially, all feelings arise from four primal emotions: anger, grief, joy and fear. Furthermore, feelings can be experienced as purely emotional in nature or as physical sensations, though distinguishing between the two can be difficult. Following, you will find examples of both emotional 'feeling' words and physical 'feeling' words, which can help you identify your own feelings.

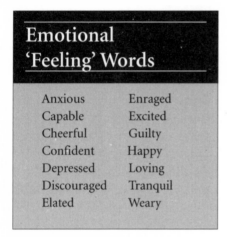

Emotional 'Feeling' Words

Anxious	Enraged
Capable	Excited
Cheerful	Guilty
Confident	Happy
Depressed	Loving
Discouraged	Tranquil
Elated	Weary

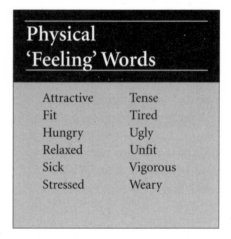

Physical 'Feeling' Words

Attractive	Tense
Fit	Tired
Hungry	Ugly
Relaxed	Unfit
Sick	Vigorous
Stressed	Weary

If you have difficulty recognizing or acknowledging your feelings, you are not alone. Many of us hide our true feelings or ignore the messages they send us because we believe that showing our feelings is a sign of weakness, or we were conditioned to believe that certain feelings are not acceptable. But feelings have a unique life force of their own. They are driven by powerful biochemical energies, and those energies must be channelled in healthy and appropriate ways. Not accepting or acknowledging your feelings (particularly the negative and uncomfortable ones) and keeping them locked inside may ultimately affect both your health and your behaviour. Unacknowledged feelings are at the core of most unhealthy habits. So let's take a closer look at the energy that drives our feelings.

The Energy of Feelings

Every feeling triggers a physiological response in the body. This happens because changes in emotions are directly linked to chemical changes in the brain that result in the production of neurotransmitters. These biochemical substances travel throughout the body and affect the cardiovascular, central nervous, immune and musculoskeletal systems.

We are all familiar with the rapid heartbeat, shallow breathing, cold sweats, hot flushes and tingling extremities that accompany fear, panic, anxiety and extreme stress. Many of us are also familiar with the facial flushing and chest tightness that occur when we are angry and our blood pressure rises. Those who struggle with depression are familiar with the emotional mood swings, sleep disturbances, food cravings, and general aches and pains that characterize that condition. On the other hand, we also know the pleasure of feeling emotionally balanced and in harmony with the world. When we are happy, we feel better, look better and cope better with the situations life throws our way.

A more common response to feelings that we can't acknowledge or feel we can't control is the development of unhealthy habits or actions that 'smother' those feelings. At the root of health and social problems, such as drug addiction, smoking, over-drinking, overeating, road rage and physical abuse (to name just a few), is the inability to 'own' or 'digest' our uncomfortable or negative feelings and to find constructive ways of channelling our energies. With overeaters, for example, grief and anger are often swallowed along with the unhealthy foods. Someone who is dealing with sadness and says, 'I feel like eating a container of ice cream,' is sending out a powerful statement. Sugar and cream may indeed pacify uncomfortable feelings, but this person may also be trying to bury her sorrows.

When you acknowledge your emotions, however, you allow yourself to feel their power and meaning and you release them in healthy and controlled ways, rather than suppressing them with an unhealthy action or habit. Acknowledging and releasing your feelings doesn't necessarily mean you have to act on them. Repeatedly and violently venting your anger, for example, whether verbally or physically, is almost always counterproductive. In fact, if you experience your feelings as too powerful to understand or control, a professional therapist or counsellor can help you through the process. Actually, anger can be a source of positive powerful energy that can serve you well if it is properly released.

I'm not saying that negative feelings are bad or less important than positive ones. Negative feelings, including anger, anxiety, guilt, envy and disgust, are normal feelings. It is what we do with those feelings that determines our well-being. Often, not discharging our feelings constructively can be at the root of our unhealthy actions and habits.

> *We all carry it within us: supreme strength, the fullness*
> *of wisdom, unquenchable joy. It is never thwarted, and*
> *cannot be destroyed.*
> —Huston Smith

Actions = Habits

A habit or action is the last link in the Habit Chain reaction. It begins with a triggering event that produces negative or positive thoughts, which in turn create negative or positive emotional and physical feelings.

If those feelings are negative, the action we take—most often an ingrained habit or behaviour that has become almost unconscious through repetition over time—is an attempt to ignore or soothe the bad feelings. In some cases a habit can actually arise as a coping mechanism to avoid positive feelings, such as the fear of success. As in Tom's story, the initial action or habit (eating sweets to deal with anger) created a vicious cycle whereby new thoughts and feelings emerged that produced other unhealthy actions (giving up on his new diet).

How do you begin to break the cycle and change unhealthy habits into healthy behaviour? Observing your bad habits, calmly and non-judgmentally, is the first step, but a difficult one for many people. Grit and determination are also key ingredients to success. Luckily, many valuable tools are available to help you make positive changes more easily.

How to Change Your Unhealthy Habits

In order to change your unhealthy habits into healthy behaviours, you must adopt the four essential ingredients for successful change:

- ◊ Motivation
- ◊ Awareness
- ◊ Knowledge
- ◊ Patience

Motivation

Since you are reading this book, I assume that you have the motivation to change. But that old axiom is worth repeating here: you have to *want* to change in order to succeed. Transforming unhealthy habits into healthy ones takes time and courage, planning and determination. Letting go of old feelings and comfortable ways of coping, however unhealthy, can be difficult. Your personal motivation for change and your unique brand of determination to 'stick with it' are the first ingredients of successful change. To help you stay on track, set your goals and keep in mind how much happier you will be when you conquer your destructive habits. As long as you keep striving to make a positive change each week, you can think of yourself as successful!

Awareness

Some of you may be aware of your unhealthy habits already. Others of you may not have stopped to think about this concept of unhealthy versus healthy behaviour. The second ingredient of successful change is becoming increasingly aware of your unhealthy habits. One way to practise awareness is to carefully observe your daily behaviours with a non-critical eye. Practising awareness can be a revelation. Some of your habits may have become so routine you don't even notice yourself doing them.

Use The Habit Diary at the end of this chapter to help you 'track' your habits throughout the day. It will also help you recognize what you are doing and how you are feeling when you engage in these habits. The diary is especially helpful in tracking behaviours that have become so routine that you do them almost unconsciously. Remember not to be too hard on yourself during this learning process. (For example, you may notice that you always eat two desserts on days when you are exhausted. Using a non-judgmental approach, say to yourself, 'I must need that extra sweet for some reason, and I'm going to watch this habit and learn why.') You'll discover that you probably had good reasons for developing some of your habits in the past, but you'll also become gradually aware that it's time to let them go. As you need your old habits less and less, you will learn to substitute new habits and behaviours in their place.

Knowledge

You need two types of knowledge to succeed in changing unhealthy habits and behaviours: knowledge of self and knowledge of skills. You gain self-knowledge by quietly observing your habits and the situations when they most often occur. Observing the thoughts, self-talk and feelings that lead to an unhealthy habit provides you with the raw material of personal transformation. Use it to change your thoughts and self-talk surrounding a specific situation, and take control of your actions instead of reacting to your feelings. Knowing you can transform your reactions will help you open the door to new healthy behaviours.

The second type of knowledge you need is the new skills for overcoming unhealthy habits that are discussed in this chapter. They include using affirmations, substituting new behaviours for old ones and building up your sense of self-worth.

Patience

The final ingredient for successfully changing old habits seems like a simple one: patience. But lack of it has undone many a good intention. You must accept that changing old, ingrained habits that get in the way of your new healthy lifestyle takes time, and perhaps a good deal of it. During this time, be patient with yourself. Consciously observing old, unhealthy behaviours and using your new knowledge to slowly change them into new behaviours is an organic process that ultimately produces lasting change. But you may have to experiment with several new behaviours in the beginning, as did the Active Wellness participant described on the next page.

> ## ❖ Karen's Story ❖
>
> Karen began with very small changes when she first tried to break her habit of eating sugary, fattening desserts and treats at the office. Whenever Karen was bored at work, she would go to the cafeteria and buy a doughnut or a piece of cake. When she decided to change her eating behaviour, she experimented with several alternatives. First, she tried walking around her office building when she felt the urge for sweets. Or she went to the water fountain for a drink instead of visiting the cafeteria.
>
> This change worked for her most of the time, but occasionally she still had the urge to go to the cafeteria. When she looked at this behaviour more closely, she realized that she wasn't going to the cafeteria for the sweets, but for a diversion when she was bored or tired. Now when she visited the cafeteria, instead of buying a sweet, she would opt for tea or a salad. She kept the cafeteria as a diversionary 'break' from the routine of her job, but she changed her behaviour when she got there. With this change, she stopped eating sweets and began losing weight, her primary goal.

When you begin the process of transforming your old habits, the changes you make may seem small at first. But no change in a healthy direction is insignificant. For that reason, you should congratulate yourself for any steps, however tiny, that take you in the direction of good health. Taking pride in even the smallest of changes reinforces your new healthy behaviours and encourages you to keep repeating them and enlarging upon them. Sooner than you think, they will become permanent parts of your Active Wellness lifestyle. And your motivation and determination will serve as anchors through this process of change, as will the new skills described below.

> *Put your heart, mind, intellect and soul even to your*
> *smallest acts. This is the secret of success.*
> —Swami Sivananda

Using Affirmations to Your Advantage

Affirmations are short, positive sayings that can encourage and empower you as you make healthy changes in your life. They also help to counteract any negative feelings that might inhibit you from moving forward and reaching your goals. On the next page are examples of some affirmations that have worked for many Active Wellness participants. Repeat them to yourself over and over during difficult times to help keep yourself on a positive track. Write them down on small index cards or post-its and put them where you can see them every day: the bathroom mirror, the door to your bedroom or the dashboard of your car.

Active Wellness Affirmations
◆ I am doing the best I can.
◆ I deserve time to focus on myself.
◆ I am intelligent.
◆ I love who I am and I don't need to change.
◆ I am a good person.

You can also make up your own personalized affirmations, using the guidelines provided below. Or try using some of the uplifting quotes scattered throughout this chapter as your affirmations. You can even use a line from a favourite commercial, such as Nike's 'Just Do It!'

When you start your day with a positive affirmation, you bring positive energy into the rest of your day and into all of your endeavours, including the process of changing unhealthy habits into healthy ones. Take a moment to write down your affirmations in the space provided on the following page.

Checklist for Creating Affirmations
◆ Believe your affirmation to be true.
◆ Use positive words and phrases, so your affirmation makes you feel good!
◆ Use the present tense.
◆ Use positive phrases that are in direct opposition to your old, negative self-talk. If you're used to thinking 'I always fail,' transform that into 'I am a winner!'
◆ Make your affirmation easy to remember.

My Personal Affirmations

◇ _____

◇ _____

◇ _____

◇ _____

*Progress always involves risks. You can't steal second
base and keep your foot on first.*
—Frederick B. Wilcox

Substitutions for Your Old Habits

Changing an old habit takes time. Often it is easier to learn a new behaviour than to undo an old one, to replace an unhealthy habit with a healthy action. For example, if your unhealthy behaviour is to turn to sweets when you are unhappy or angry, try turning to something else: a hot drink, music, a bubble bath or a good movie. Or turn to a different kind of food: fruit instead of biscuits or a tasty cereal instead of pancakes with butter and sugar.

Often we rely on our unhealthy habits for immediate gratification as a response to our feelings. Your best alternative behaviour in the short term may be to quickly do something that is easy and accessible: calling a friend or family member; taking a walk or drive; or visiting the nearest shopping centre to pamper yourself with a frivolous purchase. Listening to special music or a book on tape while walking or jogging is a favourite activity of many Active Wellness participants.

You can also turn your behavioural changes into long-term benefits that go beyond good health. Try establishing a reward system for yourself. Every time you practise your new healthy habit, for example, give yourself 50p. At the end of every month, take the money you have saved and treat yourself to a gift: a new shirt, a bouquet of flowers or a new CD.

Take a minute now to consider healthy substitutions to some old habits you're trying to change. Write them down in the space on the next page or, if you'd like to carry them around with you, on an index card or in a pocket diary. A list may seem simplistic, but it is actually a great tool when you're trying to make changes, because looking at your list forces you to stop and think before you act. When you create new healthy substitutions, they should be as satisfying for you as your old habits, or they will not be effective.

Substitution List for My Old Habits

Old Habit: Healthy Substitution:

◊_____   ◊_____

◊_____   ◊_____

◊_____   ◊_____

◊_____   ◊_____

◊_____   ◊_____

*Addiction to alcohol is alcoholism. Addiction to
perfection is perfectionism.*
—Rachel Naomi Remen, MD

Being Human Means Making Mistakes
As you make healthy changes in your life, remember to go easy on yourself. Abandoning old, ingrained habits that have served you well for years is hard work. Thinking that you are not 'OK' if you don't succeed immediately, or do something perfectly, is wrong—if not downright counterproductive. Remember, success is when you continue to try, and failure is when you give up.

I tell all of my Active Wellness clients that they are expected to make mistakes. Great learning comes from making mistakes. And if you are constantly worried about doing something wrong, more of your energy is devoted to worrying than it is to learning new information and making healthy changes.

Being human means making mistakes and not being perfect. In fact, perfectionism and self-criticism do little to help you make the healthy changes that are integral to a life of Active Wellness. Instead, you need to gently encourage yourself with positive thoughts and affirmations. Turn setbacks into new opportunities. Many mistakes have been turned into great successes, as the following story aptly illustrates.

After we created the popular Active Wellness Luscious Fat-Free Chocolate Truffle, we inadvertently added extra skimmed milk to the recipe. Although we were afraid the recipe wouldn't work, the truffle was even creamier and richer-tasting than it had been with the original recipe. By making an oversight in the original recipe we were able to create an even better product!

A person who is always striving to be perfect, and have everything, misses the opportunity to experience the feelings of hope, yearning and achievement. It is important to take the time to stop and appreciate the process of life and the feelings that come with it. Often, what we want comes to us more easily when we stop worrying about it.

When you can stop and feel whole, just as you are, with your imperfections and limitations, you can be at peace with yourself and begin the real work of making changes that last a lifetime. Life is not meant to be a trap where we live constantly on guard. We are meant to enjoy life and the day-to-day process of learning to be healthy human beings. As you change your thoughts and feelings and uncover the unconscious forces that get in the way of your conscious objectives, you will begin to achieve some of your goals. You'll begin to accept more and more who you are and where you are. Only you can decide what's important for you and how you're going to get it. And if that sometimes means you have to toot your own horn and be selfish about your needs, so be it!

Change Can Be Scary, but . . .

Remember that any effort to improve is worthwhile. If you are having trouble moving forward and taking those first steps towards change, ask yourself several questions:

> ◇ 'If I take action, what is the best thing that can happen because of my efforts?'
> ◇ 'If I take action, what is the worst thing that can happen because of my efforts?'
> ◇ 'If I don't take action, what am I getting from keeping my old behaviour?'

Often the worst thing that can happen isn't so bad—and the chance you take toward healthy change is more than worth the risk, especially when the benefits you reap are a lifetime of wellness and well-being.

In this step you've learned how to transform bad habits into healthy actions and behaviours by changing your thoughts and habits. In Step 5, you'll learn how to add physical fitness to your Active Wellness programme .

e

The Habit Journal

	Before Your Habit	After Your Habit
What Are You Doing?		
What Are Your Thoughts?		
What Are Your Feelings?		
Action		

STEP 5

Your Personal Physical Fitness Plan

If we could give every individual the right amount of
nourishment and exercise, not too little and not too much,
we would have found the safest way to health.
            —Hippocrates, 460 to 377 BC

Physical fitness is a key component of your Active Wellness programme. By incorporating physical activity into your life, you can have an impact on your mind, body and spirit. This one aspect of your programme can increase longevity, help prevent illness and disability, reduce feelings of stress and ageing, strengthen physical and mental endurance and enhance feelings of self-control and self-esteem. Combined with a proper eating plan, physical activity can also boost your energy level and help you efficiently use your nutrients. To develop your personal physical fitness plan, you will assess your current fitness level, choose an exercise regimen that is tailored to fit your needs and lifestyle, and learn how to integrate physical fitness into your daily routine. Begin by examining the general benefits of exercise.

The Many Benefits of Exercise

People who exercise regularly get sick less often and experience fewer episodes of depression, anxiety, fatigue and discouraging emotions. Conversely, a lack of physical activity is associated with diseases such as osteoporosis, heart disease, diabetes and obesity. The numerous physical, mental and emotional benefits of exercise are listed in the charts on the opposite page.

In addition to all the physical, mental and emotional benefits, regular physical exercise can also aid in slowing down the ageing process, helping you to look and feel younger. In fact, the Tufts University Center for Aging has identified 10 physical 'markers' associated with the ageing process, all of which you have the power to modify through physical exercise. They include:

⬧ Lean Body Mass
⬧ Strength
⬧ Basal Metabolic Rate (BMR)

⬥ Body-Fat Percentage
⬥ Aerobic Capacity
⬥ Blood Sugar Tolerance
⬥ Total and HDL Cholesterol Levels
⬥ Blood Pressure
⬥ Bone Density
⬥ Body Temperature Regulation

Clearly, exercise is just as important as eating right, and is a vital part of your overall wellness programme. If you want to lose weight and increase your energy—as most of my Active Wellness clients do—you have to exercise. Although some people think they can accomplish both of these goals through good nutrition alone, a regular physical exercise programme, along with proper nutrition, is the only way to permanently increase your energy level and lose weight. It is extremely difficult to succeed in keeping weight off over the years if you don't engage in some type of regular physical activity. In fact, over 90 per cent of the people who maintain weight loss have integrated a regular fitness routine into their lifestyles Therefore, there is no time like the present to think about how you can incorporate physical activity into your lifestyle!

Physical Benefits of Exercise

Strengthens the Heart
Improves Lung Capacity
Increases Metabolic Rate
Increases Muscle Strength
Improves Cholesterol Levels
Lowers Blood Pressure
Facilitates Digestion
Increases Flexibility and
  Endurance
Increases Bone Density
Helps Control Blood Sugars
Helps Control Weight
Enhances Immunity

Mental and Emotional Benefits of Exercise

Enhances Self-Esteem
Improves Concentration
Reduces Stress
Promotes Positive Mental Attitude
Promotes Emotional Stability
Increases Mental Energy
Improves Sleep Patterns
Increases Sense of Well-Being
Reduces Negative Emotions
Relieves Anxiety and Tension
Relieves Depression and Fatigue
Improves Quality of Life

Overcoming Our Sedentary Natures

Overcoming an aversion to exercise is the first hurdle that the majority of Active Wellness participants have to face. Most people average only 50 minutes of regular physical activity a week, when in fact they should be exercising an average of *200* minutes a week, or 30 minutes a day. What many people don't realize is that those daily 30 minutes do not necessarily have to include vigorous exercise regimens such as jogging or step aerobics to be beneficial.

Lifting your grandchild or baby on a regular basis, weeding your garden, walking your dog and mowing the grass all count as physical exercise. You may be surprised to learn that walking through your neighbourhood every morning or evening can greatly enhance your level of physical fitness and emotional well-being. All you need to get started is a comfortable pair of walking shoes. Once you get started with your regular routine, you may find you enjoy physical activity so much, and feel so good, that you'll move on to more challenging exercises.

Unfortunately, our technologically top-heavy lifestyles, dominated by modems, motors, keyboards and remotes, don't encourage physical movement. In fact, they discourage and even constrain it. Our minds may be racing faster than ever, but our bodies are slowing down. Physical inertia has become the norm, and inertia is a powerful state with a delicious tendency to perpetuate itself.

In addition to this, we have a multitude of excuses for why we can't exercise, from disliking sweat to thinking we need a health club membership to believing we're too out of shape to get started. But by far the most frequent excuse I hear from Active Wellness participants is: 'I just don't have the time to exercise.' Ironically, the truth is that once you make time for exercise, exercise will create more time in your life. You'll need less sleep, have more energy, work more efficiently,and become more productive, all of which make more free time to do the things you enjoy the most.

If you are willing to hurdle the inertia barrier and make the time for regular physical fitness in your life, tremendous physical, mental, and spiritual benefits will be your reward. So, begin by designing your personal fitness programme.

Beginning Your Personal Fitness Programme

As with your customized eating plan, your physical fitness plan is unique to your own needs, interests and abilities. As you begin to put the components of your programme together, it is essential to follow these two general guidelines:

- ◇ Start slowly, particularly if you have been leading a sedentary lifestyle or have specific health concerns.
- ◇ Be realistic about what you can initially accomplish at your current level of fitness.

The following Health History Questionnaire and the Assessment of Current Physical Fitness Level on page 132 will help you stick to these guidelines. Answering the questions on both forms will help you develop an exercise programme that takes into consideration any health limitations you may have, as well as your current level of fitness. By combining your health parameters with activities you find pleasurable, you will develop your own individualized plan for fitness.

Although exercise can benefit anyone at almost any age, you do not want to push yourself too hard in the initial stages of your programme, particularly if you have not been active lately. You'll enjoy your fitness regimen more by avoiding injury and frustration.

Health History Questionnaire

	Yes	No
1. Do you now have, or have you ever had, a history of heart problems, chest pain, or stroke?	___	___
2. Do you now have, or have you ever had, high blood pressure?	___	___
3. Do you now have, or have you ever had, high blood cholesterol?	___	___
4. Do you now have, or have you ever had, any chronic illness or condition?	___	___
5. Do you now have, or have you ever had, difficulty doing physical exercise?	___	___
6. Have you ever been advised by a doctor not to exercise?	___	___
7. Have you had surgery within the last 12 months?	___	___
8. Are you now pregnant, or have you been pregnant within the last 3 months?	___	___
9. Do you now have, or have you ever had, a history of breathing or lung problems?	___	___
10. Do you have any muscle, joint, or back disorders?	___	___

continued on next page

	Yes	No
11. Do you have diabetes or a thyroid condition?	____	____
12. Do you smoke or have you smoked within the last year?	____	____
13. Are you currently overweight (more than 20 per cent above your ideal weight)?	____	____
14. Are you 40 years of age or older?	____	____

If you answered 'yes' to any of the above questions, you should consult your doctor before beginning this or any exercise programme. Certain clinical conditions, including diabetes, heart disease and metabolic disorders, require advice from a doctor before initiating any exercise programme. And while individuals at any age can begin moderate exercise programmes, men over age 40 and women over age 50 who plan to start an exercise programme should consult a doctor first.

Assessing Your Current Physical Fitness Level
Whether or not you need to consult your doctor, you can design your fitness programme now, then show it to him or her before you begin. Before you do that, however, you need to assess your current level of physical fitness, regardless of any current or past medical conditions. The following fitness assessment questionnaire will help you put together a realistic, safe and gratifying exercise programme that will be tailored to your current physical capabilities.

Assessment of Current Physical Fitness Level

Occupation and Daily Activities
1. I walk at least one-half mile on most days (i.e., to and from work or my shopping area). _____ (1 pt.)

2. I usually take stairs rather than using lifts or escalators.   _____ (1 pt.)

3. The type of physical activity involved in my job or daily household routine is best described by the following statement:

   a. Most of my workday is spent doing office work, light physical activity or household chores. _____ (0 pts.)

b. Most of my workday is spent doing moderate physical activities, brisk walking or comparable activities. _____ (4 pts.)

c. My typical workday includes several hours of heavy physical activity (shovelling, lifting, etc.). _____ (9 pts.)

Leisure Activities

1. I do several hours of gardening each week. _____ (1 pt.)

2. I fish once a week or more. (Must involve rowing a boat; sitting on a riverbank does not count.) _____ (1 pt.)

3. At least once a week, I participate for an hour or more in vigorous dancing, such as line or Latin dancing (or another activity that requires continual movement). _____ (1 pt.)

4. I play golf at least once a week without using a golf cart. _____(1 pt.)

5. I often walk for exercise or recreation. _____ (1 pt.)

6. When I feel bothered at work or at home, I use exercise as a way to relax. _____ (1pt.)

7. Two or more times a week I perform calisthenic exercises, such as sit-ups and push-ups, for at least 10 minutes per session. _____ (3 pts.)

8. I regularly do yoga or stretching exercises. _____ (2 pts.)

9. I participate in active recreational sports such as tennis and handball:

    a. Once a week _____ (2 pts.)
    b. Twice a week _____ (4 pts.)
    c. Three or more times a week. _____ (7 pts.)

10. I participate in vigorous fitness activities such as jogging, swimming, aerobic exercises or cycling for at least 20 continuous minutes per session:

    a. Once a week _____ (2 pts.)
    b. Twice a week _____ (4 pts.)
    c. Three or more times a week. _____ (7 pts.)

Total Score: _____ points

Review the chart below to determine your current physical fitness level.

Assessment of Current Physical Fitness Level		
Score	Activity Level	Effect on Fitness
0 to 5 points	Sedentary	This amount of exercise is insufficient and will lead to a steady decrease in fitness. Improvement is needed.
6 to 11 points	Light	This amount of exercise increases fitness somewhat, but will not maintain adequate fitness levels in most persons.
12 to 20 points	Moderate	This amount of exercise maintains an acceptable level of physical fitness.
20+ points	Very Active	This amount of exercise maintains an active superior level of physical fitness.

Source: Adapted with permission from the University of South Carolina Columbia Human Performance Laboratory.

Comparing the Different Activity Levels

The Physical Fitness Chart on the opposite page will give you a better idea of the types of exercises that are included in each activity level: 'sedentary', 'light', 'moderate', 'active' and 'very active'. You can also see approximately how many calories you can burn per minute at each level. There are more calories burned per minute at a higher level of activity, because these exercises require more effort from the body.

However, if you are trying to burn calories for weight loss or to maintain your weight, it is less strenuous on the body to burn calories by exercising for longer periods of time at a lower intensity (low impact). Low-impact exercises also help reduce your risk for injury and are easier to sustain for a longer duration. Fast walking at moderate intensity is an excellent example of an exercise that is low impact—the more you walk, the more calories you burn, and the more fit you become. You may be surprised to learn that your everyday activities, such as strolling and hoovering, can contribute to the amount of energy (calories) your body uses every day and to your overall level of fitness. You may want to take a minute while you are reviewing the chart to estimate about how many calories you burn throughout the week—include walking to and from your car as well as your routine exercise. A goal for weight loss is to aim to use 300 calories in energy for activity each day—this will help you burn the excess storage fuel (fat) you are trying to eliminate.

Activity Level (Intensity)	Activities	Calorie Expenditure (Men)	Calorie Expenditure (Women)
Sedentary	Lying; resting; sitting; sitting while performing light desk work	1 calorie/ min.	1 calorie/ min.
Light	Ten-pin bowling; fishing; golfing; horse-back riding; strolling; hoovering; stationary light cycling; standing while performing light work	2-5 calories / min.	2-4 calories/ min.
Moderate	Dancing; fast walking; hiking; light swimming; pleasure cycling; racquet sports; leisurely roller-skating/rollerblading	5-8 calories/ min.	4-6 calories/ min.
Active	Aerobic dance; basketball; canoeing; jogging; walking uphill with weights; fast cycling; fast swimming; downhill and cross-country skiing; competitive racquet sports; rollerskating/ rollerblading	8-10 calories/ min.	6-8 calories/ min.
Very Active	Fast-paced jogging; cycling; downhill and cross-country skiing; speed walking; swimming; basketball; football; racquet sports; mountain climbing; rollerskating/rollerblading; wrestling	10-13 calories/ min.	8-10 calories/ min.

The Physical Fitness Chart

How Much Does It Take to Burn Off...			
Food Type	Approximate Calorie Count	Walking 3 mph	Jogging 6 mph
1 Slice of Bread	80	11 min.	6 min.
1 Large Bagel	400	1 hr. 30 min.	50 min.
1 Cheese Pastry	350	70 min.	35 min.
1 Ice-Cream Sundae	300	1 hr. 15 min.	40 min.
1 2-oz (60 g). Brownie	270	30 min.	15 min.
1 3-oz. (90 g) Muffin	300	1 hr. 15 min.	40 min.
1 Chocolate Chip Cookie	140	40 min.	20 min.
1 1-oz. (30 g) Bag of Crisps	150	45 min.	25 min.

Modified from Table 8.5, Relationships Among Respiration, Heart Rate, and Caloric Expenditure for Different Degrees of Physical Activity (in adults) Data from *Nutrition, Weight Control and Exercise* (3rd ed.) by F. Katch and W. McArdle, 1988, Philadelphia: Lea and Febiger.

We are under-exercised as a nation. We look instead of play. We ride instead of walk. Our existence deprives us of the minimum of physical activity essential for living.
—John F. Kennedy

Designing Your Personal Fitness Plan

Once you understand your current fitness level and your personal health limits, you can formulate the foundation of a realistic and reasonable plan. Before you begin putting together the specifics of your fitness programme, you should be aware of the following general exercise guidelines, which have been established by the American College of Sports Medicine (ACSM) and the American Council on Exercise:

- ◊ Every adult should accumulate 30 minutes or more of moderate intensity physical activity over the course of most days of the week. Activities that can contribute to the 30-minute total include walking upstairs, gardening, raking leaves, dancing and walking part or all of the way to and from work. The recommended 30 minutes of physical activity may also come from planned exercise or recreation, such as jogging, playing tennis, swimming and cycling.
- ◊ People who are already very active should aim to perform aerobic activities at 60 to 80 per cent of their maximum heart rate, three to five times per week, for 15 to 60 minutes per session.
- ◊ Resistance training for all major muscle groups is also recommended at all activity levels.

The Fine Art of Pacing Yourself

You are the best judge of how much and how often you can exercise and at what intensity level. Keep in mind, however, that if you try to exercise too much too soon, you may damage your body by injuring your muscles. Therefore, remember to increase your physical fitness gradually, by pushing yourself only slightly beyond your comfort zone. Your workout or activity should feel somewhat challenging, but never painful or unduly uncomfortable. You may feel stiff for the first few days after beginning an exercise programme. However, this feeling should quickly disappear. If stiffness or pain persist, you should contact your doctor.

You should exercise at your own pace. Whether or not you increase your activity level depends on your personal goals. Within your personal plan, you have a choice about your goals for achieving fitness. You can choose one of the two objectives listed below for each component of your fitness programme.

Maintain Your Fitness Level at a Moderate Range: Once you achieve a moderate level of intensity, you are reaping the physical and health benefits of exercise—as long as you maintain your weekly routine of at least 3 to 5 times a week for your aerobic workout and stretching and 2 or 3 times a week for your strength training. By maintaining this level you will obtain health benefits, but not necessarily increase your strength, flexibility, stamina and aerobic capacity. At a moderate level, you will burn a steady number of calories each week, which can contribute to weight loss or weight maintenance, maintain your lean body mass and maintain your level of physical health.

Increase Your Strength, Flexibility and Stamina: With this goal you will be continually striving to improve your abilities in one or all three components of your programme—aerobics, stretching, and strength training. This is a helpful goal if you want to increase the calories you are burning, increase your lean body mass, prevent bone loss and improve your strength, stamina, aerobic capacity and ease of movement.

If you are already moderately active and you want to increase your strength and endurance, you'll need to challenge yourself more. If you are walking briskly for an hour three times a week, for example, try adding a fourth day of some other moderate level of activity such as dancing to increase your stamina and add variety to your routine. If you are a runner and you're trying to increase your level of fitness, you may want to challenge yourself by adding a quarter of a mile to your run every week or two. The important thing to remember is to challenge yourself gradually over time. This gives your body time to increase cardiovascular fitness, muscle strength, and endurance with less chance of injury. When working out, it is also good to vary your exercise when you can; this will help you work different muscle groups and keep all your muscles fit.

As you work out, if your goal is to work towards attaining a higher level of fitness, you want to be aware of points in your programme where you reach a plateau of effort in your fitness regimen. The plateau will be a sign that you are staying at your current level of exercise. You should challenge yourself by pushing just a bit more beyond that plateau. In this way, you can continue to increase your aerobic capacity and strength, and focus your efforts on obtaining your optimal fitness capacity.

❖ Rose ❖

When Rose began her Active Wellness programme, one of her personal goals was to begin exercising.* Since she was at a light-intensity level, her first goal was to increase her intensity to the moderate-intensity level, to reap the benefits of physical activity and to help herself lose weight and strengthen her heart. With this in mind, Rose began to walk one mile every other day. At first it took a half hour, since she was at the light-intensity level. Then as she began to become more fit, she was able to complete the mile in 15 minutes. She was now at the moderate-intensity level; from there she increased her length of time, eventually reaching 45 minutes of moderate-intensity exercise. Before she knew it, her heart was stronger and her weight was steadily dropping by 1.5 lb (0.7 kg) a week. Rose chose to stay at the moderate level of activity, because she was comfortable with that intensity of exercise.

---

*Caution: If you have a history of cardiovascular disease or other limitations, you should get approval from your doctor before increasing your level of activity.

How to Challenge Yourself
You can increase your physical endurance during exercise in three ways:

- ❖ By increasing the *frequency* of the exercise (how *often* you do it).
- ❖ By increasing the *intensity* of the exercise (how *hard* you do it).
- ❖ By increasing the *duration* of the exercise (how *long* you do it).

As you begin your personalized fitness programme, it is very helpful to understand how to integrate the above components of frequency, intensity, and duration into your plan.

The best way to raise your fitness level is to focus on increasing just one of the above components at a time. For instance, if you walk 30 minutes a day (duration), three to five days a week (frequency), on flat terrain (intensity), you may want to increase the duration of your activity after two weeks: start walking 35 minutes a day, three to five days a week on the same terrain.

What you don't want to do is increase your duration at the same time as you increase the intensity of the walk (by changing to an uphill terrain, for example) or the frequency of the walk (by adding an extra day to your regimen). You may tire out too soon or get injured, leaving you more discouraged than motivated.

Sometimes people who have been sedentary for a long time suddenly decide to get in shape and start exercising intensely every day. By the end of the first week, every muscle in their body aches and they have to stop exercising to give their body time to heal. This can start a self-defeating cycle of stopping-and-starting exercise. Once you stop a routine, even briefly, you may have a hard time getting motivated to start again. I cannot emphasize enough that at the outset of your fitness programme you should establish reasonable and realistic goals for yourself and begin exercising gradually and moderately as you increase your ability.

As we move on, we'll take an in-depth look at each of the activities that comprise your fitness plan. Use the Personalized Exercise Programme (P.E.P.) Worksheet at the end of this chapter to help you design a realistic and enjoyable weekly fitness plan.

⁙ Laurie ⁙

Laurie had decided that her fiftieth birthday present to herself would be a hiking trip. However, she knew she wasn't in shape for it. Laurie's goal was to increase her strength and stamina. Laurie began at a light-intensity level, walking to and from work. Gradually she increased the speed at which she walked and then her effort level by walking on the treadmill at an incline. Six months later she had reached the active-intensity level category where she could walk uphill carrying a backpack, without a problem. She also lost an average of 2 lb (0.9 kg) per week!

The Personalized Exercise Programme Worksheet

Throughout the remainder of this chapter, you will be asked to refer to your Personalized Exercise Programme Worksheet on page 161. This worksheet will be used to record information that will help you develop your personalized fitness programme. Use this worksheet as your exercise 'guide'. It can be changed, as you progress, to reflect your increased level of physical fitness and new exercise goals. To develop the best exercise programme, begin at your current level of fitness and with your current fitness goals. You can record your initial fitness goal and current activity level at the top of your P.E.P. worksheet.

Your Five Fitness Plan Essentials

The five basic activities that comprise your exercise programme are:

⬦ Warm-Ups
⬦ Aerobic/Cardiovascular Workout
⬦ Cool-Downs
⬦ Strength Training/Muscle Toning
⬦ Stretching Exercises

Using your current activity (intensity) level as your starting point, this chapter will explain how to put together sets of warm-up, stretching, and cool-down exercises to complement your aerobic/cardiovascular workout and strength training/muscle toning routine. In addition to learning how to choose the best exercise for yourself, you will learn the appropriate frequency, intensity, and time for each type of exercise.

Your intensity level determines the base of your aerobic conditioning programme. You will integrate your warm-up and cool-down and stretching programme into your aerobic routine. The last component will include muscle toning and strength training. You may find that you are at a different level with each component of your programme. If this is the case, then you may want to make one of your goals to balance them. You should try to not increase your level in one aspect of your programme (i.e. aerobics) before you have added strength training and stretching to your weekly routine. In the Appendix are exercise starter programmes where you'll find suggested rates of progression for each type of exercise in your plan, so that you can challenge yourself and increase your level of fitness, if that is your goal. A healthy balance of the three components to strive for as a minimum is:

⬦ Aerobic Exercise: 3 to 5 times a week
⬦ Strength Training: 2 to 3 times a week
⬦ Stretching: 3 to 5 times a week (after aerobic exercises or as an isolated component)

Warm-Ups

Warm-ups are essential because they prepare your body for the more rigorous demands of the aerobic and strength training exercises that will follow. When your body is at rest, prior to beginning your workout, your muscles are receiving only a small percentage of the blood that is circulating throughout your body. Warming up increases blood flow to the muscles, which literally 'warms' them. This makes the muscles more pliable and flexible, which helps protect your body against unnecessary injuries and muscle soreness. Warm-ups also allow your body's temperature to adjust gradually to the increased blood flow that occurs during a more vigorous exercise.

Warm-ups should be done for 10 minutes prior to exercise. Many times your warm-up routine can consist of the same type of activity that you do for your aerobic exercise—just at a slower or more leisurely pace. Walking and low-intensity cycling are great warm-up exercises. They target most of the major muscle groups, allowing you to begin slowly and to ease into your workout. At the end of your warm-up, your body will be well primed for your aerobic or strength training activities.

Take a moment to record your warm-up routine on your Personalized Exercise Programme Worksheet. Refer to The Physical Fitness Chart on page 135 to choose your warm-up activity. The one you choose should be at an intensity level that is one level lower than your current fitness level. For example, if you exercise at a moderate intensity, you will begin your warm-up at a light intensity. Only if you are at a light-intensity level, should your warm-up be the same as your current activity level.

Aerobic/Cardiovascular Workout

The word *aerobic* means 'with oxygen'. Aerobic exercise, properly done, utilizes oxygen to improve the fitness of your heart and lungs. Your heart is a muscle, and one of the best ways to keep it in shape is with aerobic activities that strengthen the heart muscle just as they strengthen the other muscles of the body. *Aerobic fitness* refers to the ability of your heart and lungs to effectively deliver oxygen-carrying blood to large groups of working muscles during sustained and continuous physical movement.

Aerobic activity is a great way to burn fat. When a large supply of oxygen reaches your body's cells, your body burns fat more effectively by using the fat as energy to fuel your muscles. Your fat-burning ability increases as the duration of your aerobic exercise increases and your level of fitness improves. It takes 20 minutes of continuous exercise before fat is available as a fuel source for your body. The more fit you are and the longer you exercise, the more calories and fat you will burn.

For those of you who are just beginning a fitness programme and cannot begin exercising at a high level of intensity, rest assured. You can also burn calories and fat during low-intensity exercises, which is a huge step in the right direction along the path to wellness.

Choosing an Aerobic Activity

The best aerobic exercises have the following two parameters in common:

- They utilize the large muscle groups of the body (the legs, buttocks, chest and arm muscles).
- They involve continuous and repetitive movements.

If your favourite exercises fulfill these two requirements, keep up your routine! Any activities that fit this description are considered aerobic activities. If you are not sure whether an activity is aerobic, check the Physical Fitness Chart on page 135, or refer to the list below, which includes the more common and challenging aerobic activities.

Choose the aerobic exercises that you enjoy doing the most and record them on your Personalized Exercise Programme Worksheet opposite 'Selected Aerobic Activities'. If you don't want to take an aerobics class or you can't get to a gym, brisk walking is a fine way to begin your aerobic exercise programme.

Once you've chosen the type of aerobic activities you enjoy, the next step involves determining your pace or the intensity you intend to exercise.

Common Aerobic Activities

Brisk Walking	Dancing
Jogging	Continuous Rope Skipping
Rowing	Rollerblading
Cycling	Swimming
Cross-Country Skiing	Stairmaster Workout
Roller Skating/Ice Skating	Hiking
Step Aerobics	Stairclimbing

Setting Your Aerobic Pace

Exercise intensity is measured in two ways. One is how fast your heart beats during an activity. The other is how difficult you perceive the activity to be.

To determine how fast your heart should beat during aerobic activity, you need to calculate your Maximum Heart Rate (MHR) and your Target Heart Rate (THR). Your maximum heart rate is the 'maximum' number of times your heart can physically beat per minute during exercise. It is the threshold point for your heart, beyond which it becomes too difficult for your body to exercise and you will be forced to stop. No one should exercise at their MHR, because it is too intense. Instead, it is best to exercise at a percentage of your maximum heart rate, or target heart rate. When exercising aerobically, the point at which you achieve the greatest fitness benefit is referred to as your Target Heart Rate . Your target heart rate is a goal range of how many beats per minute your heart should beat during aerobic activity.

> **Warning:** No one should exercise at their maximum heart rate (MHR).

Research shows that the best way to achieve fitness is to perform aerobic activities within your THR range. Your THR range is between 60 and 80 per cent of your maximum heart rate.

For healthy individuals exercising at a moderate level of intensity, the goal is to reach and maintain a THR range between 60 and 80 per cent of your maximum heart rate. For very sedentary people who are beginning a fitness programme at a low level of intensity, the goal should be to reach your THR range slowly over time.

Active or highly active people (i.e. athletes and avid exercisers) may work slightly above their THR range (to a high of 90 per cent of their maximum heart rate). However, if you are training to exercise beyond your THR range, you should seek advice from a trainer, coach, doctor or sports-medicine professional.

You can achieve the most benefits from exercise when you reach and maintain your target heart rate at a goal of 60 to 80 per cent of your maximum heart rate during 20 to 60 minutes of exercise, 3 to 5 days per week.

Determining Your Target Heart Rate

The first step in determining your target heart rate is to assess your maximum heart rate. If you have had a stress test or a thorough fitness test within the last month, you may have been given your MHR at that time. You can use this as your MHR number. If you don't know your MHR, here's a simple calculation:

$$MHR = 220 - \text{your age}$$

For example, if you are 40 years old, your maximum heart rate is 180 beats per minute, or 220 − 40 = 180. Determine your maximum heart rate now and record it on your Personalized Exercise Programme Worksheet.

To calculate your Target Heart Rate range, multiply your Maximum Heart Rate by .60, which represents 60 per cent of your Maximum Heart Rate:

MHR x .60 =_____ (This is the lower number of your THR range, measured in beats per minute.)

MHR x .80 =_____ (This is the upper number of your THR range, measured in beats per minute.)

For example:
A 40-year-old man would have a maximum heart rate of 180.
180 x .60 = 108 (This would be the lower limit of his THR range.)
180 x .80 = 144 (This would be the upper limit of his THR range.)

When this man exercises aerobically, he will try to achieve a THR of 108 to 144 beats per minute. At his target heart rate range (108 to 144 beats per minute), he will ensure that he is exercising hard enough to achieve maximum aerobic benefit.

Now, determine your Target Heart Rate range and record it in the space provided on your Personalized Exercise Programme Worksheet.

> *Note: If you are highly active you can adjust the upper limit of your target heart rate to take into account your higher fitness ability. Do this by multiplying the upper range by .90 (90 per cent) instead of .80 (80 percent).*

How to Measure Your Target Heart Rate
It is important to know how to measure your heart rate while you are exercising so that you can be sure that you're within your Target Heart Rate range during your aerobic workout. You can do this by locating your pulse and counting your heart beats. After you have warmed up and have been exercising aerobically for 5 minutes, lightly place your index and middle fingers on the side of your neck below your jawbone, or on the inside of your wrist. When you feel a steady pulse, count the number of beats (or pulses) for 15 seconds. Multiply this number by 4 to get your heart rate. This number should fall within your Target Heart Rate range. If it is lower than your THR range you may need to increase the intensity of your activity a little or speed up. If the number is above your THR range, you are working out too hard and may need to decrease your intensity or slow down.

> **CAUTION:** If you have a heart condition or are on blood pressure medication, your heart rate may be lower than these calculations. Consult your doctor before determining your THR range.

Putting Your Aerobic Programme Together
You have determined the type of aerobic exercises you like and the intensity (THR) and now it's time to decide how many days a week you will exercise and the duration of each physical activity session. There are three factors to consider:

⬥ Your personal aerobic fitness goals
⬥ Current level of fitness
⬥ Realistic and reasonable expectations

Your Personal Aerobic Fitness Goals

Your personal goals will guide your decision about how you will proceed with your aerobic programme—whether you will focus on increasing your fitness level or merely maintaining it. For instance, if you want to lose a few pounds, any increase in activity will be helpful; aerobic exercise will help you burn more calories and decrease your percentage of body fat. If you are content with doing a minimum amount of exercise to stay fit and keep your heart and muscles toned, reaching and maintaining the American College of Sports Medicine (ACSM) recommendations of a moderate level of activity at your target heart rate, a minimum of 20 to 60 minutes per day, 3 to 5 times a week, is enough. Below are guidelines to help you determine your aerobic fitness goals, based on your current activity level.

Realistic Expectations for Different Levels of Aerobic Fitness

If you are just beginning to 'move' and be active, you are at a sedentary or light activity level for your aerobic programme. It is important for your health to work toward gradually increasing your activity level to achieve at least a moderate level of activity. The guidelines on the next page and in the appendix will help you establish a routine to increase your physical ability. By increasing your physical activity you will be able to maintain or lose weight easier and improve your physical and mental well-being. Before you know it, you'll feel more fit and this will increase your ability to do many other types of activities without tiring as easily.

If you already do aerobic exercises regularly 3 to 5 times a week, you are at a moderate, active or very active activity level. Since you have achieved the ACSM requirement, you have a choice. You can either maintain this level of aerobic intensity and work at incorporating stretching and strength training at the recommended minimum sessions per week, or, if you want to increase your overall physical fitness level, you can begin to work towards a higher level of aerobic activity. If you have not integrated the components of stretching and strength training, it is advisable to work these into your programme first, before you increase your aerobic activity level. You'll find sample strength training and stretching exercises on pages 157-160.

By balancing aerobic fitness, muscle strength and flexibility in your personal exercise programme, you will achieve a better balance of physical fitness. If you are working at gradually increasing your activity level, use the guidelines that follow. Remember to start at your present activity level and work your way up to the next level from there.

Setting Time Aside to Exercise

It is very important to establish realistic weekly goals that you can achieve. The only way to achieve your aerobic goals is to initiate your plan into your weekly schedule. By setting aside a time of day in your daily schedule that is convenient, you can begin to establish a commitment to fitness.

Many Active Wellness participants are very busy with work and family commitments. The most successful strategy is to fit your exercise into a time of day when you have the least number of distractions. You may choose to exercise by walking to and from work, first thing in the morning, at lunchtime or right before dinner. The key to keeping on schedule is to establish your routine into your daily life's activities. Before you know it, others will expect you to take that time for yourself and begin to plan around your schedule.

When you begin your exercise programme, gradually increase your workout intensity and frequency until you reach the goals you have set for yourself. Once you are at your chosen level of physical fitness, you should work to maintain that level without feeling pressured to push yourself towards a level that is too high for you. Follow the general guidelines below to plan your aerobic programme.

Sedentary or Light Activity Aerobic Guidelines

If you have been sedentary or fairly inactive don't worry about reaching your target heart rate when you first start your exercise programme. Start your moderate exercise routine with 10 minutes of warm-up exercises. Begin your programme with physical activities that increase your heart rate slightly but do not feel strenuous or exhausting. Light intensity activities include such things as leisurely walking, taking the stairs instead of the lift, housework, table tennis or gardening. For the first week of your programme, try to do 10 minutes of light physical activity every day. During the second week increase your activity to 15 minutes. Thereafter, increase it by 5 minutes each week, until you have reached a goal of 50 to 60 minutes of light physical activity at least five days a week. You may also do a combination of varying short-term activities that add up to your 50- to 60-minute total per day.

As you progress each week, your endurance and stamina will increase. You will gradually move up to the next level of exercise (moderate intensity) where you can achieve a new level of maximum aerobic benefit.

Moderate Activity Aerobic Guidelines

Exercises that fall into the moderate activity category include brisk walking, jogging at an easy pace, moderate aerobics, cycling at a medium pace, swimming, hiking, and cross-country skiing at a leisurely pace. At this point you should start trying to work within your target heart rate range.

Start your moderate exercise routine with 10 minutes of warm-up exercises. During the first two weeks of your programme, try to do 20 to 30 minutes of moderately intense aerobic exercise three or four days a week. After two weeks, add five minutes a day to your aerobic routine every two weeks until you reach a maximum duration of 50 to 60 minutes, which may be broken into two 25- to 30-minute sessions a day. Once you can comfortably maintain this level of exercise, gradually increase the frequency of your workouts to four or five days a week. Follow each exercise session with 5 to 10 minutes of cool-down exercises. At this stage, you will have reached a healthy level of fitness, and, depending on the personal fitness goals you have established, you can either maintain your aerobic routine or move on to higher intensity activities.

Active Activity Aerobic Guidelines

Exercises that fall into the high intensity category include activities such as jogging, swimming, heavy aerobics, cross-country skiing and cycling—all performed at a rapid pace.

If you are just beginning to exercise at the high activity level, you'll want to gradually incorporate the higher intensity exercises into your routine, without changing the number of days per week you exercise. Begin your aerobic routine with 10 minutes of warm-ups, followed by your aerobic activity, then 5 to 10 minutes of cool-down activity. For the first two weeks, perform your aerobic exercise for 15 to 20 minutes, three or four days a week. Then, every two weeks, begin adding 5 minutes a day to your routine until you reach a maximum duration of 45 minutes a session of intense aerobic activity. Once you are able to exercise at this level, you can increase your exercise sessions to five days a week. Or you can choose to maintain your aerobic sessions to four days a week and focus on using the remainder of the week for strength training and stretching.

If you are already exercising at high intensity for 45 minutes a session, five times a week, you can increase the length of your sessions by 5 minutes every two weeks. This is helpful if you are training to be an endurance athlete. It is advisable to consult your doctor and a trained exercise professional such as an exercise physiologist before you start a training programme. When you are training it is important to pay attention to your body's signals of fatigue and exhaustion.

When you have determined your initial intensity level, record it on your Personalized Exercise Programme Worksheet. Now, select the days of the week that you want to exercise and record the name of the activity you will be doing each day on your Personalized Exercise Programme Worksheet (P.E.P.) under the heading 'AerobicActivity'. (On the days you don't want to work out aerobically, just leave those spaces blank.) As you progress you can change your P.E.P. to reflect your new routine.

Strive for Balance but Remember to Pace Yourself

At all exercise intensity levels, vary the type of exercise you do. Variety is important for several reasons: It keeps up your interest, challenges your body in different ways, and also works your muscles differently to promote balanced, total body fitness. But whatever exercises you do, don't push yourself too hard or attempt a workout regimen that is too difficult for your body's current fitness level. Strive to find your personal comfort zone when exercising and stay within that zone until you are physically and mentally ready to move up to a higher level of exercise intensity.

Finding Your Comfort Zone: Perception of Exercise Difficulty

Regardless of your calculated fitness level, only you can determine your comfort zone within your target heart rate range. Do this by 'listening' to your body while you are exercising. You should never experience physical discomfort or pain. You should feel able to complete your exercises comfortably, within the recommended time frame, without having to stop and rest.

A good rule of thumb when you are exercising aerobically is to make sure you can say a full sentence without gasping for air while you are exercising. If you can't, your body is not receiving enough oxygen and you may be working out too intensely for your current level of fitness. If you feel flushed or dizzy, this can also be a sign that you are exercising too intensely. Keep in mind that the best aerobic benefit comes from moderately intense exercises performed within your target heart rate range (between 60 and 80 per cent of your maximum heart rate).

Remember that in order to achieve maximum fitness benefits, exercising for a longer time at a lower intensity is better than exercising for a shorter time at a high intensity. With this moderate type of exercise regimen, it won't take long to improve your aerobic fitness.

One word of caution: If you are just beginning a fitness programme and find that you reach your maximum level of exertion before you have finished exercising or that you tire very quickly, you may be pushing yourself too hard. Resist the urge to push yourself beyond your personal comfort zone. Otherwise, you may cause yourself serious injury. If your body cannot tolerate the exercise intensity at which you are working, you may experience some serious physical reactions. Below are some general signs of exercise intolerance.

General Signs of Exercise Intolerance

If any of the symptoms listed here occur during or after exercise, consult your doctor or go to your nearest medical facility as soon as possible.

⋄ Pain or pressure in the chest, the arm or the throat during or immediately after exercise. If this occurs, go to the nearest casualty department. These may be signs of a heart attack.

⋄ Substantial increase in shortness of breath with exercise.

⋄ Dizziness, lightheadedness, sudden lack of coordination, confusion, or fainting.

⋄ Sudden burst of rapid heartbeats or sudden slowing down of a rapid pulse.

⋄ Nausea or vomiting.

⋄ Unexplained weight changes.

⋄ Any of the following signs of dehydration:

Early signs	Severe signs
⋄ fatigue	⋄ difficulty swallowing
⋄ loss of appetite	⋄ stumbling
⋄ flushed skin	⋄ clumsiness
⋄ heat intolerance	⋄ shrivelled skin
⋄ lightheadedness	⋄ sunken eyes and dim vision
⋄ dark urine with a strong odour	⋄ painful urination
	⋄ numb skin
	⋄ muscle spasms
	⋄ delirium

Cool-Downs

This vital component of your physical fitness programme—cooling down—is often overlooked. Gradually cooling down allows the cardiovascular system to return to normal levels and should follow all of your aerobic workouts. This is especially important if you have a heart disease risk, are older, or are just starting an exercise programme, because cardiac complications can occur when an exercise is stopped abruptly. Cool-downs allow the heart rate to safely decrease to normal levels and prevent blood from pooling in the lower extremities, where it can cause reduced blood pressure, dizziness and, in some rare cases, lead to cardiac arrythmias.

Use the same exercise you choose as your warm-up for your cool-down, but perform it for 5 to 10 minutes at a decreasingly slower pace. You can also cool down by slowing down the pace of your current exercise. After cooling down, it is advisable to stretch your muscles to decrease possible muscle soreness and stiffness. You can use the exercises on pages 159-160 as a guide for cool-down stretches. Look at your P.E.P. worksheet and notice the space for cool-downs in the aerobic section. For each day that you do an aerobic workout, be sure to include a cooling-down session immediately after.

Adding Your Strengthening and Stretching Routines: Learning to Be a Cross-Trainer
The best overall fitness programme balances aerobic (cardiovascular) activities with other activities that promote strength (muscle tone) and stretching (flexibility). Cross-training is the term used to describe this exercise balance, which is featured in the fourth and fifth components of the Active Wellness fitness programme—strength training and stretching.

Strength Training/Muscle Toning

Strength training activities strengthen and tone muscles through weight or resistance exercises. Strength training workouts involve short periods of intense physical activity, such as weightlifting, resistance-band exercises and calisthenics (sit-ups and press-ups). In strength training you exercise with progressively heavier weights or increased resistance to develop physical endurance and increase the strength of your muscles and skeletal system. This training can have a profound effect on your physical strength, your appearance (by increasing your lean body mass), your metabolism, and your risk of injury.

Muscles utilize energy to produce movement. Think of muscles as the engines of your body. With strength training, you can increase the size and strength (mass) of your muscle fibres, which in turn makes any physical activity or movement easier.

Unfortunately, unless you perform regular muscle toning exercises, you will lose up to a 0.5 lb (0.25 kg) of muscle every year of your life after the age of 25! On the other hand, strength training at any age can prevent muscle loss. And the more muscle mass you have, the greater your body's metabolic rate and the more calories you burn. Both men and women can increase their muscle mass by about 3 lb (1.4 kg) by following a standard ten-week strengthening programme.

Strength training is also one of the proven ways to reduce the risks associated with osteoporosis, because strong muscles can support the bones more effectively. Strength training also slows the ageing process, improves posture and balance and increases energy, strength and stamina.

*The human body has the performance capability of a Ferrari,
and the durability of the Chevy. Although we need to put ourselves
through the human equivalent of an all-out lap at Le Mons from
time to time, we can also idle along for 30 years before we start
having serious maintenance problems. No machine was ever
designed to compare with this combination of performance
and durability.*

— Arnold Schwarzenegger

Getting Started with Your Strength Training Programme

Strength training exercises are performed using free weights, resistance machines such as Nautilus or Universal equipment, resistance bands and tubing, or your own body weight as resistance.

Active Wellness strength training exercises are provided on pages 157-158. However, I strongly advise that you see an exercise specialist before you begin strength training to ensure that your posture and positioning are correct when you work out. Exercise specialists, such as exercise physiologists, are available at most health clubs and YMCAs, or you can hire a personal trainer to come to your home. It is worth the investment in time and money to work with a trainer once or twice before starting out on your own. He or she can observe your form, make modifications to your programme, and help protect you against any injury. Alternatively, you can rent or buy a strength training video to work out with, or take a strength training class.

The Components of Your Strength Training Programme

The key to performing strength training exercises properly is to use progressive resistance (weights) to build muscle. Schedule your strength training exercises at least two days per week. It is best to have a day between your strength training workouts to give your muscles a chance to rest. Take a moment to write in your strength training programme on your Personalized Exercise Programme Worksheet. As with your aerobic routine, you should always warm up before beginning your strength training exercises.

After completing your warm-up for at least 10 minutes, start by doing 8 to 12 repetitions (known as a set) for each of 8 to 10 exercises, which have been designed to condition the major muscle groups of your body. If you can't do a minimum of eight repetitions for each exercise, you may be using too much resistance/weight. If this is the case, decrease the weight or resistance until you can comfortably do 8 to 12 repetitions. If you are just beginning, do not use weights or resistance bands for your first session. See how you feel just by using your own weight as resistance, and follow the movements indicated in the programme.

Also, remember to work all the muscle groups, as the programme at the end of this chapter outlines, so that no one muscle group becomes stronger than another. For instance, if you do sit-ups to strengthen your stomach muscles, remember to strengthen your back muscles as well, otherwise your stomach muscles can affect the spine and contribute to tightness or lower back pain, pulling your body out of alignment from an imbalance of muscle strength.

> **Tip:** Breathe while doing strength training. Exhale on exertion and inhale when returning to starting position.

In general, aim to perform two or three sets (of 8 to 12 repetitions) for each exercise, giving yourself a 30- to 60-second rest between each set. Each set should be done in a slow, controlled fashion that allows you to maintain your breath throughout the exercises.

When you can perform three sets of an exercise comfortably and with good form, try varying your set patterns, your tempo, and the different muscle groups you focus on. Once you can complete two or three sets comfortably, you can increase the weight/resistance you are using (by approximately 5 per cent), to continue to increase your muscular strength. With a sensible, intelligent and progressive strengthening programme designed for your body, you reap the rewards of increased energy, strength, and stamina very quickly. Plus, there's a hidden bonus to strength training—not only do you become stronger, but you become leaner. Refer to the strength training exercises on pages 157-158.

The Hidden Bonus of Strength Training

By combining both aerobic exercise (which burns fat) with resistance/weight training (which increases muscle), you can improve your overall percentage of lean body mass, which is the ratio of fat to muscle throughout your body. In fact, focusing on reducing 'fat mass' and increasing 'lean mass' may be a better fitness focus than setting a weight goal.

Fitness trainers and medical technicians have elaborate methods for determining the ratio of lean muscle mass to fat mass, including the Skinfold Assessment Test, Underwater (hydrostatic) Weighing, and the Bioelectric Impedance Technique. After obtaining your measurements, refer to the chart below to assess your body fat content. While these measurements can be helpful, you should be able to see the results of your efforts (a decrease in fat mass and increase in muscle mass) just by looking at your body and noticing the way your clothes fit. If you prefer, you can follow the guidelines provided on page 51 for measuring your body fat.

Body Fat Content

Description	Men	Women
Essential Fat	2-5%	5-10%
Goal Percentage for Optimal Health	12-20%	20-30%
Obesity	>25%	>33%

Take a moment to record on your P.E.P. the days that you'll be weight training. As with your aerobic programme, leave the days blank if you're not going to weight train. Feel free to change your programme as you increase your fitness level, so it reflects your progress and continues to meet your changing needs and goals.

Stretching and flexibility exercises are the perfect complement to aerobic fitness and strength training. Let's take a brief look at how to do stretching exercises and at how they benefit the body.

Stretching Exercises

Stretching exercises are the best way to improve and maintain your body's flexibility and balance. Many people neglect this component of physical fitness because they don't realize the importance of improving the range of physical motion (flexibility) and maintaining the suppleness of muscles, joints and connective tissue. Stretching exercises also enhance your fitness routines by making it easier and safer to move, bend, and lift without injury and fatigue. Stretching also helps to relieve stress by releasing muscle tension.

Flexibility refers to the ability of muscles, joints and connective tissue (the material that links muscles and joints together) to move through a full range of motion and extension without stiffness or pain. Some people are naturally more flexible than others, but with patience and practice everyone can improve their flexibility.

Stretching, or flexibility, exercises were once thought of as 'warm-ups', or what you did before you started your 'real' exercise workout. This is definitely not the case. In fact, you need to warm up before you do any stretching/flexibility routines.

You can take stretching or flexibility classes at many gyms, health clubs and YMCAs. Other physical activities, such as ballet, yoga and t'ai chi, are also considered stretching exercises. A basic stretching routine that includes stretching exercises for all of the major muscle groups is provided on pages 159-160. I recommend that you do formal stretching exercises for 30 to 60 minutes at least twice a week. However, when stretching is done correctly, it is very gentle on the body and can be done every day. It is a great idea to add 10 minutes of stretching exercises after you have completed your aerobic and strength training workouts since your muscles will already be warmed up, more flexible and primed for stretching.

Enter the days you will do your stretching routine on your P.E.P. worksheet. Notice the space for stretching that has been left after your aerobic workout and your strength training workouts. This is to remind you that it is a good idea to stretch after all your workouts, if you have the time. Also, please notice the space that has been left for 'warm-ups' before your stretching routine. This is to remind you to be sure to warm up for at least 10 minutes prior to stretching. You should never stretch your muscles without warming up first. If you do, your muscles will not be flexible and they will resist your efforts to lengthen by tightening up. Stretching 'cold' muscles is an invitation for injury!

The key thing to remember about stretching is that you should never force a stretch or try to bounce up and down to achieve a stretch. The correct way to stretch is to aim for a sustained and comfortable stretch without straining while breathing deeply and with your attention focused on the muscle you are working on. Forcing a stretch can activate the 'stretch reflex', where a signal is sent to the muscle to shorten and contract to keep it from being injured. Ironically, if you stretch too far, you will actually tighten the muscles you are trying to stretch and lengthen.

When you are stretching correctly, you should feel just a mild tension as the muscles and connective tissue elongate. This should not be painful. The feeling of mild tension should decrease as you hold the stretch for 10 to 20 seconds. When you complete your stretch, ease off and return to your starting position. Repeat each stretch 3 to 5 times. The goal here, as always, is no pain and great gain.

Special Exercise Guidelines for Specific Health Conditions

If you have any of the following health conditions, it is important to follow the general guidelines below and consult your doctor before you begin or change your exercise programme.

	Exercise Prescription	Exercise Precautions
Hypertension	**Aerobic Exercise** Frequency: 4 or 5 exercise sessions per week Duration: 30 to 60 minutes Target Heart Rate: 40 to 80% Maximum Heart Rate *High intensity and isometric activities should be avoided.* **Weight Training** Weight training should involve low resistance with high repetitions.	Consult a doctor because your medication may impact on your heart rate and level of aerobic intensity.
Peripheral Vascular Disease	**Aerobic Exercise** Frequency/duration: Begin with 20 minutes twice daily (or less), with a goal of increasing to one 40- to 60-minute session. **Weight-Bearing Activities** Weight-bearing exercises are beneficial. Non-weight-bearing activities provide less resistance,	Make sure resistance training is consistant with your level of fitness; be careful not to increase intensity before you are strong enough to maintain your workout.

	enabling you to exercise for a longer period of time. *Do not hesitate to take intermittent rest periods if needed.*	
Diabetes	Exercise Daily Duration 20 to 30 minutes per session to achieve glucose control at a minimum. Maximize duration to burn calories if overweight.	Monitor blood glucose before and after exercise. You may need to add a carbohydrate snack before or after exercise to maintain blood sugar at normal levels. Be cautious of dehydration in hot weather.

ACSM's Guidelines for Exercise Testing and Prescription 5th Edition. Williams and Wilkins, Baltimore, MD. A Waverly Company, 1995.

Feet: The Last Word

Sole Searching: What Shoe to Wear?
Your feet support your entire body. In turn, they must be properly supported, especially during exercise. Be certain to use the correct exercise shoe for your foot and for the type of exercise you are doing. Well-fitting shoes give your feet room to expand during a workout; allow 0.5 in (1 cm) of space between the tip of the exercise shoe and the end of your longest toe. Also, look for shoes with toe boxes that are wide and high enough to allow you to wiggle your toes.

Shopping for exercise shoes or trainers can be overwhelming—with many styles to choose from, one for every sport and each with specific features. To help you narrow your selection, focus on exercise shoes or trainers designed for the activity that you do most. Use the chart on the next page to help you determine what type of shoe to buy and with which features.

Types of Exercise Shoes and Their Features

Walking Shoes:	Forefoot Flexibility and Cushioning
Running Shoes:	Cushioning, Heel Counter and Traction
Aerobic Shoes:	Forefront Flex Grooves, Cushioning and Lateral Support
Cross-Training:	Lateral Support, Cushioning, and Traction
Basketball:	Lateral Support, Cushioning, Heel and Forefoot Cushioning
Tennis:	Lateral Support, Durability, Traction and Cushioning

> **Tip:** Replace running and walking shoes after every 300 to 500 miles of use. Replace aerobic and tennis shoes after every 150 to 200 hours of use.

Replacing Your Old Exercise Shoes

If you have tendonitis, heel pain, leg pain, blisters, calluses or pain in the balls of your feet, your shoes may not be providing adequate support. You should check your exercise shoes for structural wear and tear, including whether the rubber in the heel has narrowed, the cushioning has diminished, or the shoes bend inward or outward. Buy new exercise shoes if any of the previously mentioned problems exist.

The end of Step 5 is a great place to take a breather and look at how much you've accomplished so far on your Active Wellness journey. You've looked at your personal health fitness profile and set some long- and short-term goals for yourself, many of which you are already well on the way to achieving. You've started an optimal eating plan and begun an encompassing physical fitness programme that will strengthen your body, mind and spirit. As we move on to Step 6, we'll learn to recognize and manage the triggers that sabotage success.

Strength Training Exercises

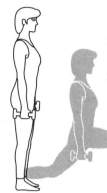

1. Lunge: Standing with feet shoulder width apart, step forward with one leg. Hold your chest high and look forward. Bend your front leg to a right angle, making sure your knee is in line with your ankle, without allowing your other knee to touch the floor. Repeat 10 to 12 times on the same leg. Switch legs and repeat. (Light weights are optional.) *Breathing:* Exhale as you lunge, inhale as you return to the starting position.

2. Side Leg Lift: Begin with your feet together, holding onto a wall or a chair. Raise one leg to the side, making sure you're standing straight. Keep your hipbones straight and keep a straight leg with toes slightly turned inward throughout the exercise. The supporting leg should be slightly bent. Lift your leg up and down 10 to 12 times and then repeat with the other leg. *Breathing:* Inhale when you lift your leg, exhale when you bring it back to meet your supporting leg.

3. Leg Lift: Sit tall with your back straight and chest lifted. Place your legs out in front of you. Bend the supporting leg. Lift your leg 5 to 8 inches from the floor, then slowly lower your leg to about an inch off the floor and repeat. Keep your foot and knee pointed upward throughout the exercise. Repeat with the other leg to complete the sequence. Exercise each leg by lifting it 10 to 12 times. *Breathing:* Exhale as you lift, inhale when you bring your leg down.

4. Abdominal Curl: Lying on your back, with your hands behind your head, cross your feet and bring them up, keeping your lower back on the floor. Keep your knees over your abdomen. (If you prefer, you can keep your feet on the floor with knees bent.) Lift your head up to the base of your shoulder blades (using your stomach muscles), then return to the starting position. Do not strain your neck, use your hands as a support. Repeat 10 to 12 times. *Breathing:* Inhale as you lift up, exhale as you return to the starting position.

5. Lower Back (Prone Head and Leg Lift): Lie down on your abdomen with your arms by your sides and your hands facing forward. Begin with your chin on the floor. Slowly lift your head and one leg off the floor, lifting your leg from the hip. Repeat this exercise with one leg at a time; repeat each leg 10 to 12 times. *Breathing:* Exhale as you lift, inhale when you return to the starting position.

6. Push-Ups: Lying on your abdomen, push your body up with your hands; keeping your back straight from your knees to your head. Keep your neck in line with your spine. Contract your abdomen. Repeat push-ups 10 to 12 times or as many as you can accomplish. *Breathing:* Exhale as you push up, inhale when you come down.

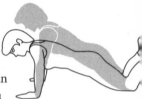

7. Bicep Curls: (with resistance bands) Stand tall with feet shoulder width apart; place one end of the band under one of your feet and hold the other end of the band with the hand on the same side of your body. Grip the band so there is no slack. Place your elbow close to your body, with your hand facing upward. Curl your arm forward slowly. Pause and return to the starting position. Repeat with each arm 10 to 12 times to complete the sequence. *Breathing:* Exhale as you lift, inhale as you lower.

8. Side Lateral Raises: (with resistance bands) Stand with your feet shoulder width apart and one end of the band underneath one foot. Grip the band with the hand on the same side of your body. Raise your arm up and away from the side of your body, until you reach just below your shoulder. Pause and slowly return to the starting position. Repeat 10 to 12 times with each arm to complete one sequence. *Breathing:* Exhale as you lift, inhale as you lower.

9. Tricep Press Down: (with resistance bands) Place the band around your neck. For comfort, you can place a towel under the band. Grasp the band with both hands, making sure your arms are parallel to the floor and facing inward. Stand straight. With your arms bent at a 90-degree angle, lower both arms so that they face the floor. As you lower your arms, rotate your hands so they face behind you when your arms are straight; pause and bring your arms back to the starting position, slowly. Repeat with each arm 10 to 12 times to complete the sequence. *Breathing:* Exhale as you lower, inhale as you lift.

Stretching Exercises

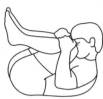

1. For Your Back: Bring both legs toward your chest, as shown in the diagram. Curl your head toward your knees and hug your legs to your chest. Hold for 10 seconds; when you release this stretch, straighten out both legs so they are lying on the floor and bring your hands and head back to rest on the floor. Repeat this stretch 3 times, or as many times as it feels good to you.

2. For Lower Back and Hips: Lying on the floor, place both arms to your sides. Bend one knee to a 90-degree angle (see diagram) over the other leg that is straight. Turn your head in the direction opposite your bent leg. Using the arm that is on the same side as the bent leg, pull your bent leg down toward the floor until you feel a comfortable stretch in your lower back and hip. Do not force a stretch if it is painful. Hold this stretch for 30 seconds; check to make sure both of your shoulders are on the floor. Repeat the same stretch using the other leg. Repeat the sequence a minimum of 3 times.

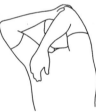

3. For Shoulders, Arms, and Upper Back: Place one arm behind your head. Hold the bent arm with your free arm (see diagram). Gently pull down on your bent elbow until you feel a stretch. Repeat this with your other arm. Hold the stretch for 15 seconds. Repeat the sequence a minimum of 3 times.

4. For Legs and Hips: Place one leg forward so that your knee is in line with your ankle. Rest your other knee on the floor with your back leg and foot out behind you (see diagram). Holding this position, shift your weight so that you move your hip downward until you feel a stretch. The movement should be gentle. When you feel the stretch hold this position for 30 seconds. Repeat with your other leg in front. Repeat the sequence a minimum of 3 times.

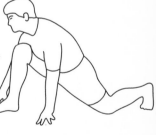

5. For Groin and Hamstrings: Sitting on the floor, place both of your feet together or as close together as they can go. Holding your feet, pull forward from your hips—not your back—until you feel a stretch. Hold this position for 40 seconds or less if you feel pain. Repeat 3 times at a minimum. Be careful not to bounce when you are in this position.

6. For Back, Shoulders, and Arms: Sitting on your bent legs, reach forward as far out as you can, with your arms stretched out over your head (see diagram). For a better stretch, keep your arms straight and press down on the palms of your hands gently.

7. For Lower Back, Hips, Groin, and Hamstrings: From a standing position, bend your knees slightly and then bend forward from your waist—hanging your arms over your head and let your head go, with your crown facing the ground. Reach as far to the floor as you can. Hold this position for 30 seconds, do not bounce. Stand up straight, keep your knees slightly bent and repeat the sequence a minimum of 3 times.

Personalized Exercise Programme Worksheet

Current Activity Level: **Goal Activity Level:**

Initial Fitness Goal:

Target Heart Rate Range:

Selected Aerobic Activities:

Maximum Heart Rate:

Days of the Week	Warm-Ups (check off the days you do aerobic activities)	Aerobic Routine		Strength Training Routine	Stretching Routine	Cool Down/ Cool-Down Stretching (check off the days you do aerobic activities)
		Aerobic Activity	Exercise Time			
Monday						
Tuesday						
Wednesday						
Thursday						
Friday						
Saturday						
Sunday						

STEP 6

Learning to Recognize the Triggers that Sabotage Success

Nothing can grow unless you devote attention to it.
—Gayle Reichler

In Step 4 we focused on the negative and uncomfortable thoughts, self-talk and feelings—triggered by an event or a circumstance—that often perpetuate our unhealthy habits. We also learned that changing our thoughts and self-talk can change our feelings and help us transform those unhealthy habits into healthy behaviours.

Learning to change our responses to triggering events is well within our power, but it is just one side of the equation for turning unhealthy habits into healthy ones. The triggers themselves are often beyond our control or not so easy to change. Having to work late, attend a family reunion, mollify an angry boss, change careers or deal with an unruly teenager, to name just a few examples, are not only triggers for unhealthy habits, but facts of life for many of us.

Step 6 will teach you how to better deal with the varied triggers that life throws your way. It will give you a variety of tools to help you prevent those triggers from sabotaging your Active Wellness lifestyle. Let's start by defining what is meant by 'triggers'.

What Are Triggers?
Like a catalyst in a chemical reaction, triggers are stimuli that ignite changes in our behaviour. Frequently they cause us to react in habitual and conditioned ways with behaviours that we adopted early in life, often unconsciously, as coping mechanisms. A trigger can come from an external or environmental source, such as people, places, and things. Or a trigger can come from an internal source that is physiological or emotional. Whether external or internal, triggers may be positive or negative, and we can respond to them in either positive or negative ways. Here the focus is primarily on triggers that elicit negative behaviours—however pleasurable they may feel! Once you identify your unique triggers, you can develop ways to short-circuit their effect on you and on your health.

Identifying Your Triggers

Environmental Triggers: People, Places and Things

Environmental triggers include anything you are exposed to that is physical. They include sensory stimuli or 'cues' that you can see, hear, touch, smell or taste. Loud noises or crashing sounds may trigger anxiety or anger, while touching something soft and warm may trigger feelings of comfort and security. When you walk into a cinema and smell popcorn, you experience an environmental stimulus—similarly with the sweet smells from a bakery that start your mouth watering. Either of these stimuli may trigger you to eat when you really don't want to, or to eat the wrong things. Television is also an external stimulus that can lull you into a state of passivity and prevent you from exercising or practising relaxation techniques.

Social events, such as holidays, dining out with friends and reunions, are also triggering stimuli. Indeed, just the thought of having to attend certain events or family get-togethers can set you off on an old behaviour pattern or way of thinking. Particular people in your life also often serve as external triggers, and they can present interesting challenges to your healthy lifestyle. Without even knowing why, you may find that being around certain people encourages you to engage in old habits that you have been trying to avoid. Perhaps these people trigger uncomfortable feelings in you that make you want to reach for your old, compensating habit. Or perhaps they engage in activities that tempt you to return to an old behaviour.

If you find yourself in either circumstance repeatedly, you may be giving other people unintentional and unwitting power over your life and your health. Sometimes 'avoidance' is the best response to physical triggers. You may have to stay away from certain people, places and things while you are giving up old habits and adapting to a new and healthier lifestyle. Avoidance does not have to mean you do away with something for ever. Once you've learned how to control a trigger, you can reintroduce those people, places and things into your life.

For many people, foods (particularly sweets) set off the most triggers that interfere with maintaining a healthy weight. Sweets are especially insidious because they often trigger a desire for more of the same thing. This can be less a matter of will power and more a matter of biochemistry. Elevated blood sugar levels created from eating sugars and carbohydrates made with refined flours can cause a chemical reaction in our brain known as the serotonin response. Serotonin, a 'feel good' biochemical, produces feelings of calm and well-being. This desire to pacify yourself with sweets and carbohydrates is doubly strong if you grew up with these types of 'comfort' foods as a child.

At the same time, refined carbohydrates can help us to feel good; they give us a short-term sugar 'high' that the body may need for one reason or another. Unfortunately, the same sugar levels drop drastically in just a few hours, leaving the body feeling fatigued, emotionally down, and craving another 'high'.

Case Histories: Environmental Triggers

When Jane first started her Active Wellness eating plan, she always had a difficult time refusing dessert when she was at a restaurant. This was particularly difficult at restaurants where she saw desserts displayed in a case or on a table before she was seated, an environmental trigger that sabotaged her eating plan. Compounding that, her boyfriend proved to be an additional environmental trigger. He always encouraged her to eat dessert, because he knew she really wanted it.

As hard as Jane tried to stick with one serving of dessert a day, restaurants remained a problem. For Jane, not eating something after she had dinner was too difficult, because she had been brought up to always have dessert after a meal. However, once she recognized her double triggers, she began to take actions to change her behaviour. At first, she would order a dessert, but share it with others at the table. Soon, Jane stopped ordering dessert altogether and had fruit instead. She developed a new and pleasurable association with fruit by linking it to her memories of holidays in the Caribbean.

Another Active Wellness participant, Lisa, created more environmental obstacles to going to the gym and exercising than she did to food and sticking to her eating plan. And her obstacles were many! If it was raining, she decided that getting in and out of her car was too much of an effort just to go and exercise. If she went home after work before going to the gym, she would often turn on the television and become engrossed in a show, and before she knew it, she felt it was too late to go to the gym.

Since developing a regular exercise routine was one of Lisa's primary goals, she needed to start practising avoidance of her obstacles. Lisa made a commitment to herself to go right to the gym after work, regardless of the weather. Before long, going to the gym became a positive experience with associated pleasures: she developed new friends, felt terrific about following through on her commitment to herself and was delighted by the changes she saw in her body. It didn't take long before Lisa began to look forward to going to the gym every day.

Physiological Triggers

Low blood sugar, fatigue, pain and stress are the most common physiological triggers that affect us physically, mentally, and emotionally, often making us feel 'out of control'.

Low blood sugar occurs when blood glucose levels drop. This drop may cause a person to feel dizzy, hungry, cranky and tired, which may trigger a craving to eat anything in order to feel better. People with diabetes are especially susceptible to the triggering effects of low blood sugar, as are some people who exercise strenuously on a regular basis, but don't eat enough carbohydrates to sustain proper muscle functioning. Eating small snacks between meals and before exercise can alleviate this problem by helping to keep blood sugar at a constant level.

A low blood sugar level is just one example of a physiological trigger that arises from an internal change in the body. Extreme fatigue is another, often sending a message to the body that it needs to eat to increase stamina. Pain and stress are two other physiological triggers that can signal the nervous system to produce biochemicals that have significant physical and emotional effects on the body. Endorphins, which are associated with pain relief, are one such substance. Noradrenaline, which is associated with the stress response, is another.

Some people are more susceptible than others to the various internal chemical reactions that influence stress, pain, anxiety and hunger. These same people may thus be more sensitive to the biochemical-like effects of certain foods that mimic those chemical reactions. They often crave such foods unconsciously.

For example, normal and elevated levels of serotonin, a biochemical produced in the brain, promote feelings of calm, well-being, and satiation. At low levels, serotonin is associated with feelings of anxiety and distress and can trigger hunger. My work with clients has shown that some people are more sensitive than others to the serotonin-like effects of refined carbohydrate foods: They invariably crave bread, sugar and pasta for their pacifying effects.

Case History: Physiological Triggers

Margaret's daily routine consisted of waking up at 5.30 a.m. to exercise for 30 minutes, commuting more than an hour to her office, working from 8.00 a.m. to 6.00 p.m., and then commuting back home. She often did not return home until 8.00 p.m. At that point, Margaret would always find herself craving sweets without knowing why. What she soon discovered was that fatigue was triggering food cravings.

Margaret's body naturally needed fuel to keep up its gruelling schedule, and sugar is the fastest-acting form of fuel. But the effects of sugar don't last long, producing a self-perpetuating cycle of artificial 'highs and lows' that encouraged Margaret's sugar cravings. The more highs and lows she experienced, the more fatigue she felt. Finally, Margaret arranged to do some stress management techniques during her lunch break to help her relax and unwind during the day. At night, she consciously committed herself to getting more sleep. The better rested and more relaxed she became, the less she craved sugar.

Emotional Triggers

Both positive and negative feelings can act as emotional triggers. Although we often assume negative emotional triggers, such as fear, anger and sadness are the ones that tend to perpetuate unhealthy behaviours, positive feelings can also be emotional triggers. Events or situations that make us feel we have lost control, succeeded, failed, increased responsibility or been forced into making a major decision, are some examples of emotionally charged circumstances that can trigger emotional feelings. When faced with such feelings, we often choose to avoid or 'bury' them. Instead of facing up to them, we latch on to old habits or behaviours that produce compensating pleasurable feelings.

Case Histories: Emotional Triggers

Anita, an Active Wellness participant who lived alone, felt loneliest in the evenings when she sat at home by herself. This was an especially difficult time for her because she had recently lost her husband, and they had always shared the hours after dinner together. Alone and lonely, Anita found it very hard not to snack after dinner. Food became the antidote for her loneliness. Once she understood that feeling lonely was a trigger for overeating, Anita was able to substitute new actions to alleviate her loneliness, ones that didn't involve food. She would call her sister or her friends whenever she felt particularly lonely, which helped her avoid overeating in the evening. Soon Anita was easily able to lose weight and achieve her Active Wellness primary goal.

Kathy was an administrative assistant in a law firm. Her bosses were overstressed people who would often take out their anxiety by yelling at her. Kathy got very upset, and her immediate reaction was to crave chocolate. She would purchase a bar of chocolate at the office vending machine or some chocolates at a nearby shop. Eventually, Kathy always kept chocolate nearby. Chocolate, as it so happens, contains a substance called phenylalanine, which helps promote positive feelings.

Kathy was particularly sensitive to the positive effects of chocolate, but also aware that she was using it as a crutch. She didn't like feeling 'out of control'. She decided to practise avoidance and introduce some substitute behaviours. First she removed all of the chocolate from her desk, which eliminated one obstacle to good health. Then she began an exercise programme that helped her reduce the stress she felt during her workday. Finally, Kathy switched to fruit as a snack instead of choco- late. Not only was this a great substitute, but it was a positive change in her overall wellness plan, since she hadn't been eating enough fruit in her diet.

Slowly but surely, Kathy began to feel better both physically and emotionally. She felt less out of control. As she gained greater control and a new perspective on her job situation, she was able to choose a dif- ferent job in a better environment. Kathy was astonished to discover that this move did away with her chocolate binges completely!

Using Food to Combat Negative Triggers

Food is a prime example of a mood-altering substance that we frequently turn to for comfort. In fact, different types of foods are associated with different feelings. 'Crunchy' foods can alleviate feelings of stress, while creamy and smooth foods are calming and soothing. Indeed, the act of feeding ourselves, in and of itself, is a healthy and highly nurturing activity. It was one of the first ways we connected with the world and knew we were loved. We literally cried and we were fed.

As adults we also use food to feel better, and we can do it in healthy ways. Although calculating just how much effect food has on our overall mood is difficult, food defi- nitely is a contributing factor. As mentioned above, one of the reasons why chocolate is soothing and pleasure-enhancing is that it contains phenylalanine, a compound that is a precursor of the biochemical noradrenaline. Noradrenaline acts as an antidepres- sant and memory enhancer. But you don't have to turn to chocolate when you need some antidepressant action: cottage cheese, bananas and soya products also contain phenylalanine. For a more extensive list of sources of phenylalanine, see the chart on the next page.

Similarly, foods high in tryptophan, an amino acid derived from proteins, can increase the amount of serotonin in the brain. Serotonin can alleviate moodiness, induce sleep, promote calmness and stimulate the immune system. For a list of sources of tryptophan, see the chart on the next page. (Note: In order for tryptophan to enter the brain and do its job, it requires the presence of carbohydrates. Remember to eat your carbohydrates along with your tryptophan-rich foods!)

Adding more of the foods that are high in phenylalanine and tryptophan to your diet may help alleviate mild depressive symptoms and combat anxiety and stress. Of course, if certain foods cause you to experience negative mood changes, you should avoid them altogether. No food permanently solves your problems or eliminates triggers. But eating the wrong kinds of foods just for their pacifying effect can sabotage your healthy lifestyle. If you are particularly susceptible to food cravings, especially cravings for sweets, a better alternative to eating is drinking water or flavoured herbal tea from a 'sipper' bottle. Sipping from a bottle is very satisfying and self-nurturing, echoing the comfort and nourishment we received through feeding as infants. I recommend you try it, particularly if you are trying to lose weight.

Foods Containing Phenylalanine

Apples	Eggs
Avocado pears	Herring
Baked Beans	Milk
Bananas	Peanuts
Beef	Pineapple
Carrots	Soya beans
Chocolate	Spinach
Cottage Cheese	Tomatoes

Foods Containing Tryptophan

Alfalfa	Eggs
Baked Beans	Endive
Beef	Fish
Broccoli	Milk
Brussels Sprouts	Soya beans
Carrots	Spinach
Cauliflower	Sweet Potatoes
Celery	Turkey
Chicken	Turnips
Cottage Cheese	Watercress

The above food lists are adapted from *Mood Foods*, by Dr. William Vayda, Ulysses Press.

Taking Control

You can learn how to manage your response to triggers proactively (rather than reactively), even though you may not be able to change, or even predict, all of the triggers that occur in your life. *Elimination, avoidance* and *substitution* of triggers are your primary tools for good trigger management. Using these tools can help you control your triggers. As you become more aware of the reasons behind your actions, you'll be able to control your triggers without needing tools. The first step in taking control of your triggers is to isolate and identify them.

> *Nothing reaches the intellect before making its appearance in the senses.*
> —Latin Proverb

Identifying and Recording Your Triggers

Take a moment to write down your personal triggers in the spaces provided below. Think of anything that acts as an obstacle to your Active Wellness programme. It could be an environmental trigger, such as walking past the vending machine at the office, going to dinner with friends who insist on dining in unhealthy restaurants, or having to attend a family dinner. You may also have emotional and physiological triggers: frustration and anger at work or extreme fatigue because you don't take time to relax.

Write any triggers you can think of in their respective categories below. Remember that you don't have to have a trigger for each category; your particular triggers may fall into only one or two of the three categories. After you've recorded your triggers, you'll learn how to use the tools that can help you manage them more effectively.

Environmental Triggers: People, Places and Things

◇ _____

◇ _____

◇ _____

Physiological Triggers

◇ _____

◇ _____

◇ _____

Emotional Triggers

◇ _____

◇ _____

◇ _____

Managing Your Triggers: Avoidance, Elimination and Substitution

Avoidance

Avoidance is a legitimate strategy for managing triggers when you are just beginning to let go of old habits and adopt new ones. In the simplest of terms, you may need to stay away—as much as possible—from any people, places and things that trigger the impulse to return to old, unhealthy behaviours. This may include some friends and family members, at least on a temporary basis, as well as certain restaurants, pubs, social gatherings, family get-togethers and even television.

Review your trigger lists above. Then, in the space provided on the next page, write down those triggers you can reasonably avoid on a short-term basis while you are beginning the work of changing your unhealthy habits.

Triggers to Avoid

◇_____

◇_____

◇_____

When avoidance isn't possible, sometimes outright elimination is the only solution.

Elimination

Elimination refers to getting rid of something that has a negative effect on you and your wellness plan and keeping it out of your lifestyle for good. For example, to stay on your Active Wellness eating plan, you may need to eliminate certain foods and beverages from your kitchen shelves and your shopping list. To maintain your fitness plan, you may have to use your lunch hour to exercise once in a while or give up working late one night. To get enough sleep so you can maintain your entire Active Wellness schedule, you may have to videotape a film you want to see and watch it at another time. This time, look over the triggers you listed above, and then in the space below write down any triggers you want to eliminate from your lifestyle right now.

Triggers to Eliminate

◇_____

◇_____

◇_____

Substitution

Sometimes you can't avoid or eliminate certain triggers in your life. However, if you're aware of how you traditionally respond to those triggers, you can prepare yourself ahead of time. Preparing ahead helps you manage triggers better by enabling you to create a new substitute behaviour or response. In fact, when you are 'unlearning' old behaviours and habits, 'reconditioning' yourself by substituting something similar to, but healthier than, your old behaviour is often easier. I call this reconditioning technique 'trigger substitution'. Here are some examples of actual substitutions used by my Active Wellness clients.

Trigger Substitution Examples

Trigger: Needing to order dessert in a restaurant.
Substitution: Ordering fruit for dessert instead.

Trigger: Taking coffee and snack breaks at the office.
Substitution: Drinking herbal tea instead.

Trigger: Not exercising because of too many commitments.
Substitution: Exercising at home in the morning or at lunchtime
at work.

Now take a few minutes to think about some of the triggers in your life that you can't avoid or eliminate, but that you would like to manage better by substituting healthier responses for them. In the space provided below, write in three of the triggers that are most troublesome to you, using the examples above as a guide. Next, think of some realistic actions or behaviours that you can substitute for your old trigger-behaviour. Keep your substitution actions simple, direct and easy to do, so that they strengthen your commitment and motivation to change.

Your Trigger Substitution List

Trigger 1: _____

Substitution 1: _____

Trigger 2: _____

Substitution 2: _____

Trigger 3: _____

Substitution 3: _____

Identifying your triggers and devising strategies for managing them better are essential tasks for reinforcing and maintaining your new, healthy habits. With time, commitment and simple repetition, your new behaviours and trigger management techniques will become second nature. Your trigger strategies will help you avoid sabotaging yourself with your bad habits. As you become aware of your triggers, it is helpful to think about why they appeared in your life, how they make you feel and what they mean to you. Over time you'll be able to better manage your responses. 'Time' is the operative word here. Before you reach the point where you believe you have mastered your old behaviours and feel comfortable with your new ones, you are bound to make some mistakes along the way.

Managing Setbacks: Tools for Self-Empowerment

To Err is Human . . .

If you are like most of my clients, you are probably going to experience some difficult and challenging days during your Active Wellness journey—days when all your good efforts seem to be falling short of the mark. Despite your best intentions and hard work at changing old behaviours and learning healthier ones, you may reach a plateau or face an obstacle that makes moving forward with your wellness goals seem impossible. Perhaps you will have a particularly hard week at work, go through an illness or face a series of stressful situations. Whatever the trigger is, you may unexpectedly hit the proverbial brick wall along the path to good health. Suddenly, reverting back to old and comfortable habits, however unhealthy, may seem inevitable, if not downright attractive.

First, Avoid Negative Self-Talk

As illogical as it may seem, having a minor 'slip' can precipitate an unproductive dialogue of negative self-talk. Take your Active Wellness eating plan as an example. A minor diet setback, such as ordering a rich and fattening dessert in a restaurant or devouring the crisps and nuts at the bar while you wait for a table, can begin a relentless barrage of negative self-talk. Once you feel that you have 'failed' at one of your smaller goals, you may be tempted to give up on your wellness plan entirely, perhaps believing yourself incapable of truly eating healthfully and losing weight. Many of my clients have faced similar crossroads with nutrition, physical fitness and stress management during their own wellness journeys. You're not alone—you're only human!

Second, Respect Your Mistakes

In terms of taking control of our health, each of us has a personal 'Waterloo'—a breaking point or testing point at which we feel so defeated and powerless that we are tempted to throw in the towel completely. One moment we are strolling confidently along our wellness path, the next moment we stumble and find ourselves falling into a deep hole that seems to offer no way out.

If you find yourself 'slipping' at this or some future point in your wellness journey, take heart. Many have been there before you and gone on to become great successes. Changing lifelong behaviours that have stopped working for you is hard and courageous work. Give yourself credit for your hard work, and forgive yourself for any small setbacks.

Remember that whenever you are learning anything new, you may have to take a few steps backward to reassess your progress and your techniques before you can move more confidently forward to success. Minor failures are an integral part of the learning process. The important thing is to avoid getting 'stuck' for too long when you have a slip or two. Missteps and stumbles are important junctures in your programme, and how quickly you handle them may make the difference between long-term success or self-defeat, lifelong wellness or chronic bad health. When you 'feel' stuck, this can be an important clue about a major roadblock you may have to face and understand, in order to move forward. By overcoming these roadblocks you will feel stronger and more confident.

Four of the most empowering techniques for managing slips and temporary roadblocks are optimism, distraction, disputation and flexibility. Let's take a look at each technique.

Optimism

Dr Martin Seligman, one of the foremost researchers in behavioural change, champions the vital role that optimism plays in our lives in his excellent book, *Learned Optimism: How to Change Your Mind and Your Life*. He points out that optimists are more likely to possess increased motivation, elevated moods, a sense of well-being and better physical and mental health. They are also superior achievers in work, school and sports.

Optimism is the ability to see things in the most positive light and to believe that one's efforts will have the best possible outcome. Clearly, optimism is a good offensive strategy for many situations in your Active Wellness programme. Faced with a particular obstacle or choice along your wellness journey, ask yourself: What is the worst thing that can happen if I am optimistic in this situation? By using optimism to manage behavioural triggers or other obstacles to good health you will only further your wellness goals. Of course, you run the risk of feeling a little disappointed if you are optimistic and still 'fail'. But as D. Seligman suggests, optimists tend to fail less because of their positive attitudes, and therefore they face disappointment less often.

I offer one warning, however. If the worst thing that can happen is dangerous or unhelpful to your situation, using optimism is not a good idea. For example, an individual who is out of shape or has a pre-existing heart condition, but tries to run as fast and as hard as he can because it's good for his health and he's feeling strong and energetic is not making a wise optimistic choice. This individual's optimistic approach is admirable, but he may ultimately do harm to his health and well-being.

Dr Seligman has devised a comprehensive questionnaire for assessing your level of optimism and its counterpoint, pessimism, around a variety of life situations. A shortened version of that questionnaire is on the next page. When you are relaxed and comfortable, take 15 minutes to answer the questions and calculate your optimism score.

> *Life is not governed by will or intention. Life is a question*
> *of nerve, and fibres, and slowly built-up cells in which*
> *thought hides itself, and passion has its dreams.*
> —Oscar Wilde

The Optimism Quiz

Read the description of each situation below and vividly imagine it is happening to you. Then check off the answer that most resembles how you would respond to the situation. Even if you don't like some of the responses offered, choose the one that most closely reflects your way of thinking. Don't choose the one that you think is 'right' or that you think other people would choose.

1. **The project you are in charge of is a great success.**
   A. I kept a close watch over everyone's work. _____1
   B. Everyone devoted a lot of time and energy to it. _____0

2. **You and your partner make up after a fight.**
   A. I forgave him/her. _____0
   B. I'm usually forgiving. _____1

3. **You get lost driving to a friend's house.**
   A. I missed a turn. _____1
   B. My friend gave me bad directions. _____0

4. **You've been extremely healthy all year.**
   A. Not many people around me were sick, so I wasn't exposed. _____0
   B. I made sure I ate well and got enough rest. _____1

5. **You forget your partner's birthday.**
   A. I'm not good at remembering birthdays. _____1
   B. I was preoccupied with other things. _____0

6. **You get a flower from an admirer.**
   A. I am attractive to him/her. _____0
   B. I am a popular person. _____1

7. **You run for a community office and you win.**
   A. I devoted a lot of time and energy to campaigning. _____0
   B. I work very hard at everything I do. _____1

8. **You miss an important engagement.**
   A. Sometimes my memory fails me. _____1
   B. I sometimes forget to check my diary. _____0

9. **You run for a community office and you lose.**
   A. I didn't campaign hard enough. _____1
   B. The person who won knew more people. _____0

10. **You host a successful dinner.**
    A. I was particularly charming that night. _____0
    B. I am a good host. _____1

11. **You stop a crime by calling the police.**
    A. A strange noise caught my attention. _____0
    B. I was alert that day. _____1

12. **You buy your partner a gift, and he/she doesn't like it.**
    A. I don't put enough thought into things like that. _____1
    B. He/she has very picky tastes. _____0

13. **You gain weight over the holidays and you can't lose it.**
    A. Diets don't work in the long run. _____1
    B. The diet I tried didn't work. _____0

14. **Your stocks make you a lot of money.**
    A. My broker decided to take on something new. _____0
    B. My broker is a topnotch investor. _____1

15. **You win an athletic contest.**
    A. I was feeling unbeatable. _____0
    B. I train hard. _____1

16. **You fail an important examination.**
    A. I wasn't as clever as the other people taking the exam. _____1
    B. I didn't prepare for it well. _____0

17. **Your boss gives you too little time to finish a project, but you get it finished anyway.**
    A. I am good at my job. _____0
    B. I am an efficient person. _____1

18. **You lose a sporting event for which you have been training for a long time.**
    A. I'm not very athletic. _____1
    B. I'm not good at that sport. _____0

19. **Your car runs out of petrol on a dark street late at night.**
    A. I didn't check to see how much petrol was in the tank. _____1
    B. The petrol gauge was broken. _____0

20. **You lose your temper with a friend.**
    A. He/she is always nagging me. _____1
    B. He/she was in a hostile mood. _____0

21. **You are penalized for not paying your income-tax on time.**
    A. I always put off doing my taxes. _____1
    B. I was lazy about getting my taxes done this year. _____0

22. **You ask a person out on a date and he/she says no.**
    A. I was a wreck that day. _____1
    B. I got tongue-tied when I asked him/her on the date. _____0

23. **A game-show host picks you out of the audience to participate in the show.**
    A. I was sitting in the right seat. _____0
    B. I looked the most enthusiastic. _____1

24. **You save a person from choking to death.**
    A. I know a technique to stop someone from choking. _____0
    B. I know what to do in a crisis situation. _____1

Scoring the Optimism Quiz:

1. Total all the points from questions 1, 2, 4, 6, 7, 10, 11, 14, 15, 17, 23, and 24.
   Enter the total here: _____

2. Total all the points from questions 3, 5, 8, 9, 12, 13, 16, and 18 through 22.
   Enter the total here: _____

Subtract the total on line 2 from the total on line 1. Enter the result of your overall score here: _____

If your overall score is:
    Greater than 4: You are very optimistic.
    3 or 4: You are moderately optimistic.

2: You are average.

1: You are moderately pessimistic.

0: You are very pessimistic.

Copyright 1998 Dr Martin E. P. Seligman. All rights reserved.

Learned Optimism

Whatever your score on the Optimism Quiz, the most important point to remember is that both optimism and pessimism are learned belief systems, and therefore can change. You can unlearn your pessimistic tendencies that Dr Seligman calls learned helplessness and teach yourself to adopt an optimistic attitude toward life. With practice, pessimists can become optimists. Developing a sense of humour and flexibility in the face of certain obstacles (techniques discussed later in this chapter) are great ways to fan the flames of optimism.

When you are optimistic, you are more likely to believe you are capable, competent, and in control of your life. You find it easier to make the small changes that have an incrementally positive influence on your health. And success at your small health goals further promotes self-confidence and feelings of competence, so that you can move forward with your programme to achieve your larger, primary health goals. Over and over again, research points to the fact that the more optimistic you are, the healthier you are —just more evidence that the mind has a powerful influence over the body!

> *If I had my life to live over, I would start barefoot earlier in the spring and stay that way later in the autumn. I would go to more dances. I would ride more round-abouts. I would pick more daisies.*
> —Nadine Stair

In addition to optimism, according to Dr Seligman, two other powerful techniques may help you manage outmoded beliefs and behavioural triggers. They are helpful when you hit a brick wall along the wellness path and feel especially dejected, unmotivated or unsuccessful. He calls these techniques distraction and disputation.

Distraction

Distractions are words, phrases or actions that help you stop focusing on an unhealthy behaviour or negative trigger and refocus on your healthy goals. You can distract yourself with a word, phrase, thought, picture or visualization, to name just a few distraction tools. Anything that distracts your mind in a positive and empowering way can function as a distraction technique.

For example, stop reading and begin thinking about biting into a soft, chewy chocolate chip cookie that is still warm from the oven. The sweet taste and warm dough are soothing to your mouth and emotions. Now, stop thinking about the cookie and begin thinking about what it would be like to bite into a wedge of a fresh, tangy lemon. The tart taste of the lemon may even make you cringe. Did you make a face when you visualized this image?

Visualization is one method of distraction. Taking action is another. To distract themselves from a negative trigger, some Active Wellness participants get out of the house or office, take a walk, and imagine themselves in their favourite place. Affirmation-like phrases also make good distractions. Other participants use a word or phrase to distract themselves, such as Stop!, or Not Now!, or I want to reach my goal! You can even use a picture of yourself, your family or a favourite holiday spot as distractions from a negative trigger.

Under each trigger below, write any type of distraction you can think of to help yourself combat negative triggers and old behaviour patterns. Feel free to use the triggers you noted in your Trigger Substitution List. But don't take it too seriously—remember the power of humour to act as a distraction tool.

Your Trigger Distraction List

Trigger 1: _____

Distraction 1: _____

Trigger 2: _____

Distraction 2: _____

Trigger 3: _____

Distraction 3: _____

Humour As a Distraction

Humour may be especially helpful when you are too hard on yourself or take yourself too seriously. Finding the humour in an event, even a negative one (and there is humour in almost everything!), helps remind you that minor mistakes and setbacks are not the end of the world, even when they feel like it.

We can use humour to gain perspective on our personal triggers and obstacles. Looking for humour in a situation that we usually find difficult and humourless may force us to develop a new viewpoint that leads the way to greater self-understanding and better health. For example, if you tend to be obsessive-compulsive, the cartoon on the next page is terrific for helping you laugh at something you may usually take too seriously.

Research indicates that having a good laugh is very therapeutic. Laughter gives your immune system a boost by increasing an infection-fighting substance known as immunoglobulin A. Laughing may also increase your pain threshold and even stimulate the release of endorphins that create feelings of euphoria. Laughter is a great stress

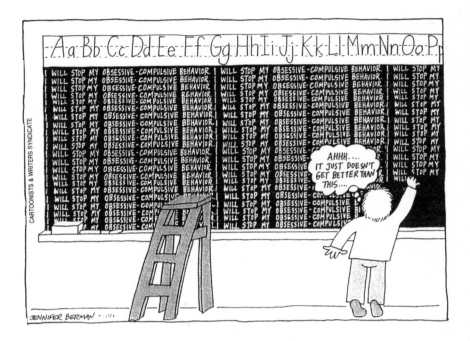

reliever, lifting our mood and reducing pretension and restraint. After a good laugh, you may even find yourself saying: Look at me. Here I go again, dallying with my old habit. Silly me. I am going to find a way out of this.

If you want to use laughter as an alternative trigger option, try clipping funny cartoons and stories from newspapers and magazines to carry with you. Look at them when you are faced with a negative trigger or obstacle, and have a good laugh. It's a fun and effective way to change negative behaviour and self-talk.

Disputation

Disputation is another way to confront unhealthy behaviour and self-talk and to better manage negative triggers. In its most literal sense, disputation means to mentally debate or question your negative beliefs and preconceived notions by looking at their origins and validity. It's important to ask yourself how your old beliefs have served you and how you can change them to serve you better. Ultimately, through self-debate and awareness, you prove to yourself that your old ways of responding to triggers and obstacles are wrong.

Although avoidance and distraction are excellent techniques for dealing with triggers and obstacles to good health, learning to dispute your old attitudes and replace them with new beliefs provides more lasting and long-term results. Our old learned beliefs and behaviours, repeated over time, create powerful but often subconscious attitude traps that we may too easily fall into when faced with changing our unhealthy behaviour. These attitude traps often 'tell' us that we can't succeed, that we can never change, that change is too hard, and that we will ultimately fail. Such attitudes can seriously sabotage our wellness journeys.

However, disputing and dismantling those attitude traps by creating opposing and positive counter thoughts is an essential step in creating new and healthier belief systems in which success becomes your rightful heritage. From your new beliefs you can develop new 'self-talk' that can also help steer you away from your old habits. While your new beliefs may feel foreign to you at first, you will learn to welcome and embrace them, because eventually they will help you cope with change in more positive ways.

Take a moment now to review the list of triggers you wrote earlier in the chapter and consider some of the old beliefs that are attached to your triggers and trigger behaviours. Look especially at personal attitude traps around change, success and failure, and good health. Try to dispute some of the beliefs that are attached to your trigger behaviours. Ask yourself: Where did this belief originate? Whose voice is attached to this belief? Do I have to go along with it? Can I prove it wrong?

Begin the process of disputing those beliefs and dismantling those attitude traps—trigger by trigger. Think about creating new belief systems that are based on what you've learned here and on your experiences with healthy change. Write these new beliefs down. To accompany your new beliefs, try creating positive counter thoughts that take the power out of old attitude traps. For example, if one of your old beliefs is 'I can't ever lose weight; I never can stick to a diet,' try replacing it with 'I love myself and will do anything to take good care of myself.' If television is a big distraction in your life, one example of a negative belief system might be 'I watch television and don't exercise because I'm lazy.' Dispute and dismantle that thought and replace it with something like 'I'll enjoy relaxing more after I've had a good workout at the gym.'

Disputing your old beliefs and dismantling old attitude traps opens the door to real change and a lifetime of healthy behaviours. Using the examples above and the one below, write some of your most persistent attitude traps in the space provided. Then create possible, positive counter thoughts to them.

Attitude Traps and Counter Thoughts
Example:

Attitude Trap: The only reason I am losing weight is because I am following this book.
Counter Thought: I am losing weight because of my own efforts. I can continue to eat in a healthy way for as long as I choose. It's up to me.

Attitude Trap	Counter Thought
◇ _____	◇ _____
◇ _____	◇ _____
◇ _____	◇ _____
◇ _____	◇ _____

Remember that your counter thought should be positive and self-empowering; it should place the responsibility for success squarely on your shoulders. Accept that you are the one expending the energy and doing the hard work to achieve your goals. Remember, also, to reward yourself for your good efforts. Remaining flexible and open to all of the creative options at your disposal is another important tool in managing negative triggers and unhealthy behaviours.

Flexibility

By remaining flexible and open about changing your old beliefs and devising healthy substitutions for negative thoughts and actions, you are teaching yourself to think creatively and proactively. This applies to many situations, not just those that involve health and wellness. Your self-confidence and commitment, together with your chances for long-lasting success, all grow stronger through flexibility.

Most importantly, flexibility gives you choices and teaches you to react quickly and appropriately for the situation at hand. When you are faced with major triggers and behavioural obstacles, you need to decide fast whether optimism, distraction, or disputation is the best way to manage the moment. Optimism almost always works from an emotional point of view, and is effective in combating attitude traps. When it comes to dealing with physical behaviour, however, distraction is often the best and quickest route away from a sabotaging trigger. Disputation, a more intellectual process, may have to be put on the back burner until you have some time for quiet reflection. In other words, distract first and dispute later!

Use Alternative Trigger Options to Manage Life Events

Earlier in this chapter, I asked you to write down three major triggers that could sabotage your Active Wellness programme. At the same time, I suggested that you come up with a substitute behaviour for each.

Now I'm going to ask you to think about your most difficult negative triggers that are related to your health. These may include triggers that originate at home, at work, at social events or with friends. What they all have in common is that they precipitate negative behaviours, self-talk and internal attitudes that you would like to take control of and change.

Use an index card or a piece of paper for each trigger, write it across the top of the card or paper. Then think of as many optional behaviours as possible to counteract this trigger. Refer to all the tools discussed previously in this chapter. Don't limit yourself! Try to think of anything you can do as a substitute behaviour, within legal limits, of course! In my Active Wellness programme, I call these 'Alternative Trigger Cards'. I encourage my clients to create as many cards for as many triggers as they can, and then to carry the cards with them wherever they go—in their briefcase, wallet or purse.

I encourage you to do the same. When faced with reacting to a trigger or obstacle, envisioning your alternatives is sometimes difficult. But you can review your alternative trigger cards on the spot and experiment with any of the substitute behaviours you have written down. To help you set up your card system, an example alternative trigger card, complete with substitute behaviours, appears below.

Alternative Trigger Card

Trigger: I eat whenever I am bored at work.

Alternative Options:
Write down a list of things I want to do for myself and do one.
Ring or e-mail a friend for a quick hello.
Read a magazine article or surf the Internet.
Eat something from my eating plan.

Change is difficult and you deserve a pat on the back for all of your efforts. Acknowledging your good efforts and hard work is very important. Reinforcing your sense of accomplishment and self-worth strengthens your chances of reaching your long-term goal. Remember to reward yourself as well, with something positive, luxurious, or self-nurturing. You deserve it!

Moving On
Stress is one of the most potent triggers that we all encounter. Not knowing how to manage all the stressors in our lives can seriously affect our physical, mental and emotional health. Step 7 is devoted entirely to managing stress—the fourth major component of the Active Wellness programme. In the meantime . . .

Bloom where you are planted.
—Unknown

STEP 7

Healthy Ways to Manage Stress

For fast-acting relief try slowing down.
—Lily Tomlin

You just missed your exit on the motorway. Someone in the car behind you is honking his horn. You have a deadline at work. The house is a mess. You have a cold. The bills are higher than usual this month. You have to race to catch your train. You spend the day worried about a loved one. Or you're expecting a baby. You're getting married. You're training for a marathon. Your youngest child is going off to college. You just got a big promotion.

Big or small, happy or sad, unexpected or routine, any of the events just described can trigger stress in your body, mind and spirit. You can't see, hear or smell stress, but eventually you feel it—as anxiety, exhaustion, moodiness, sleep disturbances, headaches, shortness of breath, a racing heart or a stiff neck, to name just a few of its symptoms.

Although we cannot control what stresses us, we can learn how to respond to stress, so that it does not affect us negatively. Since all change causes some degree of stress, stress is an unavoidable part of our lives. The symptoms of stress can impact on all aspects of our lives: eating patterns, digestion, mood, sleep, energy and immunity to disease. While not all stress is bad—in fact, some stress is necessary for us to function and survive—adverse stress can take a terrible toll on your overall health.

In this step we focus on managing our adaptive responses to the type of stress that has a negative impact on us physically, mentally or emotionally. Learning how to respond to negative stress will help you bring balance to your life. You'll learn a variety of techniques and coping skills to help you combat the effects of adverse stress and integrate stress management as a permanent part of your Active Wellness programme.

So, How 'Stressed Out' Are You?

Defining Stress
Stress is difficult to define or even recognize, because stress means different things to different people. What you regard as stressful, another person might find invigorating or challenging. For example, a job loss may plunge one individual into feelings of

worthlessness and depression. Another individual might see a job loss as a chance to reshape his or her career and move on to more interesting and rewarding work.

Our responses to what we perceive as stressful are unique; they are our physical, emotional and psychological responses to a situation, event or stimulus. Often stress is perceived as threatening or challenging to our personal well-being, family, loved ones, finances, work or social standing.

Determining Your Stress Index

The physical and emotional damage caused by stress can make us miserable, but, oddly enough, we often aren't even aware that we are under stress. The signs and symptoms of stress, together with the habits and attitudes we adopt to cope with it, are so familiar and commonplace to us that we simply accept them as part and parcel of our lives.

How high is your Stress Index? Find out by completing the brief questionnaire below.

Stress Index Questionnaire

Do You Frequently:	Yes	No
1. Neglect your diet?	___	___
2. Try to do everything yourself?	___	___
3. Blow up easily?	___	___
4. Seek unrealistic goals?	___	___
5. Fail to see the humour in situations that others find funny?	___	___
6. Act rude?	___	___
7. Make a 'big deal' of everything?	___	___
8. Look to other people to make things happen?	___	___
9. Complain that you are disorganized?	___	___
10. Avoid people whose ideas are different from yours?	___	___
11. Keep your emotions inside?	___	___

Do You Frequently:	Yes	No
12. Neglect exercise?	——	——
13. Have few supportive relationships?	——	——
14. Use sleeping pills and tranquillizers without a doctor's approval?	——	——
15. Get too little rest?	——	——
16. Get angry when you are kept waiting?	——	——
17. Ignore stress symptoms?	——	——
18. Put things off until later?	——	——
19. Think there is only one right way to do something?	——	——
20. Fail to build relaxation time into your day?	——	——
21. Gossip?	——	——
22. Race through the day?	——	——
23. Spend a lot of time complaining about the past?	——	——
24. Fail to get a break from noise and crowds?	——	——

Total your score: Count 1 for each 'yes' answer and 0 for each 'no' answer.

Your score: _____

What Your Score Means:
1-6: There are few hassles in your life. Make sure, though, that you are not trying so hard to avoid problems that you are also shying away from challenges.

7-13: You've got your life under fairly good control. Work on the choices and habits that may still be causing some unnecessary stress in your life. The suggestions in this chapter should help.

14-20: You're approaching the danger zone. You may well be suffering stress-related symptoms and your relationships could be strained. Think carefully about choices you've made and take relaxation breaks every day. Read this chapter carefully and follow the suggestions to better manage your life.

Above 20: Emergency! You must stop now, rethink how you are living, change your attitudes and pay careful attention to diet, exercise and relaxation. There are many suggestions in this chapter that can help you live a healthier, happier life.

Adapted from the Stress Index, courtesy of the Canadian Mental Health Association, Saskatchewan Division.

Although the effects of stress in our daily lives may seem unavoidable, we can learn many techniques to offset the damage done by stress. For one thing, take a look at how you personally respond to stress and then make conscious choices about changing your stress-coping methods. You can also use any of the techniques described later in this chapter to enjoy the benefits of healthful stress management.

What Are Your Stressors?

The situations, events, or stimuli that trigger a stress response are called stressors and they fall into three main categories.

Cataclysmic Stressors

Cataclysmic stressors include natural or man-made disasters such as hurricanes, earthquakes, fires and tornadoes. While they can be devastating events that cause acute stress in the short term, they occur infrequently.

Background Stressors

Background stressors include 'environmental' stressors of a repetitive or routine nature that we feel we cannot control. They include, among other things: a neighbour's barking dog or blaring music; long commutes and traffic jams; a high-pressure career or a monotonous, dreary job; and constant background noise at work or at home.

Because they are part of our daily lives and not always easy to recognize or acknowledge, background stressors are potentially very damaging, gradually gnawing away at our sense of well-being.

Personal Stressors

Personal stressors include threatening or challenging situations, events or stimuli that impact on us in a highly personal manner. They might include: the death of a loved one; having a baby; the loss of a job; the breakup of a marriage; buying a home; personal injury or illness; a major career move; nursing an ill parent or partner; or coping with an abusive partner or boss. Personal stressors often demand the most from υ

in terms of coping and adapting, which makes them particularly detrimental to our physical and emotional health.

Personal stressors are usually broken down into five distinct types, but a great deal of overlap occurs among the types. Further, what starts out as one type of personal stressor may rapidly evolve into another. Retirement, for example, is an emotional stressor that may eventually evolve into an intellectual stressor.

The Five Types of Personal Stressors

Physical Stressors. Anything that causes physical discomfort or forces the body to continually adapt or cope is a physical stressor. Chronic pain and sudden or chronic illness are examples of physical stressors.

Emotional Stressors. These include significant life events such as a divorce, death of a loved one, loss of a job, retirement or 'empty nest syndrome'. Emotional stress often leads to anxiety, depression, moodiness and poor physical health.

Intellectual Stressors. Common short-term, intellectual stressors include giving a major speech; taking final exams; or facing a complex problem that requires sharp, rational thinking when one simply is not up to it (for instance, doing one's income taxes). It is also intellectually stressful when you're not using your mind to its full capacity, as in retirement or underemployment. Intellectual stressors may leave us feeling mentally or emotionally overwhelmed and unable to problem-solve effectively.

Social Stressors. Social stressors occur when one feels unduly pressured by certain groups (such as family, co-workers, or friends) to conform to their standards, beliefs or behaviours. Anger and resentment are common reactions to social stressors.

Spiritual Stressors. Any serious challenge to one's long-held personal, religious, or moral beliefs is a spiritual stressor. Anger, anxiety and confusion are common responses. By examining your own personal stressors, you can begin to observe how you respond to stress and then make conscious choices about changing your stress-coping methods.

> *The only courage that matters is the kind that*
> *gets you from one moment to the next.*
> —Mignon McLaughlin

Understanding Stress and How We Deal with It

How we respond to stress and how it affects our health depends on three factors: its intensity, its timing and its duration.

Intensity of the Stress

Stress can be mild or severe. Assigning these labels to certain stress responses is difficult because the intensity of stress depends on your ability to adapt when confronted with a situation. The death of a loved one can clearly cause severe stress, but a person with strong coping abilities handles even a devastatingly stressful situation better than an individual with no coping skills. A seemingly mild stressful situation, such as losing one's car keys, may be a minor nuisance for one person, while throwing someone else into an emotional tailspin that ruins his or her day.

Timing of the Stress

You may find it more difficult to cope if a stress occurs after you have suffered a long line of previous stresses. Also, if stress occurs when you are dealing with an illness, it can have more serious repercussions than if you are healthy.

Duration of the Stress

Stress may also be acute (short term) or chronic (long term). A sudden and extremely threatening event or stimulus that appears for a short time is considered acute stress. A loud explosion close-by, a near-miss on the road, a sudden blackout, a suspicious crash downstairs while you are sleeping—all are examples of potentially acute stress.

Whether mild or severe, any stress that continues over a long period of time is considered chronic stress. Taking care of someone who is ill is an example of chronic stress; always worrying about money or coping with a high-pressure job are 'milder' forms of chronic stress.

If you feel like every day is its own crisis, you may be suffering from chronic stress, which could be greatly harming your body.

Signs of Chronic Stress

- Irritability; fatigue
- Pounding heart
- Inability to concentrate
- Sweating
- Migraines; frequent headaches
- Nervous laughter
- Clumsiness; increased accidents
- Neck or lower back pain
- Clenched jaw; grinding teeth
- Increased use of alcohol and drugs to relax
- Difficulty sleeping; insomnia; bad dreams
- Nervous twitches
- Short fuse
- Feelings of anxiety, tension, moodiness
- Shallow breathing; shortness of breath
- Rapid speech

The sidebar on page 189 and below illustrate both the signs of chronic stress and the long-term effects that can occur when chronic stress isn't managed properly.

The 'Fight or Flight' Response. Threatened with a stressor, the brain triggers the release of hormones that gear the body up to defend itself—either by fighting ('fight') or by running away ('flight'). These hormones spur body cells to release stored carbohydrates, fats and proteins for energy to fuel the body. The circulatory system floods with adrenaline and nutrients. Metabolism increases and all energy is switched to the muscles and brain. Muscular strength, physical endurance, mental clarity and reaction times are greatly enhanced to ensure the survival of the body.

The list of physical responses goes on. Heart rate and blood pressure increase, so

Long-Term Effects of Stress

Stress Response	Long-Term Effect(s)
Storage energy mobilized for use by muscles	Eventual fatigue; no excess energy available for storage
Elevated triglycerides, fats, and glucose (sugar) in the blood	Increased risk for elevated triglycerides, cholesterol, and diabetes (for those at risk)
Increase in blood pressure	Greater chance of forming plaque in arteries and developing chronic hypertension
System shutdown of digestion	Peptic ulcer; indigestion
Other system shutdowns (reproductive; tissue building)	Lack of ability to reproduce; loss of libido; decalcification of bones
Depression of immune response	Decreased disease resistance

that the blood can transport nutrients and adrenaline as quickly as possible. Breathing also increases, to help transport oxygen to the muscles at a greater rate. Body temperature rises to promote sweating. Digestion, sex drive, bone and tissue growth, and the immune system are suppressed to further conserve unneeded energy and channel 'survival' energy to the muscles and brain.

These adaptations create a superb survival device of the human organism. Under normal circumstances, we are well equipped to handle a threatening situation. After a short-term acute crisis has been dealt with, the body quickly returns to normal functioning. When stress becomes chronic, however, and the body doesn't get a chance to return to normal, serious damage can occur.

The Benefits of Managing Stress

◇ Increased energy
◇ Looking and feeling young
◇ Increased power of concentration
◇ Increased feeling of happiness
◇ Increased awareness
◇ Improved sleep
◇ Enhanced performance
◇ Ease and efficiency in daily activities
◇ Improved sense of self-acceptance
◇ Improved flexibility

Studies supported by the US National Institutes of Health (NIH) suggest that chronic stress may have significant effects on physical and emotional health. With chronic stress, the body remains in a modified but continual state of 'fight or flight' readiness. Brain chemistry and the circulatory and immune systems never quite return to their normal functioning. Over time, this organic imbalance may cause chronic anxiety, depression, moodiness and serious illness, including heart disease.

Managing Stress and Restoring Your Body's Balance

Changing Your Attitude and Your Stress-Coping Methods
If you can alter your psychological and physiological reaction to a stressor, you can help reduce the impact of the stress response on your body. Below is a list of adaptive responses to stressors that can help you reduce the effects of the stress response. You can use the techniques you learned in Step 6's discussion on habits and triggers to help you incorporate these adaptive responses into your daily life and thus enhance your stress-coping skills.

Positive Responses to Stress
◇ Hope for the best, but prepare for the worst.
◇ Focus on the good when things are going well.
◇ Believe you are in control of your own destiny.
◇ Choose your fights carefully and determine what's worth the stress.

◇ Stop blaming yourself; find a reason for your situation that lies outside yourself.

◇ Break down an overwhelming situation into smaller, manageable pieces.

◇ Adopt a sense of spiritual optimism.

◇ Be flexible and try not to control every situation.

Changing Your Type A Personality Traits

Traditionally, the Type A personality was described as belonging to someone who was an overachiever, highly competitive, impatient, time conscious, controlling, hostile, and short tempered. Early research seemed to indicate that Type A personalities were at greater risk for heart disease.

However, subsequent studies of Type A behaviour show that only one trait, hostility, is an accurate predictor of heart disease. Current clinical studies by Dr Redford Williams at Duke University Medical School are attempting to identify the various characteristics of hostility that are most closely related to heart disease. At least one such study, conducted among lawyers, indicated that blatant aggressiveness and cynical mistrust were prime indicators of increased heart disease risk. Another important finding of the current studies is that repressing feelings of anger and hostility (as well as certain other feelings) is a strong predictor of heart disease.

The reduction in heart disease risk associated with expressing emotions is evidenced in the Dr Dean Ornish Lifestyle Program for Reversing Heart Disease. In the majority of cases, when a participant expressed themselves in group support, he or she showed a corresponding reduction in blocked arteries.

If you fit the description of a Type A personality (someone who is hostile and holds his or her emotions inside), one of the best stress management tools you can adopt is learning how to express your emotions without hostility and anger. A therapy group or individual counsellor may help you learn effective communication skills, which could help reduce your risk of illness.

Learning to Reduce Stress (and Increase Energy!)

We all have stress in our lives at different times and to varying degrees. Our bodies and bodily systems are often in modified 'stress response' or 'fight or flight' states, fluctuating between healthy balance and stress-induced imbalance.

By learning a few, improved ways to manage stress, you can help your body return to a healthy balance faster. And you'll find that the more you practise stress management techniques, the more peaceful you will feel and the more mentally focused you will become. You can perform your day-to-day activities with greater ease, a clearer mind and an increased sense of happiness. Paradoxically, by learning to manage stress and induce relaxation, you actually create healthier energy in your life.

'The Relaxation Response'

When you restore balance to your body and bring it to a relaxed state, you are inducing the 'relaxation response'. This now-famous term, coined by Dr Herbert Benson, was based on his studies at Harvard Medical School and is detailed in his book *The Relaxation Response.*

When your body is in a relaxed state, your blood pressure and heart rate are lower, your metabolism and muscle tension decrease, your body temperature drops, and your body uses less oxygen and produces less carbon dioxide. Your hormones return to a balanced level, as does your blood lactate level. (This is significant because high levels of lactate in the blood are associated with anxiety and tension.) Blood lactate levels actually return to normal levels four times faster in people who are resting or relaxing than they do in people who are agitated.

When we are in deep relaxation, even our brain waves change in frequency. During the waking state our brain emits beta waves. As we relax, beta waves change to slower alpha waves. During deep relaxation, alpha waves change to even slower theta waves (which are the brain waves during orgasm), but while you may feel deeply relaxed, mentally you are far more aware and alert.

The more you practise reaching this deep relaxation state, the easier time you have getting there. If you practise deep relaxation regularly, a general state of calmness and mental focus eventually infuses your everyday life.

Engaging in 'Relaxing' Activities Isn't Enough

In order to achieve the benefits of a relaxed state, you must be aware of activities that actually enhance this state of being. Many times my clients tell me that they relax by reading a book, going to the movies, taking walks or socializing with friends. While these kinds of activities are more relaxing than day-to-day chores and work, they do not help you experience deep relaxation.

In order to achieve the relaxation response, you need a clear mind and relaxed muscles. According to this definition, exercise alone does not help induce relaxation. Exercise can reduce stress, but it doesn't help us relax. Why? Because our bodies and minds are not at rest while exercising. In order to achieve deep relaxation, you need to use a specific relaxation technique aimed at calming your body, mind and spirit.

Specific Techniques to Relax Body and Soul

Just as there are different degrees of stress, there are different methods for managing stress and bringing your body into a balanced, relaxed state. Some techniques can be used easily—anytime, anywhere—to counteract a specific stressor. Others require a commitment of regular relaxation practice. For the rest of this chapter, the focus will be on four powerful techniques for managing stress and inducing deep relaxation:

◆ Breathing Exercises
◆ Meditation
◆ Visualization
◆ Yoga and Deep Relaxation

As you read about each technique and review the accompanying exercises, try to choose a stress management method that particularly appeals to you. We include two types of methods here: those that can be done quickly, for on-the-spot stress relief; and those that require a commitment of 30 to 60 minutes at a stretch, but provide deeper and more lasting relaxation benefits.

Choose a practice that you are comfortable with, so that you can make a real commitment. Also choose a practice that is especially suitable for your current level of stress. For example, if muscle tension is a major problem for you, yoga practice may be your best choice. If anxiety plagues you, breathing exercises and meditation may be better choices. Or you may wish to combine several practices, doing them at different times during the week. Your goal is to incorporate whatever stress management methods you choose into your regular Active Wellness routine.

> *One thing at a time, all things in succession.*
> *That which grows slowly endures.*
> —J. G. Holland

Breathing Exercises

Breathing to Manage Stress and Relax

Have you ever stopped to think about how you breathe? Most of the time we don't have to think about breathing; it's an unconscious act that our body performs automatically. The quality of our breath reflects our emotions and state of mind. Many of us have breathing patterns that include gasping in fear or anxiously holding our breath. When we are stressed, we tend to take shallow, rapid breaths.

Although there is no correct way to breathe, there are ways of breathing that can help us remain calm and relaxed. Examining how you breathe under different circumstances can help you determine when you are stressed, angry, happy, enraged, tense. Is your breathing rapid and shallow or deep and slow? Rapid and shallow breaths are associated with feelings of fatigue and stress. Count how many breaths you take in one minute. If your count falls between 16 and 20, you probably are breathing rapidly and from your chest and are under-utilizing your lung capacity. This type of breathing inhibits the uptake of oxygen—the extreme example of this is hyperventilating, which can actually trigger the stress response.

We can learn to regulate our breathing to induce relaxation by breathing diaphragmatically. Diaphragmatic breathing, which originates in the belly, helps promote relaxation. It is an easy technique to learn and one that you can use anytime you feel stressed. Diaphragmatic breathing was the way we naturally breathed as infants. When you inhale for a diaphragmatic breath, the emphasis is on the exhaled breath, rather than the inhaled breath. As you inhale, your diaphragm moves downward, expanding your lungs. As you exhale, the diaphragm contracts, compressing the lungs and forcing the old air out. This movement gives you full use of your lungs, both to take in oxygen and release carbon dioxide.

Diaphragmatic breathing is an excellent de-stressing tool and a great way to relax, whether you use it by itself as a means to calm down after a hectic day or as part of a longer yoga and meditation routine. Generally, with diaphragmatic breathing you take fewer and deeper breaths, averaging about six to eight breaths per minute—but don't hold yourself to this. Do what feels comfortable. This type of breathing isn't difficult to learn, but it takes focused energy and awareness when you're just beginning. With regular practice, it becomes habitual.

Learning to Breathe from Your Diaphragm

This simple exercise helps you learn the process of diaphragmatic breathing. Once you feel comfortable with this process, you can start to incorporate it into your regular breathing process and use it in any position, such as sitting or standing.

Step 1: Become aware of your breathing. Sit or lie down in a quiet room with your hand placed on your abdomen.

Step 2: Bring your attention to your breathing and notice if your abdomen fills with air as you inhale. On the inhalation, your belly should expand slightly on its own. Try to relax your abdominal muscles; you'll get the most effective breath from a relaxed abdomen. If possible, inhale and exhale through your nose only.

Step 3: The hand that is resting on your abdomen should rise up with your belly as you inhale and go down as you exhale. Focus on creating this effect feeling your abdomen expand and your hand rise as you inhale and then feeling your abdomen contract and your hand drop as you exhale.

If you initially find it difficult to practise diaphragmatic breathing, give yourself time. Remember that this was how you were born breathing: Eventually it will come back to you. Some of my Active Wellness clients take several weeks to learn proper breathing. Once they do, however, it becomes their favourite of the relaxation techniques, as it is easy to do and can be done anywhere.

Mindfulness Breathing As Relaxation Practice

Mindfulness breathing involves consciously focusing on your breath for a specific amount of time. You can do this for short periods of time, at various moments throughout the day, to relax yourself. Or, preferably, set aside a designated time and place to regularly practise mindfulness breathing as part of your stress management programme. Mindfulness breathing also offers a great way to start learning the practice of meditation: focusing on the breath, and the breath alone, is a common meditative technique.

Five-Minute Mindfulness Breathing Exercise

This mindfulness breathing exercise is a wonderful way to begin or end your day. Try to find a safe, comfortable place for this exercise, so you can really relax.

Step 1: Set aside at least five minutes for this breathing practice.

Step 2: Get yourself into a comfortable position, either sitting or lying down, with your arms by your sides. (Lying down is more restful to the body.)

Step 3: Close your eyes.

Step 4: Begin breathing, focusing your attention on your breath as you inhale and exhale. Keep bringing your attention back to your breath when it wanders.

Step 5: As you breathe, take long, deep inhalations and exhalations. In the beginning, you may find it helpful to count to 3 during the inhaled breath and count to 4 during the exhaled breath. By doing this, you exhale more slowly, which helps you cleanse your lungs and further relax.

Step 6: When you are ready to finish your breathing session, slowly resume normal breathing and open your eyes.

*I am seeking, I am striving, I am in it
with all my heart.*
—Vincent van Gogh

Meditation

Meditation is a way to nourish your soul and calm your mind. It is a way of taking time to focus in a quiet, peaceful and accepting manner. The practice of meditation helps to induce relaxation, enhance concentration, increase mental alertness and promote creativity.

There are many different ways to meditate. The method we highlight here, focused meditation, involves concentrating on one thing only. Another popular form of meditation that you may want to investigate is 'mindfulness meditation', which focuses one's awareness on the present moment. This type of meditation can be done anytime and anywhere, even when you are walking or eating.

Because each person has a different learning style, I've included a variety of meditation methods. For example, some people respond to visual images, while others relate better to sound. You may want to experiment before deciding which works best for you. Although you can achieve effective meditation using a variety of techniques, the most important factor for choosing a particular type of meditation is your own comfort level with the technique.

Focused Meditation

An excellent practice for inducing deep relaxation and increasing mental clarity and awareness is focused meditation. With this type of meditation, you focus on one thing, whether it's your breath, a word, a phrase, an object, an image or a sound.

When you first begin practising focused meditation, you may have difficulty staying focused on just one thing. You may feel easily distracted, as if your mind is going off in 20 different directions. With practice, however, you can learn how to remain so focused within your meditation that time seems to stand still. This happened to me when I first 'got into' a meditative state. I sat down to meditate for 10 to 15 minutes and before I knew it, I had meditated for more than half an hour.

Before you begin your meditation, plan to follow these few simple guidelines:

⋄ Wear comfortable, loose clothing or loosen your waistband and shirt cuffs.
⋄ Choose a calm and quiet place to meditate where you won't be disturbed.
⋄ If necessary, take the phone off the hook.
⋄ Establish a regular time and place for meditating every day. Many people choose to practise first thing in the morning or right before going to bed. I personally recommend meditating first thing in the morning, which helps you start your day with a clear, calm and focused mind.

Beginning Your Meditation
Sit or kneel with your spine straight. For sitting positions, you may use the floor or a chair.

For Floor Position:
Sit cross-legged on the floor with your spine straight, a hand on each knee, and palms facing upward.

For Chair Position:
Sit upright in a chair with your feet flat on the floor, spine straight, a hand on each knee, and palms facing upward.

For Kneeling Position:
Kneel on the floor with your spine straight, a hand resting on each knee, and palms facing upward.

Hand and Finger Positioning:
With palms facing upward, gently touch your thumb to your index finger. By uniting your thumb and index finger, you, in effect, 'close a circuit' and keep the flow of energy circulating throughout your body.

Breath-Focused Meditation
Close your eyes and begin deep breathing through your nose, focusing on your breath as it travels in and out of your body. If it helps you maintain your focus, count to 3 as you inhale and then count to 4 as you exhale. At first, you may find yourself easily distracted by outside noises and by your own thoughts, random images and feelings. Observe any thoughts, images, feelings and distractions that come up during meditation, but try not to become 'attached' to them. Picture them as clouds floating through your mind. Observe them calmly, but let them go and return to focusing on your breath. As you continue your meditation practice, you will find it easier to remain focused on your breath.

If you are a beginner to meditation, start out by meditating for five minutes at a time. Gradually increase your meditation time each week. By beginning slowly, you give your body a chance to become comfortable with the meditation posture and discipline. If your body is uncomfortable, you may have difficulty remaining still and focusing your mind.

You may choose to continue doing breath-focused meditation exclusively, or you may want to try another type of focused meditation.

Word-Focused Meditation

In this type of meditation, a continually repeated word or phrase (also called a "mantra") becomes the focus of your meditation. You may repeat the word or phrase silently to yourself, timing it with the inhalation and exhalation of your breath, or you may say the word or phrase aloud, but quietly. What is important is to select a word or phrase that has a strong personal meaning for you and is also uplifting and positive. Words such as 'love', 'light', 'hope' and 'relax' are excellent choices for word-focused meditation. A phrase such as 'I wish all living creatures love and kindness' is also a good choice.

Image-Focused Meditation

An object or image offers a visual focus that may help sharpen and increase your awareness. You should choose a simple object or image—a beautiful stone, a crystal, a candle, a plant or a small painting. Place the object or image about one to two feet away from you. Begin deep breathing, but do not close your eyes. Instead, focus on the object or image in front of you for a few minutes, until you feel calm and centred. Then close your eyes, if you wish, and become aware of any thoughts or images that enter your mind.

Sound-Focused Meditation

Choose an outside sound—the singing of birds, the rustling of leaves, the laughter of children—and use this sound as you focus when you begin deep breathing. Try to focus on the unique timbre and various facets of the sound. You may also choose to use a passage of music as your focus, concentrating on hearing each sound as a separate note. You can use meditation tapes, recorded natural sounds or chanting as sounds for your meditation. Do not become attached to the sound, simply allow it to pass in and out of your meditative space.

Mindfulness Meditation

This type of meditation focuses on being aware of each moment. It involves observing the things that we do or that occur in our lives moment by moment. Mindfulness meditation is a process of fine-tuning your awareness of the present and learning how to become absorbed in each moment of your life as it occurs. You can practise mindfulness meditation anywhere and anytime, such as sitting in your office, eating dinner or walking in the park.

As you focus your attention and awareness on each facet of the particular moment you are experiencing, you will begin to notice and observe things that you were not aware of before. This is a particularly illuminating exercise when done while eating.

While meditation is frequently incorporated into yoga and breathing exercises, it can also stand on its own as a means of training your mind to relax and focus. If you do not have time to meditate at home, try taking time for meditation in your office. Shut your office door and hold all calls for the time you have allotted to your meditation. It may be difficult to meditate in your desk chair. Since this is where you do your work, it's not a spot associated with relaxation. Instead, choose another comfortable spot in your office where you can sit calmly to begin meditation.

Visualization

Visualization is a technique whereby you picture a specific image in your mind as a way to change your thoughts. It can alter your subconscious, help you relax and even promote healing. Visualizing an image in your mind has a very powerful influence on your emotions, one that is far more potent than just reading or hearing about the image. It has been proven that various types of imagery affect breathing, heart rate, blood pressure, sexual arousal, hormone levels in the blood and the immune system.

Take a moment now to compare how differently your feelings are affected by the idea described in the statement below and, after that, the impression evoked in your mind by the image that follows.

> **Statement:** *It is a beautiful day.*
> Now, close your eyes, take three deep breaths, and visualize the following image.

> **Image:** *The sun is shining. The sky is blue. The air feels crisp and fresh. Birds are flying overhead.*

You probably noticed that the image was much stronger than the statement, or perhaps reading the statement caused you to instantly picture an image. The image affects how we feel; the words are a tool by which our body and our mind communicate. You are probably more familiar with the practice of visualization than you realize. For example, before trying anything new, we usually try to see ourselves doing it first. This is visualization and it is powerful, particularly when done in combination with meditation. In fact, images sent to your subconscious while you are in a meditative state are 20 times more effective than visualizations done in the conscious state.

This ability is linked to the fact that there are two sides to our brain, the left and the right, which function together. The right brain is responsible for responding to images and the left brain is the logical side of the brain. By using visualization in meditation, you can use the images that naturally come to you to tap into the right brain's 'knowledge' of the big picture of an event or feeling. This helps you discover feelings that would not have been unearthed by logical thinking alone. Discovering these hidden needs and desires, about which you may not have been aware, can be very valuable.

In fact, because visualization helps me uncover my 'gut feelings' about specific situations, it is one of my own favourite ways to meditate. When you follow your instincts, you are more connected to your inner voice and more likely to make a balanced decision between your logical side and your emotional, instinctive side. I find this very valuable in both my business and my personal life. You can also purchase guided meditations, which lead you through the visualization process and show you how to incorporate the practice of visualization within your meditation practice.

Yoga and Deep Relaxation

The practice of yoga unites the techniques of breathing and relaxation through a series of gentle stretching exercises called 'poses' or 'postures'. In fact, the Sanskrit word 'yoga' means 'union' or 'yoking'. Yoga itself is an ancient practice designed to link body, mind and spirit in a balanced and relaxed state of well-being.

To have a free and relaxed mind, we need a flexible and relaxed body. The various yoga poses do just this by relieving muscle tension and promoting physical and mental well-being. I like to think of yoga as self-massage. It is even better than having a massage partner, since once you learn the poses you can practise them anywhere by yourself. Although practising yoga is not considered a strenuous workout, I recommend that you check with your doctor before you start practising it (as you should with any new type of physical activity).

A basic yoga practice, consisting of a series of poses that targets all the major muscle groups, is explained and illustrated on the following pages. However, I highly recommend that you take a yoga class or work with a private instructor when you first start out. An instructor can teach you proper breathing techniques for each pose and can show you how to make a smooth transition from one pose to the next. When practising your yoga poses, please remember that you should not force your body into any position. Instead, try to feel a comfortable stretch. The goal in yoga is to improve flexibility, not to increase tension by exceeding your body's limits. Use your breathing to help release your muscles by inhaling and exhaling as you flex.

The order in which the yoga poses are explained is deliberate, so practise each pose in successive order. The overall organization of the poses is intended to help balance the left and right sides of your body. Set aside a specific time for your practice—60 to 90 minutes is ideal in a quiet and relaxed environment where you will not be interrupted, although 15 to 20 minutes is better than not practising at all. Also, practising yoga on an empty stomach is best.

Beginning Your Yoga Practice
Begin your practice standing tall, with your feet together and your arms by your sides.

1. The Corpse: This is a relaxation pose. Lie down on your back with your feet about 18 in (46 cm) apart and turned outward slightly. Place your arms at your sides, about 6 in (15 cm) from your hips, with palms facing upward. Close your eyes and breathe deeply—slowly inhaling and exhaling. Remain in this pose for at least one minute. While you are in this pose, use your breath to release any tension or tightness by focusing your mind on the area of discomfort and releasing it when you exhale. Hold this pose for one minute.

2. The Cat: To begin the Cat pose, slowly roll over onto your stomach with a gentle movement. Begin this pose on your hands and knees. Breathe in slowly and deeply, while you arch your back and look up—you should feel a gentle stretch, but no strain. Exhale and tuck in your head, rounding your back so your spine bends in the opposite direction. Repeat this pose 3 to 5 times, coordinating your breath with the up and down stretching of your spine.

3. The Child: Kneel with your legs together and sit back on your heels; bend from your hips and extend your upper body over your knees. Place your forehead down and your arms to your sides, palms upward. Rest in this pose for 30 to 60 seconds, then slowly sit up.

4. The Mountain: Stand with your arms by your sides, palms facing inward and feet together; balance yourself equally on both feet. Keep your spine straight and imagine your head being lifted straight up. As you stand, inhale and exhale slowly and deeply. Hold this pose for 60 seconds, or less if uncomfortable.

5. The Rag Doll: Gradually bend over, hanging your head down. Cradle one arm in the other by holding each arm with the opposite hand. Hold this pose for 30 seconds, then slowly stand up, raising your head last. Repeat this pose one more time. Return to a standing position.

6. The Tree (This is a more advanced pose—if you choose to skip this pose, proceed to Step 7, the Cobra.): Lift and bend one leg so the foot of the bent leg is resting on the opposite thigh. Reach your arms upward and over your head. Interlace your fingers—keeping your index fingers free and pointing upward. Hold for 30 to 60 seconds. Repeat with the other leg.

7. The Cobra: Bending your elbows, place your hands flat on the floor next to your shoulders. Slowly touch your forehead to the floor. Make sure your elbows are pointed toward your feet. Inhale as you push down with your hands and look up. Continue to inhale as you raise your head and chest, trying to lift only your upper body (see diagram). When you reach as far as you comfortably can go with your abdomen and chest, take a deep breath, and exhale as you slowly return to the floor. Repeat this pose three more times. When finished, rest on the floor with your head turned and your arms comfortably by your sides.

8. The Half Locust: In preparation for the Half Locust, place your arms under your thighs. Lift one leg up, pressing down with your arms for support and squeezing your buttocks. Raise the lifted leg outward and upward—lifting through your heel and toes. Press down both hips equally. Return your leg slowly to the floor. Repeat with the other leg. Repeat this sequence one more time for both legs. Hold your leg up for 30 seconds.

9. The Full Locust: At the end of the Half Locust, raise both legs together for a Full Locust. This sequence may be repeated twice. Hold your legs up for 30 seconds.

10. The Corpse: Return to the Corpse pose in Step 1. Hold for 60 seconds.

11. The Knee Down Twist: Lie on your back with

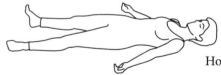

your arms extended out. Inhale and place your right foot on your left knee. Exhale, turn your head to the right, and bring your right knee toward the floor (see diagram). Release slowly, then repeat on the other side.

12. The Full Forward Bend: Sit with both legs directly in front of you, feet together and your back straight. Inhaling, slowly bring both arms straight over your head. Exhale as you bend from your hips and grab your ankles. Drop your head and neck. Hold this pose for 30 to 60 seconds. Inhale as you raise your torso to return to a seated position. Repeat this pose two more times.

13. The Corpse: Return to the Corpse pose in Step 1. Hold for 60 seconds.

14. The Shoulder Stand (This is a more advanced pose—if you choose to skip this pose, proceed to Step 15, the Bridge.): Lie on your back with your arms along your sides. Make sure that your feet are together. Inhale and slowly lift both legs until they are at a right angle to your back. Place both of your hands on your lower back, to support your body. Inhale and extend your legs straight up (see diagram). Make sure to keep your chin tucked into your chest. Hold the pose for 30 seconds, or as long as you are comfortable, and then slowly return to the relaxation pose. Take several deep breaths.

15. The Bridge: Lie on your back, knees bent, palms on the floor. Inhale as you slowly raise your pelvis and squeeze your buttocks. Press your arms and shoulders to the floor. Exhale as you lower your pelvis back down to the floor. Hold this pose for 30 seconds, breathing slowly and evenly. Repeat this pose two times.

16. The Corpse: This pose is for Body Scan and Deep Relaxation. Return to the Corpse pose in Step 1.

Body Scan: Remain in the Corpse pose and continue breathing for 5 minutes. Take a minute to mentally scan your body from your toes to your head, checking for any tension. Wherever you feel tension, picture that area of your body. As you exhale, imagine the tension disappearing from that part of your body.

Deep Relaxation: Raise your legs 2 in (5 cm) from the floor, and tense them. Then release them and let them fall to the floor. Let your feet lie still as though they are too heavy to lift. Raise your right arm and clench your fist. Then spread your fingers out and release your hand and arm, letting them fall to the floor. Repeat the same movements with your left arm and fist. Then allow your hands and arms to lie still and 'be absorbed by the floor', as though they were too heavy to lift.

Raise your buttocks from the floor and tense your muscles. Then relax, allowing your buttocks to drop to the floor.

Take a deep breath. Inhale and fill your stomach with as much air as possible, then let out the air with a sigh.

Raise your back and chest from the floor and tense them. Then relax your muscles and let yourself fall back to the floor.

Pull your shoulders up to your ears and tense your neck. Then release them and let your shoulders fall back to their original position.

Crunch and tense your facial muscles, open your eyes wide, stick out your tongue, and stretch your face. Then let go and relax. Roll your neck from side to side to find a comfortable place for your head. Then allow your body to lie still. Picture a warm wave of relaxation entering at your toes and travelling up your body through your legs to your back, stomach, arms, neck, face, and jaw, finally quieting your mind in a peaceful state of calm relaxation. You may lie in this position for several minutes.

To waken your body, gently begin to move your arms and legs. Then slowly come to a sitting position. You may, at this stage, want to practise a short meditation before you resume your daily activities.

17. The Lotus: To finish your stress management routine, you can return to the Lotus pose (meditation pose) and close with a short meditation. To sit in the Lotus pose, cross your legs; bring one leg close to your body and the other leg to the opposite thigh. It's best if your knees don't touch the floor. Sit with your spine straight and your arms resting on your knees, palms faced upward. Close your eyes, inhale, then exhale slowly and begin your meditation.

> *Rest assured, anything that relaxes the body,*
> *stimulates the mind, and refreshes the spirit is*
> *healing.*
> —Betty Wood

Creating Stress-Free Living and Working Environments

Feng Shui

If you have ever been in a room that feels stuffy and tight, you probably felt uncomfortable and even drained of energy. On the other hand, in a spacious, light-filled, and airy room with a good view, you probably felt energized and happy.

Creating energy in a living or working environment is the goal of Feng Shui (pronounced 'fung shway'), the ancient Chinese art of the placement of buildings, rooms, objects and colour to promote positive energy, happiness, and prosperity. In fact, the Chinese ideogram for Feng Shui means 'under the canopy of heaven'. There are many excellent books available if you want to learn about Feng Shui in depth. Here, we are introducing some Feng Shui basics for creating stress-free home and work environments.

If you live and work in an environment that is brimming with good feeling and good energy, you probably feel energetic, creative and centred. This in turn helps you feel more productive and less stressed. In Feng Shui, the type of energy created in an environment depends on the intended use. The energy in a home environment, for example, should be calming, while the energy in a retail store should be stimulating enough to promote business.

The first step in using Feng Shui to re-energize your home or office is to look at any areas of your environment that disturb you. Is there a lot of clutter in one area? Do you have a brick wall for a view? Does your home or office feel tight and closed off? Focus on the feeling you get when you walk into your home or office: is it a good feeling or an uncomfortable one?

Feng Shui is based on the Chinese philosophy of yin and yang, whereby two separate but complementary elemental energies of the universe are constantly interacting with each other. Together, they are the components of Qi (pronounced chee), the fundamental life force that lives within everything. Yin is feminine energy and yang is masculine energy. Yin is light, yang is dark. Yin is cold, yang is hot. Yin is the earth, moon, darkness, and death. Yang is the heavens, sun, light and life. One cannot exist without the other. Both are necessary for harmonious balance.

Balance and order, based on the yin-yang dynamic, are the fundamental tenets of Feng Shui and of creating stress-free environments. Rooms are designed and objects are placed in them, based on the goal of balancing yin and yang qualities. In Feng Shui, design and placement are also dependent on geographical direction. For example, a southerly direction is associated with fortune, the colour red and summer; a northerly direction is linked to business, death, the colour black and winter; the westerly direction is associated with children, purity, the colour white and autumn; and the easterly direction symbolizes family, health, the colour green and spring.

Suggestions for Home and Office

As you walk into your home, what is the first thing that greets you? Is it cheerful or depressing? Hopefully you enter a well-lit and open environment. However, if you walk into a room and find yourself facing another wall, you may feel stifled and uncomfortable. Placing a mirror on that wall, or a painting of a landscape, opens up the environment. Adding warm light to a dark foyer brings in good energy, as does placing lights, mirrors and pictures in a narrow hallway. As you go through your home, room by room, look for areas with clutter, darkness, narrowness, or poor views.

How you decorate a room also sets a mood. If a room is cold and uninviting visitors will feel uncomfortable. When you are decorating or rearranging furniture keep in mind that it is important to leave space between furniture and to eliminate clutter.

It helps to visualize the flow of positive energy beginning at the doorway of the room. That energy then flows toward groupings of furniture, slowly meanders through the room, and then leaves via another door or window. Because positive energy enters at the door, avoid obstructing the doorway with any furniture.

For an office environment, the ideal location for your desk is facing the door, positioned far enough inside the office so that you can see the entire room from your desk. Plants and flowers contribute to the positive energy in an environment, as does a good view. Any furniture that has edges is thought to cut into positive energy in a negative way. Try to avoid having any corners from bookcases or furniture face you directly. Good lighting is important, but glaring lights should be avoided. Clear thinking is obscured with clutter, so avoid clutter or try to organize it.

If the energy in a room is active, such as in a living room, it is more yang than yin. To balance the yang energy in an active room, try using yin touches throughout the room, such as throw pillows and cooling elements such as plants. Combining dark and light colours, will also help achieve more harmonious energy and great balance in the room.

Colour

The colours you use throughout your home can greatly affect your well-being. Colour can influence appetite, the autonomic nervous system, muscular tension, and emotional reactions. Surround yourself with colours that suit your emotions. In general, many of our emotional associations with colour come from the natural world around us. For example, red is associated with fire, green with trees and blue with the sky.

Also, remember that you are striving for a harmonious balance with colour, based on the same yin-yang principle of energy used in Feng Shui. Yin colours are cooling, contrasting and astringent. They include blues, indigo and violet. Yang colours are warm, arousing and vitalizing. They include red, orange and yellow.

If you want to learn more about the use of colour to create a balanced and stress-free environment, you can find specific books devoted to Feng Shui and the use of colours for each room of your home.

Lighting

In general, a well-lighted room feels more comfortable. However, choose carefully what types of lighting you use. A glaring overhead light that is hard on the eyes is not as welcoming and soothing as a lamp with a warm-glowing bulb. Fluorescent light is much harder to live with than soft light.

The Bedroom As a Special Place

The main rule for positioning your bed is to avoid placing the foot of the bed in such a manner that your feet face the door. The Chinese refer to this as the 'death position' because traditionally the dead were placed with their feet facing the door to allow them easier access to heaven. Since sleep is so highly regarded as a time of healing, several similar Feng Shui rules apply to the bedroom. For example, mirrors shouldn't face the bed, as they could scare your spirit at night. Also, furniture with sharp edges should never be placed so that the sharp edges are pointed at the sleeping person.

Avoid clutter in order to allow the maximum positive healing energy to circulate through the room. If you are using a portion of your bedroom for storing boxes, books and extra clothing, these objects interrupt the flow of energy. Similarly, using the space under your bed for storage creates stagnant energy over your bed.

For those of you who can't avoid the placement of your bed and furniture in precarious positions, solutions to these problems are available. You can hang a crystal sphere or wind chime from the ceiling, between the bed and the door, to lessen the negative energy. Folding screens and plants also divert the flow of negative energy. And, if possible, try to create an enjoyable view to wake up to, such as a picture, plants or a pleasant view through the window.

Another tenet of Feng Shui is using 'conscious intent' to achieve your goals. Meditating right before sleep about your aspirations and goals is highly recommended. Write down your thoughts and dreams before you go to bed, which is considered a cleansing ritual in Feng Shui, and then focus on your goals right before falling asleep. By focusing on your goals and dreams just before sleeping, you are closing the day with positive energy—a great place to begin your night.

Kitchen and Bathroom

According to Feng Shui philosophy, a well-lighted kitchen enhances the flow of good energy. This concept is especially important because the kitchen is often a place where clutter easily accumulates. Try to eliminate clutter, or it may stagnate the good energy flow. That stagnant energy, in turn, affects the food you prepare and eat in the kitchen.

The bathroom is a tricky room to arrange, according to Feng Shui principles. Water, which in Feng Shui is symbolic of business, wealth and success, is also something that gets flushed out of the bathroom daily. Therefore, even more attention should be paid to the flow of positive energy in and around the room. Keep the room clean and uncluttered. The bathroom is a mostly yin environment, so adding yang touches—warm colors and candlelight—promotes balance and positive energy.

Finally, if the bathroom is facing the front door or situated near the kitchen or in the central part of your house, hang a mirror outside the bathroom door to deflect any negative energy from spilling over into these other environments.

Now that you have learned about light, colour and placement in the home to create a positive environment, let's look at scent and how the right scents can help you relax and feel calmer during high-stress times.

Essential Oils for Various Moods

Calming: Cedarwood, Chamomile, Frankincense, Geranium, Lavender, Lemon grass, Orange, Patchouli, Rosewood, Sandalwood, Ylang-Ylang

Uplifting: Basil, Bergamot, Ginger, Lemon, Lime, Lavender, Neroli, Peppermint, Rose, Rosemary

Clear Thinking: Black Pepper, Juniper, Lemon, Peppermint, Rosemary, Rosewood, Sage

Sensuality: Basil, Bergamot, Cedarwood, Frankincense, Geranium, Ginger, Jasmine, Juniper, Lavender, Lemon grass, Lime, Neroli, Orange, Patchouli, Rose, Sandalwood, Ylang-Ylang

Aromatherapy

Aromatherapy is the ancient art of using the healing power of essential oils to balance the mind and body. Essential oils are distilled from organic plant sources, including flowers and the leaves, bark and gum of trees.

Smell is a potent influence on how we feel and act. Here is one example of just how potent smell can be. When I was trying to sell my home, a real-estate broker suggested that I make baked apples when clients were coming to view my home. She explained that the scent of baked apples invariably gives a cosy and warm feeling to a house.

The right scent can trigger your brain to stimulate your endocrine and hormonal systems in positive ways that help you relax and de-stress. While more than 300 essential oils are available for home use, you should need no more than 10 to 15 different scents. Essential oils can be found in many shops, and also come in scented candle form. They offer a great way to quickly scent any room, even your bathroom. In the sidebar on the left, you'll find a list of the most popular and effective essential oils.

Oils can be used during baths or showers, in inhalers or light-bulb diffusers, or as rubs or personal perfumes. But before you begin to experiment with oils, try a patch test on your skin to make sure you do not have an allergic reaction. Also, some oils should not be used if you are pregnant or photosensitive, so read the label on the bottle carefully or consult an aromatherapist.

Essential oils are also extremely volatile, so be sure to store them in a dark bottle in a cool and dark location. When essential oils are blended with a good base oil, they can keep for several months. There are many aromatherapy books available that can help you learn how to make a variety of skin-care and home-care products from essential oils.

Sound

Finally, don't forget the auditory senses. Sounds are directly linked to our nervous system, and therefore can greatly affect our level of relaxation and stimulation.

Music therapy is an emerging field. Two excellent books on the subject are *Healing Imagery & Music* (CD included!) by Carol A. Bush and *The Sound of Healing* by Judith Pinkerton. Both books contain marvellous discussions about how various types of music affect us differently, both physically and emotionally. Loud and fast music is stimulating to our senses and increases the action of our autonomic nervous system. Slow and soft sounds are soothing and relaxing, decreasing the autonomic response and thereby helping decrease blood pressure, heart rate and respiration.

When selecting music to help you relax, one of the most important criteria is your personal reaction to the piece of music. How much you like the music is the best indicator of how well the music will make you feel and how much it will help you relax.

Music is also an invaluable aid to meditation and visualization practice. Many musical audiocassettes and CDs are designed specifically for use during meditation and visualization.

Now that you have learned the basic components of the Active Wellness programme, good nutrition, physical fitness, behaviour modification and stress management, take a breather and congratulate yourself on how far you've come on your wellness journey. As you continue practising your programme, living the Active Wellness lifestyle will become second nature to you, and the hurdles you need to jump will become smaller and fewer and far between.

One last hurdle you now have to face is how to maintain your Active Wellness programme when you're away from home, travelling on holiday or business. Let's move on to Step 8, where we tackle that very problem.

Strategies for Success Away from Home

The people who get on in this world are the people
who get up and look for the circumstances they
want, and, if they can't find them, make them.
—George Bernard Shaw

How many times have you gone off your health regimen because you went on holiday or a business trip? Not being in your usual environment makes it more challenging to remain on your new healthy routine. Travelling for work or pleasure can become an easy justification for letting go of your self-control. Then, when you return home, you may have difficulty resuming your former healthy routine.

Before you know it, three weeks have gone by and you haven't been able to get your eating, exercise and stress management under control. Beware! The 'off the programme' blues can get you down, which can be discouraging. You may feel like you have to begin at the starting line all over again. Luckily, this doesn't have to be the case.

In this step you'll learn strategies for maintaining your Active Wellness programme away from home, whether you are dining out for just one evening or travelling on holiday for several weeks. You will learn how to make your Active Wellness programme 'portable' and carry it with you into many different environments. You will also learn how to plan ahead to deal with obstacles along your wellness path, so that being away from home becomes an easier transition for you.

Dining Away from Home

Dining away from home when you're trying to follow a healthy eating plan can create some anxiety. You are no longer in control of what food is put in front of you or how it is prepared. By using several simple strategies, however, dining anywhere—while staying on your Active Wellness programme—can be easy and satisfying.

In particular, developing strategies for the challenges you face is the best way to feel secure about staying on your programme. The recommendations I've put together here come from the days when I was a chef, and from my understanding of how a restaurant really functions, from the kitchen to the dining room. Here's an insider's tip: When you dine out, you are more in control than you may think. You are the customer, and in the restaurant business 'the customer is always right.' In fact, throughout the entire hospitality industry, the primary goal is to please the guest.

'Dining out' can mean anything from grabbing food on the go to eating in a fine restaurant or on an aeroplane. But anytime you don't prepare your own meals, knowing what ingredients are in the food becomes difficult. Choosing healthy meals, therefore, is more challenging and requires a few learned skills. For one thing, realize that different strategies are needed for different environments. In a restaurant, your goal is to take control of the food you order by asking questions and making creative choices from the menu. At a friend's house or at a dinner party, you need to use different strategies to remain in control and stay on your eating plan. In this step we'll tackle each challenging dining situation one at a time, beginning with restaurants.

Dining Out in Restaurants

Dining out is a social occasion, a time to relax and enjoy the people you're with, the ambiance of your surroundings, and the flavours of various foods. All treats to be treasured! And your Active Wellness dining strategies can enhance your enjoyment of the experience by helping you choose nutritious and flavourful foods that don't leave you feeling deprived because you're trying to be 'good' and stay on your programme.

Amazingly, most Active Wellness participants report very similar experiences and challenges when they dine out. Does this scenario sound familiar?

General Guidelines for Dining Out

◇ Choose a restaurant that has a healthy cuisine, so you have appropriate and tasty menu choices.
◇ Ring ahead and speak to the chef about making special requests.
◇ Read the menu carefully.
◇ Ask questions. Make sure you know what is in your food.
◇ Remember, as the customer, you are in control of your dining experience.

You arrive at a restaurant hungry and ready to eat anything that is put in front of you. Then, as you are waiting for a table, you have a drink at the bar. This relaxes you and further stimulates your appetite. Next, you are influenced by what others in the group are ordering, and since dining away from home feels like a special occasion, you are tempted to order anything you want and eat everything on the plate. Later, leaving the restaurant, you feel uncomfortably full and guilty that you ate too much.

This doesn't have to be your experience of dining out.

Restaurant Strategies: First Things First

When you sit down at a restaurant table, one of the first things the waiter or waitress does is put bread on your table. This can be a problem if you are one of those people who cannot control themselves around a breadbasket, especially when you're really hungry. Since bread is part of the grains/starches group, you can use your Active Wellness serving guidelines and count each slice of bread as one serving. But if you do that, remember that you then have fewer grain servings to eat at dinner. Instead, why not give some of these breadbasket strategies a try?

Breadbasket Strategies

◇ If bread is one of the foods you tend to overeat, ask the server to take the breadbasket away.

◇ Don't spread anything on your bread if you can help it. Bread is typically served with butter or oil. If you use such a spread, you must count it as a fat option (1 tsp/5 ml = 1 fat serving).

◇ Ring ahead and ask the restaurant to prepare a platter of crudités (fresh-cut vegetables) for the table, to be served as soon as you sit down. This gives you something to munch on while you are waiting for your dinner.

◇ Order a favourite beverage and slowly drink this instead of eating bread while you wait for dinner.

Once the bread is served and you have your drinks, the next decision is what to eat. This is where following the Active Wellness guidelines for assessing menu entrées can help you.

How to Assess a Menu for Active Wellness Options

◇ Read the entire menu carefully, from appetizers to desserts.

◇ Determine your hunger level.

◇ Use the 'meal layering' strategy described on page 218.

◇ Plan ahead: assess how restaurant foods fit into your daily food plan.

◇ Make your selections from the entire menu. Don't limit yourself to just the items listed as main courses. Appetizers and side dishes can also make a meal.

◇ Don't assume that you know how a dish is prepared. Always ask questions about whether cream and butter are used, or whether the food is fried. (See the Dining Out Guides on pages 221 and 222.)

◇ If you want dessert but your options are limited, you can always ask for fruit.

Read the Entire Menu Carefully. When you are choosing a meal, consider mixing and matching from the entire menu, regardless of where the item is located. For example, if you want to start your meal with fresh fruit but it is listed under 'Desserts', feel free to order it as an appetizer. Think of yourself as someone on a treasure hunt as you attempt to discover all the healthy options on a menu when making your meal selection. Try to focus on foods you find satisfying and appropriate for your health needs.

To help you get started on the right track, read through the sample menu shown below. Circle all the food items that you can eat on your Active Wellness plan. At this point, don't worry whether a main course may have a high-fat sauce. Just consider whether the food itself is appropriate for your eating plan. Then, think about whether or not you can make substitutions to the meal defined on the menu, so that it is more appropriate for your eating plan. You can jot down substitution ideas that come to you when you read the menu. For example, if the pasta with fresh salmon and spinach in a cream sauce came without the cream sauce, it would be a 'legal' dish. If you're not sure about certain dishes, put a question mark next to them; you can check your answers with the dining guidelines and substitution suggestions after you finish the exercise.

Making Substitutions

Many Active Wellness participants have the best results in restaurants when they suggest the substitutions and modifications. If you want to order a main course, such as the pasta with salmon and spinach without the heavy cream sauce, you'll also want to know how to suggest making tasty substitutions or modifications so you can enjoy your meal and not feel deprived.

Most chefs will welcome the challenge of creating an appetizing meal that meets your health requirements if they are given advance notice, and if the restaurant is not encountering a particularly hectic time. On most occasions when you let the chef know your health limitations, you'll be pleasantly surprised by what you are served. But at times when the kitchen is very busy, your best bet is to give the waiter   specific instructions about how you would like the dish prepared in order to meet your requirements.

The Sample Menu choices below along with the Healthy Substitutions list on the next page will help you learn how to modify your menu selections when dining out.

Sample Menu

Appetizers and Starters
◇ Black Bean Soup with Sour Cream and Chives
◇ Hearty Vegetable Soup
◇ Mixed Green Salad with Vinaigrette Dressing
◇ Stuffed Artichokes with Mustard Dipping Sauce
◇ Grilled Prawn Skewers with Pineapple Salsa
◇ Fried Calamari

Main Courses
◇ Grilled Chicken Breast with Wild Mushroom Sauce over Wild Rice Pilaf
◇ Baked Salmon over Spinach in a Dill Cream Sauce
◇ Fillet of Flounder Stuffed with Spinach and Feta Cheese
◇ Angel Hair Pasta Primavera with Light Tomato Sauce
◇ Grilled Sirloin with Baked Potato and Mixed Vegetables

Desserts
◇ Apple Pie
◇ Chocolate Mousse Cake
◇ Tricolour Sorbet: Raspberry, Lemon, Mango
◇ Fresh Fruit

Healthy Substitutions for Menu Items

On the Menu	Active Wellness Alternative
◇ Creamed soups	◇ Stocks, vegetable soups, consommés
◇ Cream sauces	◇ Tomato-based sauces; sauces made with wine and broth as a base
◇ Chicken or seafood toppings	◇ Salsa; barbecue sauce
◇ Soured cream on potato	◇ Mustard; barbecue sauce; plain low-fat yoghurt; Parmesan cheese
◇ Salad dressing and spreads	◇ Dressing on the side ◇ Sandwiches without mayonnaise ◇ Balsamic vinegar with a little oil ◇ Mix balsamic vinegar with mustard and a packet of sugar or sugar substitute to make a fat-free salad dressing
◇ Abundance of cheeses	◇ 2 tbsp/30 g of Parmesan cheese
◇ Fried foods	◇ Grilled, broiled, or baked
◇ Pasta	◇ A tomato-, stock- or wine-based sauce

| ◇ Stuffing | ◇ Omit stuffing—it is almost always high in saturated fat. |

In the sample menu on page 215, many of the items are healthy selections. The two healthy desserts listed are the sorbet and the fresh fruit. The foods that require substitutions in order to fall within the Active Wellness guidelines include:

Appetizers: Black bean soup without the soured cream, grilled calamari instead of fried, salad with the dressing on the side, or make your own fat-free dressing *(opposite page)*. Steamed artichoke (no stuffing) with dressing on the side.

Main courses: Make sure all entrées are in wine-, tomato- or stock-based sauces without butter. All side dishes should be baked butter free and all stuffings and cheeses should be omitted.

Determine Your Hunger Level. Becoming absorbed in all the choices a restaurant offers is a common hazard. If your eyes are bigger than your stomach, you end up ordering more food than you need to satisfy your hunger. This tendency is dangerous for those who feel that they must eat everything on their plate. Ordering only the amount of food you want to eat at a given time is the wisest choice, so take your hunger level into account when you order. If you are aware of how hungry you truly feel and you consider what food options remain on your Daily Allowance Card for that day, you'll gain a better sense of how much food to order.

Some restaurants serve very large portions. So here you can typically eat half of a meal, split one with a friend, or order an appetizer as a meal. When you do receive a large portion, plan to take some home for lunch the next day, or simply leave it. Remind yourself that leaving food on your plate is perfectly acceptable: you should eat until you are satisfied, not stuffed.

Helpful Strategies to Use *Before* You Arrive at the Restaurant

If you know you will be dining late, eat a late snack around 4.00 or 5.00 p.m. to help you stay in control while you are waiting to be served at the restaurant. Foods with fibre (vegetables, fruit and whole grains) and protein hold you over longer than other foods. Good snacks include fruit, non-fat yoghurt, salad, air-popped popcorn or a healthy drink.

Plan to exercise before dinner, which will help curb your appetite.

Know what you want to order before you sit down. Ring ahead if you are not familiar with the restaurant and have a menu faxed to your office. Then make sure the restaurant serves something healthy you can eat. If you can find nothing on the menu that sounds healthy, but you must eat at this restaurant, speak to the chef before 'restaurant rush hour'. If the chef is not available, ask the dining room manager for advice.

Use the 'Meal Layering' Strategy. When you order, think about layering your meal with different courses. Meal layering helps you feel full on less food. The premise of meal layering is to use all the food groups to your advantage by ordering the lower calorie and fibre-rich foods first, prior to your main course. This is a strategy that is used at health spas, which can also be applied to dining out or eating in.

The way to meal layer is to order a light appetizer or two, followed by your main course. For example, have a light, stock-based soup and a salad with low-fat or fat-free dressing. This will help you to fill up on low calorie, healthy food. It also begins the 20-minute interval needed to signal your brain that food is now in your stomach. If you eat most of your food before the 20-minute mark, your body suddenly feels full after you may have already eaten too much. If you eat slowly, and use the meal layering strategy, you'll feel full on less food.

If you are a fast eater, you probably consume a lot of calories within the first 20 minutes of eating, especially if you start with a main course as your first course. With meal layering, a smaller main course can satisfy you because you will not feel as hungry after the 20-minute mark. Whenever you can, plan to eat this way. You don't have to wait until you dine out; try meal layering at home. You'll be amazed at how well this method of eating works, and how easy it is to arrange. Meal layering is especially helpful if you're cutting portion sizes to lose weight and are accustomed to eating large quantities of food.

Plan Ahead: Assess How Restaurant Foods Fit into Your Daily Food Plan. This rule helps you think about dining out as a part of your daily eating plan. Even though eating out at a good restaurant is a special treat, you must not forget to include the foods you eat when dining out as part of your overall eating plan for the day. For example, if you plan to order a meat, fish or poultry main course at the restaurant for dinner, you probably should avoid those foods at lunch, so you don't overload on your protein servings for the day. Focus your lunch choices on vegetarian selections such as vegetables, grains and fruit.

Make Your Selections from the Entire Menu. Don't limit yourself to only the items listed in the main course and appetizer sections. Side dishes can make a great meal! In fact, a meal can be created from anything that is listed on the menu. If it is on the menu, assume it is in the kitchen and can be ordered as an option. Following is an example of how to mix and match.

First, read over the menu carefully and look at the broad range of food selections available. Restaurants have refrigerators full of unprepared food. For example, by looking at the Sample Menu on page 215, you can see that the options for main courses include chicken, fish, steak and pasta. As healthy supplements, rice pilaf, salad, cooked vegetables, potatoes and mixed fruit are available. Healthy sauce options include tomato sauce and salsa. From all these choices, you can mix and match menu items and create your own healthy meal. Some possible options include grilled chicken breast with salsa and a baked potato, or baked salmon with cooked vegetables and rice pilaf. If you are a vegetarian, you can have the bean soup, salad and cooked vegetables with a baked potato.

If you can't find a healthy main course on the menu, ask that the item be prepared using a healthier cooking method, such as steaming, baking or grilling. Even light sautéing is better than frying. Have fun mixing and matching menu options. Who knows? You may discover a great new combination!

Don't Assume You Know How a Dish Is Prepared. Always ask questions about how your food is prepared. The Dining Out Guides on pages 221 and 222 suggest detailed questions, arranged by cuisine type. It is also important to let your server know you are concerned about your health before you ask questions about the food. This offers a possibly busy server a reason for your questions and helps him guide you to what is appropriate and available from the kitchen. Most of the time, servers try their best to answer all your questions, but sometimes they may need to go ask the kitchen staff directly. The chef is the ultimate decision maker concerning what alterations in food preparation are possible. If your health needs are critical, your best strategy is to call the restaurant early and speak to the chef personally.

Some questions you can ask your server include whether the food is baked, sautéed or grilled and whether it has butter or a butter sauce on top. Restaurants are notorious for adding butter to food in order to make it tender and moist. If you are concerned that added butter is a problem, ask them to limit all butter and oil in a dish. At restaurants, speak in terms of the ingredients, not nutritional content (fats, carbohydrates, proteins). For example, when speaking about reducing the fat used to prepare a dish, refer to the type of fat that should be reduced: butter, oil, mayonnaise or cream.

Several points are important when asking questions about food preparation. The ingredients in sauces, coatings or toppings should be a major focus, as they contain a lot of the fats just mentioned: cream, butter or oil. If you are watching your sodium intake, you should ask if the dish is salty. If you are avoiding alcohol, any sauce that is prepared with alcohol still has alcohol in it after it is cooked—the alcohol does not completely burn off. If you have allergies to certain foods, don't forget to enquire whether a dish contains the specific ingredient that triggers your reaction, such as prawns and peanuts.

Don't be shy about asking questions: you're talking about your health. If you have many health concerns and need to ask questions and take your time going over the menu, plan to avoid the restaurant's rush hours when you dine out. Those hours tend to be 7.00 to 9.00 a.m. for breakfast, 12.00 to 2.00 p.m. for lunch and 6.00 to 8.00 p.m. for dinner.

Once You Receive Your Food, Enjoy It! This point is simple. If you have taken the effort to create a meal that you feel is right for your needs because you have asked the right questions, then when the meal arrives from the kitchen, enjoy it! Even if it contains one or two ingredients that are not quite right, still enjoy it. You did your best, and with each new restaurant experience, you learn more information that you can use the next time you dine out. Also, the more you return to the same restaurant, the easier time you'll have deciphering the menu and getting your food prepared the way you want it. Each restaurant's menu presents different challenges, but the process of studying the menu and asking questions is always the same.

If You Want Dessert—Think Fruit. Dessert presents a tricky situation because many people have difficulty passing it up, particularly when with a group of people who all decide to order dessert. Desserts are usually full of sugar and fat, which is why you would be wise to avoid them. The calories can be worked into your daily food options, but the food itself is typically unhealthy.

But never fear! Some healthy dessert selections are available. Roasted or poached fruit, sorbets and low-fat ice cream or frozen yoghurt all make good desserts. If you have to eat a regular dessert, share it with one or two people. But try your best to avoid the very rich desserts.

More on Reading Menus

When you read a restaurant's menu, key words can help you distinguish healthy meal preparation from unhealthy meal preparation, as well as healthy ingredients from unhealthy ones. Use the lists *(opposite)* of these key terms, together with the Dining Out Guides opposite and on page 222, to learn how to identify ideal meal options and avoid unhealthy choices.

Key Terms for Meal Preparation and Ingredients

Healthy Preparation: Baked, Boiled, Glazed, Grilled, Poached, Steamed, Seared, in Stock.

Healthy Ingredients: Fresh, Medallions (cuts of meat that are leaner), Au Jus ('with its own juice'), Rump and Loin (cuts of meat that are leaner), Marinated (usually adds flavour without fat, but ask about the ingredients, which may be high in sodium), Beans, Pulses, Whole Grains, Vegetables, Fruit, Wine Sauce.

High Sodium Preparation and Ingredients to Avoid: Chilli Sauce, Smoked, Cured, Salted, Cold Cuts, Hot Dogs, Sausages, Pickled Foods, Salted Crackers, Snacks, Nuts, Anchovies, MSG, Soy Sauce, Miso, Meat Tenderizers, Capers, Cheese, Salt.

Dining Out Guide 1

MEXICAN

LOOK FOR: Baked, Grilled, Sautéed, Soft Tortillas (Corn or Flour), Black Bean Soup, Salsa, Salads, Gazpacho Soup, Fijitas (without Guacamole), Rice, Burrito (without Cheese)

WATCH OUT FOR: Fried, Excessive Cheese, Enchiladas, Refried Beans Flavoured with Lard, Guacamole, Fried Tortilla Crisps, Cheese Quesadilla, Soured Cream, Chorizo, Chillies Rellenos, Tacos, Flan, Sopaipillas, Nachos, Chimichangas, Fried Ice Cream

ASK: Can you make this item with half the amount of cheese? Is this dish prepared with a lot of oil? If yes, can the oil be reduced?

CHINESE

LOOK FOR: Steamed, Baked, Stir-Fried (Sautéed), Barbecued, Lots of Vegetables.

WATCH OUT FOR: Crispy, Fried, Batter-Fried, Pan-Fried, Breaded, Sweet and Sour, Egg Rolls, Spring Rolls, Peking Duck, Bird's Nest, Lo Mein, Pancakes, Combination Plate. If on a low sodium diet, watch out for the Soy Sauce and Hot & Sour Soup.

ASK: Can you prepare this without MSG? Is this dish prepared with a lot of oil? If yes, can the oil used in preparation be reduced? Can this dish have extra vegetables added? May I have the meat, poultry or fish steamed or stir-fried instead of the batter-fried or deep-fried?

FRENCH

LOOK FOR: Poached, Steamed, Roasted, Grilled, Provençal Cuisine. En Papillote, Sorbet, Vinaigrette, Au Jus, Marinated, Bouillabaisse, Demi Glacé.

WATCH OUT FOR: Crusted, Stuffed, Cheese (all types), 'Light Sauce', Au Gratin, Béchamel, Béarnaise, Hollandaise, Beurre Blanc, Crème, Crème Fraîche, Crème Brûlée, Foie Gras, Pâté, Buttery, Gratiné, Pastry (all types), Gravy, Confit, Caesar Salad.

ASK: Is this dish prepared with a lot of oil or cream? If yes, can the oil or cream used in preparation be reduced or omitted?

Dining Out Guide 2

GREEK (Middle Eastern)	
LOOK FOR:	Steamed, Baked, Roasted, Grilled, Mixed Vegetable Salads, Rice Stuffed Vine Leaves, Pita Bread (without oil or butter), Roasted Aubergine, Soupa, Seafood, Tabbouleh, Plaki, Baba Ghanoush, Shish-Kebab.
WATCH OUT FOR:	Pan-Fried, Filo Pastry, Tahini, Tzatziki (with full-fat yoghurt), Goat Cheese, Hoummus, Feta, Kasseri, Pastries (especially nuts), Lamb, Olives, Anchovies, Falafel, Locanico (sausage), Moussaka, Ice Cream.
ASK:	(If pita is served) May I have the pitta without butter or oil? Is this dish prepared with a lot of oil/butter? If yes, can the oil/butter used in preparation be reduced or omitted?
INDIAN	
LOOK FOR:	Roasted, Marinated, Soup, Tandoori, Vegetables, Rice, Chapti, Naan, Tomatoes, and Onions.
WATCH OUT FOR:	Fried, Pakora, Batter-Dipped, Samosa, Coconut/Coconut Milk, Ghee, Desserts, Cream Sauce, Lamb, Fritters, Raita (with full-fat yoghurt), Pappadams, Puri.
ASK:	Is the yoghurt sauce made with full-fat yoghurt? Is this dish prepared with a lot of oil/ butter? If yes, can the oil/butter used in preparation be reduced or omitted?
ITALIAN	
LOOK FOR:	Baked, Grilled, Roasted, Marinated, Sautéed, Polenta, Pasta, Half-Orders, Beans, Medallions, Vinaigrette, Tomatoes, Vegetables, Salads, Primavera, Fresh Clam Sauces, Mushroom Sauces, Vegetable Pizza Toppings, Seafood.
WATCH OUT FOR:	Cream Sauces, Risotto, Alfredo, Four-Cheese, Extra Cheese, Fried Aubergine, Parmigiana, Pancetta, Carbonara, Francese, Milanese, Prosciutto, Tortellini, Piccata, Ham, Olives, Pepperoni, Salami, Meatballs.
ASK:	Is the aubergine fried? Is this dish prepared with a lot of oil/butter? If yes, can the oil/ butter used in preparation be reduced? Are half orders of pasta available? Is this pizza made with part skimmed mozzarella or without cheese?

Never, never, never feel bashful about taking care of yourself by ordering healthy foods. What you eat 99 per cent of the time makes the most difference in your overall health. A slight deviation from your meal plan on your birthday or another special occasion is not terrible, as long as it only occurs occasionally (once a month at most). But if you are following a low-fat diet because you have heart disease, even an occasional high-fat meal stresses your system and can cause problems. It would be wise to play it safe and stick to your healthy eating plan all the time.

Becoming an expert at deciphering menus the Active Wellness way doesn't take long. When you dine out, the anxiety of finding healthy foods on a menu is diminished. Food becomes a pleasurable part of the whole dining experience, rather than your sole focus. And when food becomes less of an issue for you, you'll feel more in control of your overall health.

Quick Meal Strategies

Of course, some dining experiences are the 'grab, eat and run' kind. Often breakfast and lunch fall into these categories. During the day we typically run errands and do work, which leaves little time to prepare and eat meals. Eating becomes a matter of convenience. But remember that satisfaction remains important, regardless of how quickly or slowly you need to eat. And finding satisfying, quick meals is difficult unless you know where to look and what to do.

If you can't prepare your own quick meals at home, your quickest option becomes the first available food that has enough taste and bulk to satisfy your hunger. Take-out or fast-food meals become the most tempting choice in a time crunch, and good options are available. You can choose from home-delivery places, delis, fast-food restaurants, pizza shops, cafeterias and cafés.

You have two main options for quick meals. One is to opt for prepared food that is available through home-delivery services, supermarkets, and home meal-preparation services. Prepared healthy-food services or even home meal-preparation, usually done by private chefs, can provide meals that meet your nutritional specifications. When your meals are pre-made, you can bring the food with you to work for heating up, or you can sit down to a well-cooked meal at home. More supermarkets are starting to carry a line of prepared meals that include a nutrition label, so you can identify which foods meet your health needs. Freshly prepared, packaged food is becoming more popular as well.

Your other option is to locate several food sources, including supermarkets, delicatessens, take-out emporiums and pizza shops, that are close to your home or office. Following is a list of lunch foods to look for in those 'on-the-go' eating locations.

Supermarkets

Hot Foods: soups; freeze-dried soups; microwave low-fat main courses; bean spreads; wholemeal crackers or bread; roast chicken (remove the skin).

Cold Foods: salad bars (but choose salads that do not contain mayonnaise); fresh turkey; lean roast beef; ham; fresh crabmeat; fresh vegetables; pre-made salads; fresh fruit or pre-diced fruit salads; fat-free and low-fat cheese and yoghurt.

Deli Tips

Almost all of the salads at the deli contain a great deal of oil and mayonnaise, so be careful and ask about salad ingredients.

When you order a sandwich at a deli, you usually receive 4 oz (115 g) of meat. If you want less meat, ask for less. Or take part of it out, and take it home.

Delicatessens

Any bread, except white (avoid rolls); grilled chicken breast; fresh turkey breast; ham; lean roast beef; stock-, tomato- or vegetable-based soups (bean soups can make a complete meal); low-fat or fat-free yoghurt; hard boiled eggs; health salads (take from the top, since deli salads have less oil there than on the bottom); fruit salads.

Pizzerias

Regular pizza; pizza without cheese; pizza with vegetable toppings, except fried aubergine; pasta (half the order) with tomato sauce; any vegetables. (At a pizzeria, the best choice is usually pizza. Some shops now use part-skimmed mozzarella to make their pizza. Ask your local pizza establishment what they use.)

Cafés

Egg-white omelettes; sandwiches (with any bread other than white bread); turkey; chicken breast; lean roast beef; tuna without mayonnaise (try balsamic vinegar with plain tuna and you'll be surprised how good it tastes); salads; vegetable-, tomato- or stock-based soups (bean soups can make a complete meal); fresh fish; pasta with tomato sauce; lean burgers, turkey burgers or veggie burgers; fresh fruit; low-fat yoghurt or cottage cheese; cereal with skimmed milk.

Fast-Food Emporiums

Pasta with chicken or tuna and vegetables in a tomato sauce; grilled fish; skinless poultry; fajitas without soured cream and light on the guacamole; burritos with reduced-fat cheese and low-fat soured cream; salads with meat or fish added; low-fat salad dressing; grilled chicken breast; plain, lean beef burgers; baked potatos; salads with low-fat dressing. (Note: Fast-food establishments provide the smallest selection of fresh fruits, vegetables and wholemeal breads.)

One look at the calorie and fat content of this very basic fast-food order dramatically demonstrates how you could eat about half of your calorie allotment for the entire day in just one meal—and get the equivalent of 8 fat options!

Basic Fast-Food Order

Basic hamburger (with bun)	=	245 calories and 11 grams of fat
With 1 slice cheese	=	+100 calories and 9 grams of fat
With 1 tbsp/15 ml) mayonnaise	=	+100 calories and 9 grams of fat
With small portion of chips	=	+220 calories and 12 grams of fat

Total = 665 calories and 41 grams of fat

Salad Bars

We tend to assume that salads are healthy, but the truth is that salads can be just as high in calories and fat as a typical fast-food meal. If you want to approach a salad bar with nutritional savvy, follow these few healthy rules:

◇ If you like greens, choose the darkest salad greens that are offered, including romaine, leaf lettuce and spinach. Or combine them for variety.

◇ Choose any other vegetable from the salad bar that you like, provided the vegetables are not marinated in oil, dressed with mayonnaise or fried. If the items look creamy or shiny, avoid them. Good vegetable choices are broccoli, tomatoes, mushrooms, cucumbers, green peppers, carrots, cauliflower, beetroot, spinach and radishes.

◇ Look for protein sources to top off your salad, such as plain tuna (without mayonnaise or oil); chunks of chicken (without mayonnaise or oil); tofu; a tablespoon or two of Parmesan cheese or low-fat cottage cheese; or a few spoonfuls of beans.

◇ Dress your salad with low-fat salad dressing, flavoured vinegar or balsamic vinegar. If you want to make your own salad dressing, mix equal parts plain yoghurt with mustard or mix 1 tsp (5 ml) of mustard with some balsamic vinegar and a packet of sugar or artificial sweetener.

◇ For dessert, have fresh fruit.

Best Bite for Breakfast

Research has shown time and again that children who eat breakfast are more attentive and do better in school. The same is true for adults. Think of breakfast as your body's wake-up call, the first fuel of the day, which stimulates your metabolism. I often hear from my Active Wellness clients who don't eat breakfast that they find themselves hungrier later in the evening, because they didn't have enough 'fuel' throughout the day.

Eating earlier, rather than later, makes sense because our metabolism functions at a higher rate during the day. When we sleep, our metabolism decreases. This means that the food you eat late at night is not burned as efficiently as the food that is eaten during the day. In the morning, even a little something is always better than nothing.

Smart Breakfast Choices When You're On-the-Go

Cereal with low-fat or skimmed milk; instant oatmeal; non-fat or low-fat yoghurt; boiled or poached egg; plain egg-white sandwich on toast; fresh fruit; fresh yoghurt shake with berries (aka 'smoothie'); whole- grain toast with low-fat cream cheese

Note: Eating fruit provides bulk in your diet and helps prevent an increase in your hunger level throughout the morning.

Most people don't plan to fail, they fail to plan.
—John L. Beckley

Strategies for Special Occasions

Planning ahead, nutrition-wise, is key when you go to a special function or catered affair, such as a wedding, anniversary or birthday party, bar/bat mitzvah or christening. Here are some guidelines to keep you on your Active Wellness programme and enjoy yourself at the same time.

⋄ Don't go to the event hungry. For one thing, you don't know what is being served as a main course, so you might be inclined to overindulge in appetizers before the main dinner. Eat a light snack at home before leaving for the event. That way, you can eat less during the cocktail hour and focus on enjoying the conversation and the drink in your hand, rather than indulging in appetizers.

⋄ If you drink alcohol during the cocktail hour, start slowly so you can remain within your daily allowance. Try beginning with a glass of sparkling water with a slice of lime or lemon added. No one will know this is not alcoholic. Or try mixing juices together with sparkling water (half juice and half water). This drink is both tasty and healthy, and has more flavour than water with lemon or lime. You can also opt to have a weaker drink by mixing less alcohol than is the standard serving portion.

⋄ Determine whether you want to have the hors d'oeuvres for dinner or the main meal. This is not as strange as it sounds. The cocktail-appetizer part of the party usually gives you more of a selection of foods than the main meal. It is up to you whether you want to eat your dinner from the appetizers or the dinner course. One good way to determine your eating strategy is to ask a waiter what the main course will be. If the waiter doesn't know, ask him to find out on the next trip to the kitchen.

⋄ Avoid all fried, cheesy, pastry, or dough-based appetizers. Look for vegetables, sushi, sliced meat, steamed shellfish or pasta. Watch your portion sizes. Try to eat only one serving of several appetizers or make a meal of a favourite one. Don't load up on each type of appetizer. Do your best to estimate how the appetizers fulfil the option equivalents on your Daily Allowance Card.

⋄ During the cocktail hour, if you feel that none of the food being served meets your eating plan requirements, try to arrange to have a vegetarian plate made up for you. A vegetarian plate usually consists of several vegetables that are available in the kitchen, plus potatoes. Specify that you would like this served as your main course, otherwise the meal served usually includes a piece of chicken, fish or beef, with a grain or potato and some vegetables. You do not have to eat much of the meal if you don't like it. Enjoy the conversation instead!

⬦ Dessert almost always looks better than it tastes, but if you feel it's worth a try, help yourself! Opt to take only a bite or two of a dessert, and stop there. The dessert table, with its abundance of choices, provides great temptation to many people. The way to handle any large array of choices is by planning what you'll take before you approach the table. Fruit should be your first choice. If you find yourself eyeing the pastries, ask yourself if they are really worth the calories. If not, perhaps you can wait for dessert until you go home. Then enjoy one of your favourite low-fat treats—without the guilt and extra calories!

Strategies for Dinner Parties

If you're going to someone else's home to eat and they're friends of yours, your best bet is to let them know about your health needs. If everyone is bringing a dish, feel free to bring something that fits into your eating plan. If you're comfortable with your hosts, you can also offer to contribute to the dinner. This makes the meal easier for everyone involved. It puts less of a burden on the hostess, and you'll feel less anxious about the event. Some of my Active Wellness participants have been so distraught about not having a choice at a dinner party that they opted to not go to the event —an unnecessary sacrifice. You can avoid this, if you plan ahead.

Strategies for Eating on the Road

Aeroplane Dining

While travelling, most of the eating you'll do will be on aeroplanes, in hotels and in coffee shops or cafés.

Each airline has a selection of meal options that are available in any class. They include low-fat or healthy choices; low sodium, kosher, vegetarian, non-dairy vegetarian and the regular meal option. If you travel first class, you have a better opportunity for making specific requests to adapt the meal being served. In coach, you simply need to choose ahead which option best fits your requirements.

I always suggest ordering the low-fat choice on most flights. On overseas flights, you may want to stick with the regular meal because it usually offers a variety of foods, including at least one that is heart-healthy. To order a special meal, call ahead to your travel agent or the airline and place your order when you purchase your ticket or at least a week prior to your travel time. Once you have ordered your meal, try to call several days before your flight to confirm that they have your special order.

Another factor to consider when flying is the quick rate of dehydration the body experiences, which makes it important to drink as much water as you can during the flight.

Eating on the Road: Cars, Hotels, Coffee Shops, and Cafés

One of the best ways to ensure that you always have something healthy to eat while travelling is to pack your own 'travel eating kit'. The sidebar on the right contains a list of items you can purchase at the airport to carry on to the plane in case you prefer not to eat the food served. You can also keep your eating kit with you in your car or hotel room. The list is broken down into daily supplies that you may want to have on hand for a possible 'emergency' and supplies for longer trips and hotel stays.

Eating for Satisfaction

Whether you are taking a three-week car trip or dining alone in your hotel room, sometimes how you eat is just as important as what you eat. (This is true for dining at home as well!)

Travel Eating Kit

⬦ **Daily Emergency Supplies**
Packets of low-fat salad dressing
Packets of whole-grain crackers
Herbal or decaffeinated tea or
  coffee bags
A packet of dehydrated soup

⬦ **Supplies for Longer Trips**
Low-fat yoghurt
Instant oatmeal packets
Fruit
Rice cracker snacks
Bottled water
Dehydrated low-fat and fat-free
  soups in a cup

Whenever you eat, make sure that you aim for the most satisfying eating experience possible. I call this 'learning to dine like a European'. In continental Europe, meals are regarded as an important part of the day, and time and attention are devoted to them. Unfortunately in the US and Britain, especially if you work and live in a fast-paced environment, eating becomes secondary to any other activity you are doing at the same moment. Eating this way can never provide satisfaction or promote the enjoyment of the good tastes and textures of food. In order to feel as if you have eaten, you have to respect the eating experience, make time to enjoy your meals, and eat in a way that enhances the dining experience.

In many parts of Europe, if you're eating even a small meal at a coffeehouse, the waiter covers the table with a large cloth napkin, which acts as a tablecloth, and sets it with silverware, which creates the sense that you are dining properly. This and other simple dining strategies can help you feel more satisfied, and therefore more satiated, with the food you've eaten. And, when you feel satiated, you are less likely to help yourself to seconds or to binge later.

*Pleasure is the object, duty and the goal of
all rational creatures.*

—Voltaire

Simple Dining Tips to Use Anywhere

⋄ Always sit down to eat.
⋄ Make sure the eating atmosphere is as enjoyable as
  possible.
⋄ As you eat, focus on the tastes and sensations
  of your food and savour each bite.
⋄ As you eat, ask yourself the following questions:
   ⋄ Do I like the food I am eating?
   ⋄ What do I like about the food?
   ⋄ Is the flavour and texture satisfying to me?
   ⋄ Do I feel like eating more because I am enjoying
     the food so much?
⋄ Take your time when you eat, and chew your food well. The
  more relaxed you are, the better your digestion will be.
⋄ Use the meal layering strategy you learned earlier in this chapter
  to help you feel full as you eat.

Physical Fitness Away from Home

Exercising away from home is fairly simple these days because many hotels have fitness centres on site. Also, many fitness centres allow you to use their facilities for a day, if you're away from home. Easy-to-pack fitness accessories allow you to exercise in your hotel room. But wherever you go, bring along your trainers and workout attire. If there is a pool, bringing your swimsuit is also a good idea!

Making Fitness Easy

If no gym is available, be prepared to adapt your programme to your environment by locating a place to walk or jog and using some easy-to-pack fitness tools. In fact, you can liven up your daily walk or jog by taking a mini 'walking tour' through your new surroundings. All three components of your physical fitness programme—stretching, aerobics and strength training—can be adapted for practising away from home.

Stretching Away from Home

In general, a stretching routine *(see Step 5, pages 159-160)* can be done anywhere, providing you have a small space in your room. If your room doesn't have enough space, try stretching outside your room in the hallway or outdoors in the sunshine when the weather is good. If you do your stretching routine in the morning, you'll feel more alert throughout the day. Once you stretch, move on to the aerobic or strength training portion of your programme.

Aerobics Away from Home

If you can't find a gym in the area where you are staying, adapt your aerobic programme to the environment you are in. One of the easiest ways to do aerobics is to walk at a brisk pace, which can be done just about anywhere. Brisk walking for 20 minutes quickly burns approximately 100 calories—the equivalent of jogging for 10 minutes.

If you normally jog, this is an easily transportable activity, as long as you remember to pack your trainers and make sure you don't get lost in an unfamiliar neighborhood. You may also want to pack a portable radio and headphones, so that you can listen to music while you're walking or jogging. An upbeat tempo will also help you keep up your pace.

If you're travelling strictly on business, your time is more limited than if you are travelling for pleasure. Nevertheless, you may find time for one or more of the following activities: walking, jogging, going to a gym, playing racquetball, tennis or golf (briskly walking the course) and swimming.

If you're on holiday and travelling simply for pleasure, you can choose from a number of aerobic activities. These might include cycling, rollerblading, ice skating or rowing (you can rent the necessary equipment in most larger cities and towns), hiking and water-skiing.

Strength Training Away from Home

Lugging weights around in your suitcase is not a practical way to travel. You can, however, keep up with your strength training on the road by using your own weight as resistance *(see Step 5, pages 157-158)* or by bringing along resistance bands for working out. Go to a sports shop to find inexpensive resistance bands that provide the same weight resistance as free weights. Some have the additional advantage of having handles, which makes them easier to grip. These bands come with their own instruction book and set of resistance exercises.

Stress Management Away from Home

Your Active Wellness stress management programme can be done anywhere, as long as you make time for it. You'll find stress management particularly beneficial when you are on a business trip, because it helps diminish the stress associated with airline travelling, meeting deadlines, irregular hours and living out of a suitcase.

Another great stress management tool when on the road is an audio cassette tape. You can purchase specially designed meditation tapes that guide you through deep relaxation and visualization exercises.

Stress Management Routines for the Office, Train or Plane

Finally, many stress management routines can be adapted to use at work or when travelling on a train or plane. Below are some simple breathing, stretching and yoga exercises, all of which can be done while you are seated. You can do each of the exercise sets at different times during the day. You may prefer to combine all three components of the routine into one mini stress management workout, which is especially beneficial when you travel.

Breathing Exercise

Take three deep meditating breaths to relax. Repeat two or three times. You can also use a stress management audio cassette tape to practise deep breathing or listen to relaxing meditation music.

Stretching Exercises

Stretch your neck by gently rotating your head from the front to the right side, to the back and to the left side in a circular motion. First, look straight ahead, then drop your chin to your chest and allow your neck to stretch for approximately 15 seconds. Slowly move your head to the right so that your ear is touching or is horizontal to your right shoulder. Remember to stretch only to a point that is comfortable for you. Now slowly rotate your head toward the back and then continue around to your left shoulder. Repeat this stretch three times.

Gentle Yoga Exercises

Sitting yoga postures energize you and relieve some of the tension caused by work or by sitting for long periods of time. Follow the diagrams shown for each posture.

Seated Spine Twist: Sitting straight in a chair with a back, with your feet flat on the floor, place your left hand on the outside of your right knee and your right hand on the back of your seat. Look forward and gently inhale as you turn toward the right, twisting your spine as far as possible without strain and exhaling at the furthest point. Repeat this three times. Perform the exercise twisting to the left, switching hands so that your left hand is on the back of your seat.

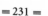

Seated Knee Squeeze: Sit straight up and forward in your seat. Breathe in and lift your right knee up toward your chest. Exhale, inhale, grab your knee with both hands, and hold your breath while gently squeezing your knee toward your chest. Exhale as you release your leg, and return it with one smooth movement back to the floor. (If you have joint problems with your knees, grab your inside thigh instead, to reduce the pressure placed on your knee.) Repeat the exercise three times. Then switch legs to perform the exercise four times.

Overhead Stretch for Shoulders, Arms, and Upper Back: Hold your right arm up and bend it behind your head, grasping your elbow with your left hand and gently pulling the elbow downward until you feel an easy tension in the shoulder or back of the upper arm. Breathe and hold the stretch for 30 seconds. Do not force this stretch. Repeat the exercise three times with each arm.

Lower Back Stretch: To end your stretches you can do a lower back stretch by sitting forward in your chair and leaning over your knees, as shown in the diagram. This releases the tension in your back. Make sure you hang your neck down to release the tension there as well. Look toward your feet. Hold this stretch for 45 seconds. Breathe throughout the stretch. When you are ready to return to a seated position, you can use the seat of your chair or your thighs for support as you push up.

End your routine by taking three deep breaths, inhaling and exhaling through your nose.

Travel never needs to be tedious again if you think of it as a special time to devote to yourself and to your health. You've nearly completed the Active Wellness programme, realized many of your short-term goals, and are well on the way to experiencing your long-term goal of lifelong wellness. It's time to take a breather, and congratulate yourself for a job well done. To reward yourself, move on to Step 9, where you will learn some new techniques for nurturing yourself and maintaining your successes.

As you travelled along the Active Wellness path, you may have noticed what happened as you applied yourself more to a specific goal: it became easier to practise your new behaviour in the short term and to achieve that goal in a shorter length of time.

Long-term changes (the ones that are meant to last a lifetime), however, require renewed vigilance, patience, and practice. As you progress and mature along the wellness path, you will continue to use your new awareness and health skills to replace unhealthy behaviours with healthy ones. But to truly feel good for life, you need some new tools as touchstones for your journey.

New Tools for a Lifetime of Active Wellness
- ◇ Commit to Yourself
- ◇ Nurture Yourself
- ◇ Use Positive Reinforcement and Visualizations
- ◇ Do a Realistic Self-Appraisal
- ◇ Set Realistic Goals
- ◇ Ask for Support and Cooperation
- ◇ Use the Strategies for Maintaining Success
- ◇ Prioritize Your Long-Term Goals

Commit to Yourself

The very act of taking responsibility for your own health actually furthers your good health. Research shows that caring, nurturing people are healthier and happier. Making a compassionate commitment to care for ourselves and others gives us a sense of purpose and enhances our self-worth and well-being. How much more powerful is a compassionate commitment to our own good health?

Nurture Yourself

Nurture yourself with rewards and self-care. Rewards can come in the form of gifts, personal treats or special events. For self-care, use the information you learned about yourself during the Active Wellness journey to replace something that is missing from your life, which may even be hurting your health.

An example of self-care involves realizing that you overeat when you are bored, lonely or stressed. One of the most nurturing gifts you can give yourself is something to help replace those feelings—and prevent you from sabotaging your eating plan. If you are lonely, join a support group or club. If you are bored, try a new hobby. If you are stressed, take a day off or treat yourself to a yoga class.

Use Positive Reinforcement and Visualizations

The daily affirmations you created in Step 4 can be used as positive reinforcements for your new wellness lifestyle. Try saying your affirmations to yourself every day and keep them displayed in your home or at your office. If you prefer, you can also buy pre-made affirmation cards or refer to inspirational books for positive sayings.

Positive reinforcement can also take the form of visualizations based on thoughts and memories. Remember how great you felt when you succeeded at riding a bike, operating a computer or putting together a stereo system? Then remember how wonderful your Active Wellness efforts felt when you completed your first day of exercise or cleaned out your cupboards of unhealthy foods. Those are big accomplishments! Remembering how it feels to accomplish something worthwhile—and picturing it in your mind—brings you closer to achieving your next Active Wellness goal.

Sometimes, remembering even negative 'achievements' can help you stay on track. Occasionally recalling how bad you felt to be out of shape, eat in unhealthy ways, or feel acutely stressed can help you stay on the wellness path—just to avoid feeling that bad again! Then use visualization to help you create an image of how it looks and feels to be successful and to achieve your goals.

Do a Realistic Self-Appraisal

Honest self-appraisal is critical to maintaining your wellness progress. How did you see yourself at the start of your Active Wellness journey? Who are you today? How capable are you of staying on course and achieving your long-term health goals?

Achieving your long-term goals takes time and patience. In order to move forward, you need to accept how far you have come. Think of your gains, no matter how small, as real progress. All your efforts may not be visible, but every change you made took effort. And every effort you've made is worth recognizing, rewarding and positively reinforcing.

Perhaps you're disappointed because you didn't achieve as much as you wanted. But any movement forward is progress, and progress is always a slow and deliberate learning process. With each step, you build upon the success you achieved in an earlier step. Bit by bit, you'll begin to weave together the fabric of a lifetime of healthy living. Without the first, small steps and slow, steady progress, your changes would never be permanent.

One helpful tool for positively reinforcing your small and large successes is to do a realistic daily appraisal of how your day went. At the end of each day, divide your experiences into several categories:

- Things you or others did that pleased you
- Things you wish you had done

◊ Things you didn't want to do but did anyway

◊ Things that you can't change

Things You or Others Did That Pleased You

Reflect on positive experiences and favourable compliments that occurred throughout your day. Cherish them. Unfortunately, we tend to accentuate the negative and forget the positive. Don't let a positive experience go by without acknowledging it and holding on to it. If someone gives you a compliment, accept it and let it make you feel good. You deserve it. When you do something that you are proud of, give yourself a pat on the back or a nurturing reward.

Things You Wish You Had Done

Learn from your mistakes and then move on. Nobody is perfect. When you've done something you wish you hadn't done, think about how you might do things differently in the future. Mistakes are an integral part of learning. They provide essential feedback when we are learning new behaviours and tasks, which makes them, ironically, vital to our going forward to eventual success. Many times, a mistake means that we're finally learning how to do something new.

Things You Didn't Want to Do but Did Anyway

Sometimes we just can't help ourselves. No matter how much we know better, we still go ahead and do or say something that is counterproductive to our good health and well-being. Our stronger desires and passions get the best of us, and we yield to temptation: opting, for example, for sticky toffee pudding instead of fresh fruit for dessert. Let those kinds of occasional slips go, forgive yourself and move on. You're not a bad person who has no will power. You're simply human and you yielded to a little temptation. Instead of beating yourself up about occasional slips and missteps, use these situations to expand your awareness about yourself regarding your true needs and wants around a particular temptation or old pattern, whether it's eating rich desserts, neglecting exercise or slipping back into unhealthy behaviours. Expanding your awareness helps you understand why you 'slipped' to begin with and gives you the confidence to move forward with a greater understanding of yourself and your behaviour.

Things that You Can't Change

Obsessing about things that have already happened or have been said, which simply cannot be changed, is a waste of time and energy. They are out of your control, so one of the best things you can do for yourself is to just let them go. A useful way to let go of such experiences is to write them down and then destroy or discard them—in effect, eliminating them from your life.

Set Realistic Goals

Were your original goals reasonable and realistic? Often we sabotage our chances for success when we set unrealistic goals or have grandiose expectations. We inadvertently set ourselves up for failure, then we channel the energy we could have used in achieving our goals into unhealthy behaviours.

In the space below, write down one of the short- or long-term goals that you set for yourself in Step 1 of your Active Wellness programme, then write down the steps you took to achieve that goal. Stop at the point where you are right now with that goal, and pay particular attention to the problems that you overcame and the obstacles that may still stand in the way of your success.

My Original Goal: _____

Steps Taken to Achieve My Goal:

1. _____

2. _____

3. _____

4. _____

5. _____

6. _____

7. _____

8. _____

9. _____

10. _____

What else do you need to do to achieve your original goals or to reach any new goals you set for yourself? You may want to use what you learned in the previous assessment to establish a new, realistic short-term goal.

The best way to succeed in your Active Wellness programme is to continue to set attainable short-term goals each week, all designed to help you achieve a long-term wellness goal. As you complete one goal, set a new one. For example, if your long-term goal is to reach your ideal weight and feel physically fit, your short-term goal that week might be to eliminate all high-calorie desserts from your diet and eat fruit instead. The next week, your short-term goal might be to drink eight glasses of water a day, without fail. The following week, your new short-term goal might be to start walking a half-mile a day after dinner.

As you tackle each new short-term goal, you will encounter obstacles—new and old—along the path to success. Use your new behaviour management skills to short-circuit those obstacles. If you're having difficulty achieving your short- or long-term goals, feel free to seek help from professionals and friends.

Eventually—and perhaps now—you'll be ready to set a new long-term goal for yourself. If you've been concentrating on eating well and exercising, you may want to move on to stress management. When you're ready, take a moment to record your new long-term goal and the new steps—short-term, weekly goals—that you'll take to achieve that goal.

My New or Current Goal: _____

Steps I Will Take to Achieve That Goal:

1. _____

2. _____

3. _____

4. _____

5. _____

6. _____

7. _____

8. _____

9. _____

10. _____

As you continue with your Active Wellness programme, consider purchasing a small notepad for keeping a list of your short- and long-term goals. Checking off your accomplishments will feel great and will reinforce your sense of success and self-empowerment.

To celebrate your progress along the Active Wellness journey, remember the word *REWARD*. It will remind you to acknowledge all your gains, small and large, and to remain committed to your programme.

REWARD = Recognize Every Win And Remain Driven

> *Be proud of your accomplishments no matter how small.*
> —Gayle Reichler

Ask for Support and Cooperation

Creating change in your life is never easy. Certainly some changes come more easily than others, but in the long run focusing on your health takes conscious effort and energy.

Accepting support and encouragement from others is one of the best ways to help yourself stay committed to your goals. Having friends, loved ones and co-workers as your personal cheerleaders and confidantes helps you stay on the Active Wellness track. Feeling appreciated and accepted for who you are during the good times helps you maintain a positive outlook during the tough times. Also, wanting to please your loved ones gives you another reason to succeed. If doing it for yourself (which is the most important reason) just isn't enough, then do it for the others who care for and believe in you so much.

Going through major changes alone is very difficult—more than it needs to be. When you have friends and family rooting for you on the sidelines and when you have people in your life who are genuinely concerned about your well-being, then making changes somehow feels easier and less frightening.

If you feel that you don't have friends and loved ones in whom you can confide, consider joining a structured support group. You can find both therapy and self-help-oriented groups that focus on both specific and general issues around health and well-being. Some self-help groups meet simply so members can support one another through a similar experience, such as having breast cancer, heart disease, diabetes, or overeating problems. Structured therapeutic groups usually are led by therapists who are specifically trained in group dynamics.

Groups can provide great support systems. They are places where you can speak freely and confidentially to others who understand your personal situation and can give you objective feedback. You feel less alone in your wellness journey and, by sharing your own experiences, others can learn from you.

You can also seek out a non-therapeutic type of support group, one that directly helps you actualize your Active Wellness lifestyle. This might include fitness groups that walk, jog or cycle together. You can also join an Active Wellness programme near your home for support in making Active Wellness a lifetime goal.

(For more information about Active Wellness please visit our website at www.activewellness.com.)

Learn How to Communicate Effectively

As you make personal changes in your life, you'll begin to see greater changes in your self-awareness, your needs and your goals. Your new perspective, though significant to you, may not always be obvious to other people. If you are looking for support and cooperation from others, you may need to make them aware of what you need.

You may be surprised by how many people want to help you, once you let them know how they can help. But no one, not even those who love you most, can help you effectively if you don't communicate what you want from them. Learn how to clearly articulate your needs and wants in a way that is truly heard and understood by others. Effective communication with others is crucial to being understood.

Effective Communication

Effective communication is an open exchange between people that promotes discussion and builds relationships. It is usually an exchange where words and manner are analogous to behaviour expressing the same feeling. The object of effective communication is to be heard and understood in order to make one's feelings and thoughts known to another. Effective communication is also reciprocal. Like an emotional *pas de deux*, we alternate between listening and speaking, empathizing and sharing.

If you look at great actors and actresses, you can see how powerful their excellent communication skills can be. In communicating the emotional life of a character, the actress uses her tone of voice, expression of words, actions and body language to let the audience fully 'know' who that character is.

An alternative way of communicating that is much less effective is 'venting'. Venting is very one-sided, emotional communication. If someone is venting, you usually feel that you can't get a word in edgewise and can't truly communicate with that person. Venting often arises from a build-up of emotions that need to be released. The storing of emotions creates an energy force that needs to be discharged—so much so that the need to release the feelings often overpowers the need to be heard.

If you find yourself constantly venting rather than communicating, you might consider this a sign that you're unable to ask for what you need or to express your feelings and needs in ways that make them genuinely 'heard'. You need to sharpen your communication skills because venting simply turns people off—and then they really don't hear you.

Communicating So That Your Message Is Heard

Effective communication, the type that helps you get what you need, involves learning to express yourself with assertiveness, which means you know what you want and how to ask for it directly. When you communicate effectively with assertiveness, others can listen more easily and you're more likely to be heard.

You want your entire message to be heard, and the entire message is composed of three main parts:

⋄ Your thoughts
⋄ Your feelings
⋄ Your request

The rewards of sending effective messages are many, including meeting your needs, increased self-esteem, less bickering and improved relationships. Let's briefly review the how's and why's of each of the components of an effectively communicated message.

Your Thoughts: Be Clear about Them. Express your view or perspective on a specific situation calmly and clearly. Give your listener your frame of reference.

> *Example*: I have read *Active Wellness*, and now I am focusing on integrating a personalized wellness programme into my lifestyle so I can stay healthy.

Your Feelings: Express Them Clearly from an 'I' Perspective. Our feelings help us to connect through empathy. Our feelings help us to understand one another, because each of us can remember a time when we had a similar feeling. The best way to communicate feelings is by taking responsibility for them, speaking from the 'I', and never placing the responsibility for how we feel on someone else (which isn't communication and only elicits a defensive and angry response from others).

> Examples of effectively communicated feelings from the 'I' position include: I feel tired; I feel frustrated; I am happy; I am glad; I was disappointed.

> Examples of placing the responsibility for your feelings on someone else include: You are not listening; You don't care; You don't understand; You're not thinking of me; You made me feel upset.

Your Request: Simply State What You Need or Want. When your thoughts are clear and you 'own' your feelings, you can simply state what you need or want effectively and unemotionally. When you combine all three communication components—thoughts, feelings, and request—together, you have an effective and powerful statement and you can communicate skilfully.

> *Example*: I have read *Active Wellness*, and I am focusing on integrating a personalized wellness programme into my lifestyle so I can stay healthy. I am very happy about my new decision. However, I am worried that I don't have the support I need. It would be very helpful to me if I could share my progress with you as I continue with the programme.

If this is not your normal way of communicating, don't worry. With practice, it becomes easier, even though initially you have to make a conscious effort to structure your sentences carefully for effective communication. If you're concerned about your listener's response, try saying your message aloud to yourself before approaching someone. You'll gain confidence and reassurance from 'practising'.

Listening: The Forgotten Component of Effective Communication

Listening effectively is as important as sending effective messages. When someone is talking to you, they may or may not be communicating effectively. If you are a good listener, however, you can 'read between the lines'. You can observe their body language and empathize with how they are feeling.

When you listen well, you truly hear the feelings that are being expressed and acknowledge them with empathy. Empathetic listening translates to compassion and support. The other person feels understood, which opens real lines of effective communication.

By combining effective listening with effective communication, you build support systems that make maintaining your Active Wellness programme easier. Such support is especially important for those times when you slip off the wellness path and have a relapse.

Use the Strategies for Maintaining Success

Nobody is perfect. We all have times when maintaining our Active Wellness programme becomes difficult. Since learning new skills takes time, energy, and practice, don't be surprised if you occasionally lapse into old, unhealthy habits. Relapses are more likely to occur in high stress situations involving arguments, job stress, social pressure, and negative emotional states.

PEACE: On your Active Wellness journey, if you find yourself heading down a crooked path that feels like an old habit or pattern, try your best to stop what you are doing at that moment and change your direction. The word PEACE can help you think through the steps to choosing a new, healthier route rather than relapsing into old behaviours.

P = Pause and take a few deep breaths
E = Experience the moment
A = Acknowledge your thoughts and feelings
C = Choose what you feel is best for you to do
E = Enjoy the choice

Here are some strategies that other Active Wellness participants have successfully used when they felt they were veering off the path of wellness.

Real-Life Strategies for Maintaining Success
- Take things one day at a time. Just because you had trouble today, doesn't mean you'll have trouble tomorrow.
- Use your new habits as substitutes for your old behaviours.
- Distract yourself with something else. Try deep breathing, meditating on a beautiful scene, writing a letter to a friend, listening to music, taking a walk, writing down new affirmations or reading a book.
- Work through your Active Wellness programme by trying to accomplish one realistic short-term goal each week. Stick with the same goal until you achieve it, then move on.
- Reward yourself for your positive efforts.
- Forgive yourself for your relapses. Relapses happen to everybody. Don't beat yourself up over them. Just regain control and move on.
- Treat yourself with love and understanding. You deserve it!
- Give yourself time to notice visible results. Let longer intervals go by— two weeks or a month—before you measure yourself, weigh yourself or do a self-appraisal.

Compassion: The Last Essential Ingredient for Maintaining Success
One of the best things you can do for yourself is to treat yourself with compassion. Compassion for yourself means you accept yourself. When you accept yourself, you'll find it easier to let go of the occasional relapse and get back on a healthy track. With compassion, you won't feel like a failure when you fall off the wellness path; you'll simply feel human, get up, dust yourself off, and start all over again.

Compassion is equal parts understanding, acceptance and forgiveness. With understanding, you seek to observe and learn about yourself with curiosity instead of criticism. With acceptance, you not only accept yourself and your strengths and weaknesses, but you respect others as well. You are who you are, and they are who they are. If you want to improve yourself by becoming stronger or leaner or healthier, that's great. However, the greatest strides in good health and well-being may finally occur only when you accept yourself as you are, anytime, in any moment. Then you find yourself centred and truly at peace. With forgiveness, you let go of mistakes.

Forgiveness means learning from the past and moving on with no regrets. Forgiveness also means that you stay rooted in the present and look forward to the future with a clean slate. Learning to sincerely forgive—yourself and others—may take time, but it is essential to good health and body, mind and spirit wellness. The opposite of forgiveness is resentment, which can eat away at our inner strength and sabotage the best of intentions. Forgiveness is liberation from resentment, and that liberation is nothing less than a dose of optimal good feeling.

> *Motivation is what gets you started*
> *Habit is what keeps you going.*
> —Jim Ryuh

Prioritize Your Long-Term Goals

To maintain your Active Wellness successes for a lifetime, you must learn to prioritize your long-term goals. Set your sights high, but be realistic. Make sure each new goal is reasonable, attainable and builds on a previous goal that you've successfully accomplished. The following list will help you prioritize your long-term goals for the future and assess where you are now. As you accumulate skills and knowledge, your learning speed will increase and you should find it easier to make small changes. Remember: you are in control. How far you travel in the Active Wellness journey is determined by what you choose for yourself and how you go about getting it. If you want to, you can do it.

Long-Term Goals Priority List
The goal(s) I have accomplished:

◇ _____

◇ _____

◇ _____

The goal I am working towards now:

◇ _____

The goals I plan to work towards in the coming months and future years:

◇ _____

◇ _____

◇ _____

All the strategies listed in this step are meant as suggestions and guides. If you have alternative solutions for helping yourself continue the Active Wellness journey, please feel free to use them. What's important is that you continue to take the road to healthy self-empowerment and a lifetime of wellness.

An Active Wellness Cooking Class

Cooking should be a carefully balanced reflection
of all the good things of the earth.
—Jean and Pierre Troisgros
from the *Nouvelle Cuisine of*
Jean and Pierre Troisgros

Contrary to what you may think, preparing healthy food that is also tasty isn't difficult. It simply involves learning a few easy techniques that you can use every time you cook. When you're preparing healthy foods, your goals should be to:

⋄ Create great tasting food that promotes good health.
⋄ Eliminate unhealthy ingredients in your cooking, such as
  saturated fats, hydrogenated fats and processed foods.

I have developed all of the recipes in this chapter under strict standards, with the help of Deborah Cohen, founding chef at Active Wellness. We are committed to preparing low-fat recipes that are as tasty and as satisfying as their full-fat counter-parts, while meeting all the nutritional guidelines to qualify as low fat and fat free. We use mainly fresh, whole foods (you are welcome to use organic ingredients if you pre-fer), and salt is only added when absolutely necessary.

The recipes are familiar favourites from a variety of cultures. Moreover, they are both flavourful and filling. The key to creating this great tasting food is to accentuate the full flavours of the fresh foods by choosing and combining the right ingredients and by using ingenious low-fat cooking techniques to bring out the full taste and tex-ture of the foods.

In this chapter, we present techniques that can be integrated into your entire cook-ing repertoire, whether you're preparing simple dinners during the week or planning an elaborate party menu for weekend guests. You'll soon be able to easily prepare pleas-ing meals that win rave reviews. You'll also be making delicious low-fat desserts that are just as satisfying as their high-fat counterparts.

The Active Wellness cooking class is organized according to the courses of a meal, from soup to dessert. Each course introduces simple techniques that you can apply to the recipes at the end of this chapter. Once you learn these techniques, you can apply them to all your favourite recipes—even those that aren't included in this book. You'll also be able to mix and match recipes with different kinds of foods to create delicious, one-of-a-kind meals for your friends and family.

First Things First: *Mise en Place*

Before you start cooking, you must be prepared. *Mise en place* is a French term that means to put everything in its place. *Mise en place* applies to setting up your kitchen for low-fat cooking; it also applies to preparing all of the ingredients prior to cooking.

Preparing the ingredients and measuring them out prior to combining them is considered your 'prep' before following a recipe. When you practise using *mise en place* in your cooking, you become more organized and the recipe is much quicker and easier to execute. Also, when you keep your larder stocked with all the basic ingredients, your shopping trips move quickly because you only need to buy fresh foods.

The following list of basic equipment and the basic larder staples list on the next page are helpful to have on hand for quick and easy low-fat cooking.

Basic Equipment

- A set of professional knives or, at a minimum, a good paring and chef knife
- Knife sharpener (steel or mechanical)
- Measuring cups (separate for liquids and dried foods)
- Measuring spoons
- Cutting board
- Food processor or hand blender
- Hand-held mixer
- Assorted small tools to make cooking easier: zester, vegetable peeler, grater, large strainer, kitchen shears, wire whisk, rubber spatulas, wooden spoons
- Timer
- Non-stick pots and pans
- Greaseproof paper
- Vegetable steamer
- Spray bottles for oil
- Storage containers for frozen foods

Basic Larder Staples

For the Cupboard:
⬥ Canned stock (vegetable, chicken, beef)
⬥ Corn flour, arrowroot or potato starch
⬥ Dried herbs, spices and fruits
⬥ Variety of grains
⬥ Variety of beans (canned or dried)
⬥ Flavoured oils and cooking oils (olive and peanut oils)
⬥ Flavouring sauces (e.g. low-sodium soy sauce, hot sauce, barbecue sauce)
⬥ Assorted vinegars (e.g. rice wine, balsamic, red wine and white wine)
⬥ Vanilla extract and other extracts of flavours you enjoy
⬥ Evaporated skimmed milk

For the Refrigerator/Freezer:
⬥ Fat-free and low-fat salad dressings
⬥ Condiments
⬥ Non-fat yogurt
⬥ Low-fat or fat-free mayonnaise
⬥ Non-fat or low-fat soured cream
⬥ Onions, garlic, hot peppers
⬥ Frozen stocks or soups
⬥ Skimmed or low-fat milk
⬥ Eggs or egg substitutes
⬥ Assorted sweeteners (e.g., honey, frozen grape
  juice concentrate, maple syrup)
⬥ Tortillas (corn or wholemeal)

A Special Note on Preparing Tasty Low-Fat Foods

When you reduce the fat in a recipe, learning how to properly compensate for the reduction in fat and still retain taste and texture is important. The key is to realize that fat has three primary functions in a recipe:

⬥ Fat carries the flavour
⬥ Fat adds moisture
⬥ Fat improves texture and provides a pleasing 'mouth feel'—the sensation
  of full, rounded flavours that linger in your mouth

Flavour Layering

When reducing or omitting fats from a recipe, pay careful attention to enhancing the flavour. In the Active Wellness kitchen, we use a strategy called 'flavour layering'. To compensate for the reduction of fat in a dish, we combine several flavours together to enhance the taste of the whole dish.

As you read through the recipes at the end of this chapter, think of ways to practise 'flavour layering' in each dish.

Soups

The base of any good soup is the stock. A stock is a flavoured broth or infused liquid of a meat, fish, poultry or vegetable flavour. A stock also works as a base for sauces, as well as the poaching and cooking liquid for grains or vegetables. In fact, a flavourful stock can be a great base for almost any recipe. You can subtly change the taste of a stock by experimenting with the different ingredients used. For example, a vegetable stock can be made sweeter if you add more carrots. Because stock is a base for many recipes, adding salt to it is not necessary.

Stocks, like soups, can be frozen and kept on hand until you need them. Freeze homemade stock in ice-cube trays for small portions, or in containers for larger quantities. Although freshly prepared stock is usually the most flavourful, you can substitute purchased canned or frozen stocks if you are short on time. Fish stock is usually difficult to find in stores, but can sometimes be found at Marks & Spencers or at a fishmonger.

On page 264 you'll find the recipe for the basic vegetable stock used in the Active Wellness dishes throughout this chapter.

Making Low-Fat Soups

You can make two types of stock-based soups: clear soups that have vegetables or meat added and heavier soups that are thickened with puréed vegetables or starch. The following techniques for stock-based soups include a clear vegetable soup and a puréed soup of white beans.

You can use the same cooking techniques to make most low-fat soups. Just a few simple steps are involved. Use the basic technique as your guide, then feel free to improvise with your favourite ingredients.

Cooking Terms

Sweat: To heat in a small amount of fat or liquid so that the vegetables sweat out their juices, but do not change colour.

Bouquet Garni: A small bundle of aromatic herbs tied together in muslin. A basic garni consists of fresh parsley stems (2), a pinch of dried or fresh thyme and a large bay leaf (or two small ones).

Mirepoix: A mixture of vegetables used to flavour foods. Traditionally, it includes carrots (25 per cent), celery (25 per cent) and onions (50 per cent), but you can alter this ratio if you wish, or include additional vegetables, such as leeks and turnips.

Basic Technique for Clear Soups (Preparation Time: 20 to 30 Minutes)
1. Sweat mirepoix in a bit of oil or stock.
2. Add the stock (the liquid base).
3. Bring it to a boil.
4. Skim the top of the soup, if necessary.
5. Add the bouquet garni.
6. Simmer for approximately 10 minutes.
7. Add the remaining ingredients and let the soup cook for about 20 minutes or until the ingredients are cooked through. If you want to add small pieces of cooked meat to the soup, add them 5 to 10 minutes before the soup is done so they just heat through but do not overcook.
8. Adjust the seasonings. Let the soup cool and remove the bouquet garni.
9. Serve, or store in the refrigerator or freezer.

Basic Technique for Puréed Soups (Preparation Time: 30 to 45 Minutes)
1. Sweat the vegetables.
2. Add the stock.
3. Bring it to a boil, then lower the heat to a simmer.
4. Add the main ingredients (beans, vegetables, etc.).
5. Add the bouquet garni.
6. Simmer approximately 20 minutes, or until ingredients are cooked.
7. Discard the bouquet garni or bay leaf.
8. Strain the soup and purée the solids to a smooth consistency. (You may also purée the entire soup in a food processor or blender.)
9. Add extra stock to thin the soup, if necessary.
10. Adjust the seasoning. Cool. Serve, or store in the refrigerator or freezer.

Salads and Salad Dressings

Think of salad dressing as a sauce for salads. Full-fat salad dressings, like full-fat sauces, can contribute a significant amount of fat to your diet: 1 tbsp (15 ml) of full-fat salad dressing equals 3 Active Wellness fat portions. By preparing the delicious fat-free and low-fat recipes in the recipe section of this chapter, you can significantly reduce the fat in your daily diet.

Instead of oil, we use yoghurt and tofu to give the dressings body. For creamy salad dressings, try low-fat yoghurt, soft tofu, or low-fat soured cream as a base. To reduce or eliminate the oil, use stocks, juices and vinegars as a base for vinaigrette-type salad dressings. Remember, salad dressing can also be used as marinades on food including lean beef, fish, chicken, tofu, tempeh and soya burgers. On pages 280-282 you'll find recipes for some salad dressing favourites from Active Wellness.

Tips for Preparing Salads

If you like salads, but can't seem to find time to chop the vegetables before your meals, several other possibilities can help make life easier. Buy precut vegetables from the produce section or salad bar of your supermarket. Or, you can make your own salad bar at home by washing and slicing some vegetables a day or two ahead and keeping them in the refrigerator. The best way to store vegetables is to:

- Keep them chilled, between 30° and 40°F (0° and 5°C)—except for lemons, potatoes, tomatoes, bananas, green pineapple and tropical produce.
- Limit their exposure to oxygen by loosely wrapping them in plastic wrap or storing them in plastic bags or sealed containers.
- Keep them in a humid environment.

When you have precut vegetables on hand, reaching for a vegetable can be just as easy as reaching for a biscuit.

Main Courses

The main course recipes on pages 270-280 are divided into two sections: Meat Main Courses and Vegetarian Main Courses. If you're a meat eater, don't forget to try the Vegetarian Main Courses as well.

Meat Main Courses

When your goal is to make a low-fat meal of meat, fish or poultry, take these points into consideration:

- Choose leaner cuts
- Choose a cooking method that maintains flavour and texture
- Use other low-fat ingredients to accompany the dish

See the Low-Fat Cooking Methods chart on the next page for helpful hints for cooking meat, fish and poultry.

> Remember, when you cook foods, their weight changes. Usually a 4 oz (115 g) piece of raw fish or chicken results in a 3 oz (85 g) cooked portion.

Low-Fat Cooking Methods

Technique	Helpful Cooking Tips
Roasting/Baking: Cooking by dry heat; place on rack so that the air circulates.	◇ Use with tender cuts. ◇ Place meat and poultry on rack to drain fat. ◇ Roasting is usually used for large cuts. ◇ If basting the food, use fruit juice, stock or wine for flavour. ◇ Roasting vegetables enhances their flavour and increases the sweetness of most root vegetables.
Grilling: Cooking by dry heat emanating from under or above the food. Generally at high temperatures and with smaller cuts.	◇ Salt meat after cooking to prevent drying. ◇ Touch test for meat when pressed: rare—soft; medium—medium firmness; well done—firm. ◇ Grill meat in aluminium foil until the last few minutes of cooking to reduce potential carcinogens. ◇ Use a marinade to flavour and tenderize. ◇ Not recommended for lean pork and veal.
Sautéing: Quickly cooking small-size foods on the cooker, using high heat.	◇ Use just enough oil or oil spray to prevent sticking. (Helpful to have a non-stick pan.) You can also sauté in a small amount of stock, wine or vegetable juice. ◇ Good way to brown food and then finish cooking it in the oven. ◇ Juices from food can be used for a sauce. ◇ Preheat pan before cooking, so food cooks at high temperature.
Stir-Frying: Cooking small pieces of food over high heat, using little fat.	◇ With stir-frying, it is easy to combine different foods together. ◇ Peanut oil is traditionally used for flavour. ◇ When cooking the food, it should be constantly stirred. ◇ Start cooking the food that takes the longest to cook first. ◇ If you add a liquid to the stir-fry, thicken it with corn flour or arrowroot.

Steaming: Cooking with moist heat by surrounding foods with steam and no fat.	◇ Food should not touch water. ◇ Excellent way to retain texture, colour and nutritional value of vegetables.
Poaching: Cooking food in a liquid bath; does not need fat.	◇ Cover about half the food with liquid in a shallow poaching pan with a lid. ◇ The liquid can be stock, juices or wine and will add flavour to the food. ◇ Used with tender cuts.
Braising/Stewing: Cooking food by searing it, then placing it in liquid to finish.	◇ Not necessary to use fat. ◇ Good for less tender pieces of meat, poultry and pork; root vegetables work well, too.

Once your food is cooked—using a low-fat technique—you can make the dish more interesting and tasty by adding flavours and textures, which can be accomplished by using sauces, crusts, stuffing, marinades and herb and spice rubs. You can also add sauces and rubs to your low-fat cooking repertoire to jazz up a simple roasted chicken breast or a plain fish fillet.

Another type of 'sauce' that adds excitement and flavour to foods is salsa. Traditional tomato salsas are easy to find in the supermarket. Fruit salsas also provide a variety of uses. They can be sprinkled as a topping, blended as a sauce or poured as a salad dressing.

Crust Toppings for Poultry, Fish, and Meats
Crusts can be made with nuts, bread-crumbs, herbs, spices, and dough. They offer a great way to seal in the food's juices to keep it moist and tender. Spice rubs are easy to make ahead, so they'll be ready when you need them.

The Chicken Roulade with Pistachio Crust recipe on page 271 describes how to use nut crusts; it also shows how much flavour and texture is added when you stuff a breast. The lowest calorie ingredients to use for stuffing are vegetables, but bread

Using Marinades and Sauces

When marinating fish, keep the fish in the marinade for approximately 1 hour before cooking. When marinating chicken and beef, keep them in the marinade for up to 4 hours before cooking. Marinades can be made ahead and kept, well covered, in the refrigerator for up to 1 week.

stuffing, dried fruit, and rice mixtures offer other low-fat options. Both techniques in this recipe are fun to learn because once you add them to your cooking know-how, you can use them to become creative and improvise with other combinations.

Rubs

A 'rub' may sound like a funny name for a cooking technique, but the term is literal. When you use spices to coat a piece of meat on both sides, those spices are called a rub. To use a rub, simply prepare the mixture beforehand and then rub it all over the meat with your hands. Let the meat stand, covered, in the refrigerator or cook it right away. Before cooking, spray both sides of the meat lightly with oil to prevent it from sticking to the grill or pan; then cook as you would if the meat were not coated.

Vegetarian Main Courses

Vegetarian cooking can be delicious, low in fat and satisfying when you use a variety of techniques that combine the basic five foods that are essential to most vegetarian diets: pulses, grains, soya products, vegetables and fruits. One of the main challenges for vegetarians is eating enough protein to meet their needs. This is easy when you focus on preparing meals that provide more concentrated sources of protein such as soya, pulses and wheat gluten.

Traditionally, vegetarians try to combine the right foods at each meal (beans with grains, for example) to make a whole protein, in order to compensate for not eating animal protein. However, eating a variety of foods throughout the day enables your body to combine the nutrients itself, so you don't have to be concerned about combining foods at every meal—just every day.

If you are a beginner at vegetarian cooking, you should familiarize yourself with the numerous types of pulses, grains and soya products on the market. The chart on the next page and the chart on pages 256-257 illustrate the cooking times for many of the beans and grains you'll find in the supermarket. The soya chart on page 258 also shows how diverse soya is as a food product.

With vegetarian cooking, you can create new and interesting recipes by focusing on different preparation and cooking techniques. You can wrap, stuff, layer, stir-fry, grill, bake, rub, marinate, sauce, steam, form and purée ingredients. The key to good vegetarian cooking is learning the best way to marry a technique to its ingredient. The combinations are endless, considering the many types of grains and pulses.

Cooking Beans			
Type	Soaking Time (Hours)	Cooking Time and Liquid Measurement per 8 fl. oz/235 ml**	Yield per 8 fl. oz/ 235 ml*
Adzuki Beans	1	1 to 1½ hours in 16 fl. oz/475 ml liquid	1½
Black-Eyed Peas, Pigeon Peas	2	1 to 1½ hours in 16 fl. oz/475 ml liquid	1½
Kidney, Barlotti, Cannellini, Fagioli, Flageolet, Pinto, White	2 to 3	1 to 2 hours in 16 fl. oz/475 ml liquid	1⅓ to 1½
Chickpeas	3	1 to 2 hours in 16 fl. oz/475 ml liquid	1½
Soya beans	Best if soaked overnight	2 hours 25 minutes in 16 fl. oz/ 475 ml liquid	1⅓
Lentils and Split Peas	none	20 to 30 minutes Lentils—12 fl. oz/ 355 ml liquid; Split Peas—16 fl. oz/ 475 ml liquid	Lentils— 1⅓ to 1½ Split Peas—1

*Yield is per 4 fl. oz (115 ml) when raw.
** The quick-cooking method for beans.

Preparing and Cooking Beans

1. Pick any stones and soil out of the beans, then rinse them under cold water. Cover with water. Use 4 pints (2.4 litres) of water per 1 lb (0.45 kg) of beans, or about three times the beans' volume in water. When you cover the beans, make sure that at least 1 in (2.5 cm) of water reaches above them.

2. Bring to a boil for 2 minutes, then remove the pot from the heat and allow the beans to soak. Remove any beans that float to the top. Note: If you prefer to do the long soak-

ing method, you can soak the beans for 12 hours (overnight) in the refrigerator. Soak them in enough water to cover the beans by at least 1 in (2.5 cm).

3. When you are ready to cook the beans, place them in the pot and add enough cold stock to cover them by about 2 in (5 cm). Turn up the heat to bring the beans slowly to a boil. Bring the liquid to a rolling boil, then turn down the heat to finish cooking the beans at a simmer. Skim off any foam that rises to the top of the pot.

4. Use the chart on page 255 to determine the cooking time. Add more stock, if necessary. The beans should be tender, but firm. If the tip of a sharp knife can easily pierce the skin, the beans are done.

Grains

When cooking grains, keep in mind that each grain has its own distinct ratio of liquid to grain. With a little practice, you'll learn that cooking grains is easy, and grains add great variety to meals. I encourage you to sample new grains; each one has its own distinctive texture and taste.

Cooking Grains			
Grain	Ratio of Grain/Liquid	Simmering Time in Liquid	Yield
Amaranth	4 fl. oz/115 ml to 4 fl. oz/115 ml liquid	30 minutes	10 fl. oz/ 300 ml
Barley Pot Barley	4 fl. oz/115 ml barley to 12 fl. oz/ 355 ml liquid	45 to 55minutes; let stand 2 to 3 minutes	16 fl. oz/ 475 ml
Cracked Barley	4 fl. oz/115 ml barley to 6 fl. oz/ 180 ml liquid	45 to 55minutes; let stand 2 to 3 minutes	3 fl. oz/ 90 ml
Buckwheat Kasha	4 fl. oz/115 ml kasha to 20 fl. oz/ 590 ml liquid	12 minutes	16 fl. oz/ 475 ml

Grain	Ratio of Grain/Liquid	Simmering time in Liquid	Yield
Corn /maize Polenta	4 fl. oz/115 ml to 16 fl. oz/475 ml liquid	30 minutes	16 fl. oz/475 ml
Millet	4 fl. oz/115 ml millet to 12 fl. oz/355 ml liquid	25 minutes	20 fl. oz/590 ml
Oats Rolled	4 fl. oz/115 ml grain to 8 fl. oz/235 ml liquid	5 minutes	8 fl. oz/235 ml
Rice Brown, White, Long grain	4 fl. oz/115 ml rice to 8 fl. oz/235 ml liquid	For moist rice—20 to 30 minutes	12 fl. oz/355 ml
Basmati	4 fl. oz/115 ml basmati to 12 fl. oz/355 ml liquid	15 minutes	16 fl. oz/475 ml
Arborio	4 fl. oz/115 ml arborio to 6 fl. oz/180 ml liquid	15 minutes	12 fl. oz/355 ml
Fragrant	4 fl. oz/115 ml fragrant to 8 fl. oz/235 ml liquid	15 to 20 minutes	14 fl. oz/415 ml
Wild	4 fl. oz/115 ml wild to 16 fl. oz/475 ml liquid	50 minutes	16 fl. oz/475 ml
Wheat Bulgur and Cracked Wheat	4 fl. oz/115 ml grain to 8 fl. oz/235 ml liquid	15 to 20 minutes	8–12 fl. oz/235–355 ml
Couscous, instant	Follow directions on package.	5 to 10 minutes	double

Soya Foods and Their Uses

Type	Uses
Tofu (Soya Bean Curd)	Tofu takes on almost any flavour. Use it diced on salads or in stews. The firmer tofu can be used as a main course with sauces and marinades.
Textured Vegetable Protein	This dried form comes in packages of various sizes. Large pieces can be added to meat stews; smaller pieces can be used in soups or sauces. It has the texture of mince and should be soaked in hot water before using it. It can be found ready-to-use and pre-seasoned at many health food shops.
Soya Bean Milk	Use like regular milk on cereals and in custards, creamy sauces or soups.
Soy Sauce, Tamari, Miso	These seasonings flavour soups, sauces, meats and marinades and are made from fermented soya beans. Note that all three are high in sodium; avoid them if you are on a low-salt diet.
Soya Flour	This ground form is used to thicken gravies and soups. It can also add protein to baked goods. In many traditional recipes, you can replace regular flour with soya flour. It does not promote rising in breads, so it should be mixed with other ingredients if rising is desired.
Soya Nuts	Roasted soya nuts make a great high protein snack. Look for the ones that have been dry roasted.
Soya Cheeses	A good source of protein in your diet. Look for the low-fat brands.
Tempeh	This fermented soya bean cake is usually combined with other grains. It is best when used with a marinade or sauce to complement the taste of the product.

What Is Seitan?

Seitan is a protein-rich food made from wheat. You can purchase seitan already formed, or you can purchase it dried and make your own forms. It is great for making meat-textured foods such as meatballs. It can also be sliced like chicken or beef for stir-frying.

Fruits and Vegetables

Fruits and vegetables come in different varieties—each with different qualities and tastes. Experiment with the produce you find at your local market. Try, among other things, different lettuces, mushrooms, tomatoes, peppers, onions, apples, pears, and melons. Cooking helps to improve the digestibility and palatability of many vegetables. Cooking fruit concentrates sweetness and softens the texture.

You have several alternatives for cooking vegetables in a low-fat fashion that retains both their flavour and nutritional value. Vegetables and fruit can be steamed, sautéed, roasted, grilled, puréed, parboiled, braised and microwaved. Following are charts for two of the smartest and tastiest ways to make vegetables: steaming and roasting. If you find yourself short on time, frozen vegetables make good substitutes for fresh.

Steaming Vegetables: Preparation and Cooking Times

General Directions: Vegetables can be steamed in a metal steamer or, if you prefer, you can try an Asian bamboo steamer.

Vegetable	Preparation	Cooking Times
Artichokes	Wash and cut off the top 1 in/2.5 cm of bud and trim the leaves, if desired. Stand in the steamer.	25 to 40 minutes until the base of the artichoke is tender.
Asparagus	Slice off rough ends before cooking; best if standing in asparagus steamer; if not, use a large pot and a metal steamer so the asparagus can lie flat.	Cook uncovered 5 minutes; covered 7 to 10 minutes.

Vegetable	Preparation	Cooking Times
Aubergine	Peel and slice. Salt the slices to remove bitterness. Let salted slices stand for 15 minutes, then rinse them well.	Steam for 3 to 5 minutes. If you are steaming aubergine in preparation for grilling or roasting, steam for 3 minutes, then place in the oven or on grill. See roasting direction on the next page.
Beans, green	Wash and snap the ends off.	15 to 20 minutes until tender.
Beetroot, small	Scrub the skin. Do not peel.	20 to 30 minutes until tender, but still firm.
Broccoli	Peel off the rough bottom stalk before cooking. Cut into smaller florets.	10 to 20 minutes
Brussels Sprouts	Wash well; cut off stems.	12 to 15 minutes
Carrots	Scrub thoroughly or peel. Cut off the ends. Chop the carrots into bite-size pieces.	12 to 15 minutes
Cauliflower	Core. Remove the outer leaves. Cut into florets.	12 to 15 minutes
Corn on the cob	Remove the husks. Wash.	Steam, covered, for 6 to 10 minutes.
Fennel	Wash well. Slice out core of bulb.	20 to 30 minutes
Greens	Wash well. Remove bad leaves.	5 to 9 minutes or until just wilted.
Mushrooms	Wipe with a damp towel or clean with a mushroom brush. Cut off the ends.	3 to 8 minutes
Okra	Wash; remove 'fuzz' with a towel. Remove the tips.	3 to 6 minutes or until tender, but firm.

Vegetable	Preparation	Cooking Times
Parsnips	Scrub well or peel. Leave whole or chop them into equal pieces	Whole: 20 to 40 minutes. If cut: 5 to 15 minutes.
Potatoes, red	Small ones are best for steaming. Scrub the skin. Cut off any dark spots.	Steam halved potatoes for 15 to 20 minutes; steam whole potatoes for 20 to 30 minutes.
Squash & Marrow	Wash and trim each end. Slice the squash horizontally or vertically into ¼-inch slices.	5 to 10 minutes

Roasting Vegetables: Preparation and Cooking Times

General Directions: Place whole, halved or sliced vegetables (sliced 1 in/2.5 cm thick) on an oil-sprayed baking sheet and bake in a preheated oven at 450°F (235°C, gas mark 8) for 30 minutes, or until soft to the touch. Specific directions for roasting vegetables are listed below.

Aubergine	Follow the directions for steaming, then place the aubergine on a baking sheet. Roast until soft to the touch.
Garlic: Whole	Place the whole bulb, positioned top-down, on a baking sheet. Wrap each individual bulb in aluminium foil and place top down on a baking sheet. Bake in a 325°F (165°C, gas mark 3) oven for 1½ hours.
Cloves	Place peeled cloves flat on a baking sheet and roast in a 400°F (235°C, gas mark 6) oven until slightly browned, 15 to 20 minutes.
Onions: Whole	Cut off ends of unpeeled onion, so it can stand in an oil-sprayed baking dish. Prick onion with a fork and place in the baking dish. Roast at 375°F (190°C, gas mark 5) for 45 to 60 minutes.

Onion: Halved	Peel and halve onions; place cut side down on an oil-sprayed baking sheet and roast in a 400°F (235°C, gas mark 6) oven for 25 to 30 minutes until browned.
Peppers, red and yellow	Place whole peppers on a baking sheet. Grill 4 in/10 cm from the heat source. Roast peppers until browned, but not black, on each side. Turn the peppers as each side is finished cooking. Cook for 10 to 15 minutes. When cool, peel skin off peppers by rubbing peppers with a paper towel.
Potatoes	First steam potatoes until barely tender. Cut large potatoes into wedges and small potatoes in half. Place in an oil-sprayed baking pan. Roast at 450°F (235°C, gas mark 8) for 20 to 35 minutes or until potatoes are browned and soft.
Tomatoes	Slice tomatoes in half and place cut side up in an oil-sprayed baking dish. Roast at 400°F (200°C, gas mark 6) for 12 to 15 minutes. Top with breading, herbs or a little low-fat cheese.

To Maintain the Colour of Vegetables:

Do not cook them in a cast-iron, coppe, or tin-lined pan. The metal alters the green chlorophyll colour. Avoid bathing them in acidic sauces for a long time. Put acidic vinegar, lemon juice or wine-based sauces on the vegetables at the last minute, or serve acidic sauces on the side. Cook fresh green vegetables in a lot of water to dilute the acid in them, or steam the vegetables.

Noodles and Pasta

Everyone loves pasta—and it's an easy item to overeat. Remember to monitor yourself if you are trying to lose or maintain your weight: 4 fl. oz (115 ml) of cooked pasta is one portion. Sometimes, a side dish of pasta in a restaurant can be 8–12 fl. oz (235–355 ml) and main course can be 16–32 fl. oz (475–945 ml)!

Pasta is fun to prepare and eat, because it comes in so many shapes and sizes. And now you can find pasta made with different protein grains. Wholemeal pasta is available in health food shops and supermarkets, as is Asian pasta made from rice and buckwheat.

Wholemeal pasta and some of the other grain pastas are higher in fibre than traditional semolina or white flour pastas. Unfortunately, the higher fibre pastas are also chewier. If you find the higher fibre pastas to be too 'different' in texture and taste, you can increase the fibre content of a regular pasta meal by mixing half of the regular semolina pasta with half of a higher fibre pasta, such as wholemeal pasta. You can also add fibre to pasta by serving it mixed with vegetables.

Desserts

Low-fat desserts take a bit of ingenuity because you need to improvise for the reduction in fat by using techniques that compensate for the rich texture, tenderness and moisture that fat adds to cakes and baked goods. Below is a chart of substitutions that can be used in baking. Feel free to try them in your favourite recipes.

Substitutions for Common Dessert Ingredients	
Ingredient	Low-Fat Substitution
Egg	2 egg whites
Butter	Oil, or fruit purées* and oil: ½ oil plus ½ apple sauce, banana purée, sweet potato purée, or silken tofu.
Soured Cream	Non-fat or low-fat soured cream
Whole Milk	Skimmed milk or 1% milk
Buttermilk	Low-fat buttermilk or nonfat or low-fat yoghurt
Nuts	Reduce the nuts by half and chop them into smaller pieces; there is more nut flavour per bite. Or reduce the amount of whole nuts and add dried fruit.
Chocolate	Use cocoa powder in place of chocolate. For every 1 oz (30 g) of chocolate substitute 2 tbsp (30 ml) of cocoa powder.
Cheese	Low-fat or non-fat cheeses

* A note about purées: When you substitute puréed fruit or sweet potato you can enhance the texture and moistness of a product. However, the decision about which purée to use is up to you. The banana carries the most flavour, so it is best used in products that have a banana taste. Use the silken tofu in recipes that have strong flavour, so that the tofu taste does not come through. The apple sauce is the lightest purée to use. The sweet potato purée adds sweetness and colour. You can also try white potato purée if you want to minimize colour.

Active Wellness Recipes

SOUPS

Always good for body and soul, soups are a delicious way to bring a wide variety of vegetables and beans to your diet. Use these recipes as a starting point for your own creative soups, incorporating favourite herbs and farm-fresh vegetables. And remember to always skim the fat from any stock—whether it's canned or homemade—before making any soup.

Basic Vegetable Stock

6 large carrots	1 large green or yellow squash
2 large stalks celery, including leaves	4 stems parsley
2 large yellow onions	2 cloves garlic
1 leek	1 bay leaf
1 large potato	4 black peppercorns
1 turnip	2 sprigs fresh thyme

1. Thoroughly wash or scrub all vegetables.
2. Peel carrots and cut into large dice.
3. Cut remaining vegetables into large dice, leaving the skin on the onions, and put into a medium to large pot, along with herbs and seasonings and cover with 3–4 pints (1.8–2.4 litres) cold water. The water should just cover the ingredients.
4. Bring the water to a light boil, reduce the heat and let the broth simmer for about 45 minutes to 1 hour, or until all the vegetables are completely soft and have rendered their flavour.
5. Strain the stock through a strainer or muslin-lined colander until all sediment is eliminated and the broth is clear and golden.

Makes eight 8 fl oz/250 ml servings.

Nutrition Facts: Calories 54, Fat 0 grams, Saturated Fat 0 grams, Cholesterol 0 mg, Protein 0 grams, Carbohydrate 12.5 grams, Sodium 38 mg

Active Wellness Portion Equivalent: Free Food

Hearty Vegetable Soup

1 14 oz (300 g) can plum tomatoes
   in their juice
2 tsp (10 ml) olive oil
1 small onion, diced
4 medium leeks, white part only, cleaned and
   sliced into rounds
2 stalks celery, diced
1 clove garlic, minced
48 fl. oz (1.5 litres) vegetable stock, or
   enough to cover vegetables
1 small head green cabbage, shredded

4 carrots, peeled and diced
4 medium red potatoes, skins on, diced
2 turnips, diced
1 tablespoon chopped fresh parsley
½ teaspoon dried thyme
¼ teaspoon dried oregano
1 bay leaf
½ lb (250 g) green beans, cut
   into 1 in(2.5 cm) pieces
Freshly ground black pepper
Pinch sugar or fructose

1. Coarsely chop plum tomatoes and set aside. Save the juice of the tomatoes.
2. Heat a large pot over medium heat, add oil followed by onion, leeks, celery and garlic.
3. Cover and cook over medium heat until vegetables are wilted, adding some stock if necessary to prevent burning.
4. Add cabbage and cook for 5 minutes, or until it begins to soften. Add tomatoes and their juice, the remaining stock, carrots, potatoes, turnips and herbs.
5. Cover and cook until carrots and potatoes are barely soft. Skim foam from surface of soup occasionally. Add green beans, and cook until just tender. Adjust seasonings and serve.

Makes eight 8 fl oz/250 ml servings.

Nutrition Facts: Calories 107, Fat 1 gram, Saturated Fat 0 grams, Cholesterol 0 mg, Protein 3 grams, Carbohydrate 22 grams, Sodium 132 mg

Active Wellness Portion Equivalents: ½ Grains/Starches and 2 Vegetable Servings.

White Bean Soup

1 teaspoon oil
1 small leek, cleaned and finely diced
1 small onion, diced
2 stalks celery, diced
3 medium carrots, diced
3 cloves garlic, minced
2 fl. oz (60 ml) white wine
3 pints (1.8 litres) chicken or vegetable stock

1 bay leaf
1 tsp (5 ml) finely chopped fresh thyme
1 tsp (5 ml) finely chopped fresh sage
1 lb (450 g) dried cannellini beans
2 fl. oz (60 ml) finely chopped fresh basil
½ teaspoon salt
1 tsp (5 ml) black pepper

1. Heat oil in large pot. Add leek, onion, celery, carrots and garlic.
2. Cook, stirring, for about 1 minute, then add the wine. Cook until the onions are soft and golden.
3. Add stock, bay leaf, thyme and sage.
4. Add the soaked beans and bring to a boil. Lower heat to medium and simmer until beans are just tender, about 1 to 2 hours.
5. Remove the bay leaf, and transfer half of the mixture, in batches, to a blender and purée.
6. Return to the pot. Add fresh basil and stir well. Season with salt and pepper.

Makes eight 8 fl oz/250 ml servings.

Nutrition Facts: Calories 204, Fat .5 gram, Saturated Fat 0 grams, Cholesterol 0 mg, Protein 12 grams, Carbohydrate 31 grams, Sodium 282 mg

Active Wellness Portion Equivalent: 2½ Grains/Starches Servings.

PASTA

When traditional pastas left Italy, they were transformed from very healthy foods into cheese- and meat-laden dishes high in fat, particularly saturated fat. The Active Wellness makeovers of two Italian classics proves that you can enjoy rich, creamy pasta with very little fat.

Lasagne Verde

This recipe is a bit labour intensive, but all the vegetable components can be made a day ahead. Actually, it is better to make this entire dish a day ahead, so that the casserole really sets and is easy to cut into portions. If you want to simplify the recipe, purchase no-cook or fresh lasagna noodles, which do not require boiling. For a lighter dish, use egg-free fresh spinach lasagne sheets.

9 dried, ready-to-cook lasagne sheets	1 large aubergine
2 large bunches spinach, about 2 lb (0.9 kg), stemmed and washed	2 large courgettes
	Cooking oil spray
24 oz (675 g) fat-free ricotta	10 oz (30 g) button mushrooms, sliced
1 oz (30 g) freshly grated Parmesan cheese	½ oz (15 g) minced fresh parsley
	Freshly ground black pepper to taste
½ teaspoon freshly grated nutmeg	24 fl oz (750 ml) low-fat tomato
1 tsp (5 ml) salt	sauce

1 oz (30 g) chopped fresh basil
1 tsp (5 ml) fennel seed
1 tsp (5 ml) dried thyme

1 tsp (5 ml) dried oregano
6 oz (180 g) shredded non-fat mozzarella

1. Preheat the oven to 350°F (175°C, gas mark 4).
2. Place the spinach with the water still clinging to its leaves in a hot frying pan and cook until just wilted. Let cool slightly, squeeze out excess moisture and chop fine.
3. In a large bowl combine the spinach with the ricotta. Add the Parmesan and nutmeg and season with ½ teaspoon of salt. Set aside, covered, in the refrigerator.
4. Peel the aubergine and cut lengthwise into ¼ in (0.6 cm) thick slices. Peel the courgettes and cut lengthwise into ¼ in (0.6 cm) thick slices. Spray a large baking sheet with cooking oil spray. Spread the aubergine and courgette slices on the sheet and bake until tender but not too soft, about 10 to 15 minutes. Set aside.
5. Spray a non-stick frying pan with cooking oil spray and heat over medium heat. Add the mushrooms and sauté until browned. Season with the parsley, the remaining ½ teaspoon salt, and a light sprinkling of pepper. Set aside.
6. In a large pot of boiling, salted water, cook the lasagna noodles until *al dente*. Drain.
7. Spread 1 cup (8 fl oz/250 ml) of the tomato sauce in the bottom of a 9 x 13 in (23 x 33 cm) lasagne pan. Line the bottom of the pan with 3 cooked lasagne sheets.
8. Spoon half of the ricotta mixture over the sheets, spreading it evenly to within ½ in (1.25 cm) of the sides of the pan. Top with the courgette slices.
9. Sprinkle half of the basil, fennel, thyme and oregano over the courgettes. Cover with 3 more sheets and press down lightly.
10. Spread the remaining ricotta over the sheets. Place the aubergine slices on top and sprinkle with the remaining basil, fennel, thyme and oregano. Spoon the mushrooms on top. Cover with the remaining sheets.
11. Spoon the remaining 16 fl. oz (500 ml) tomato sauce over the top of the pan, completely covering the top and edges so they will not burn while cooking. Sprinkle the mozzarella on top.
12. Cover the pan with aluminium foil and bake for 40 minutes. Remove the foil and bake for another 10 minutes, or until the top is lightly browned.
13. Let cool for 15 minutes before slicing.

Makes 6 servings.

Nutrition Facts: Calories 488, Fat 11 grams, Saturated Fat 6 grams, Cholesterol 32 mg, Protein 38 grams, Carbohydrate 38 grams, Sodium 770 mg

Active Wellness Portion Equivalents: 3 Dairy, 3 Vegetable and 2 Grains/Starches Servings.

Lite Fettuccine Alfredo

8 fl oz (250 ml) part-skimmed or fat-free
  ricotta
5½ oz (160 g) freshly grated
  Parmesan cheese
20 fl oz (625 ml) skimmed milk
1 oz (30 g) arrowroot or corn flour
5½ oz (160 g) fat-free Parmesan
  cheese

Pinch of freshly grated nutmeg
1 tsp (5 ml) salt
Freshly ground black pepper to taste
12 oz (375 g) fettuccine
1 tsp (5 ml) olive oil
2 tbsp (30 ml) chopped fresh flat parsley

1. Blend the ricotta with the grated Parmesan cheese in a blender or food processor.
2. In a saucepan, whisk the milk and the corn flour or arrowroot. Heat over medium-high heat, stirring, until the mixture thickens and comes to a boil, about 10 minutes.
3. Transfer the mixture to a medium-size metal bowl or to the top half of a double boiler and whisk in ricotta mixture and fat-free Parmesan. Season with nutmeg and salt. Add freshly ground pepper to taste.
4. Place the sauce over hot water in the double boiler to keep warm while you cook the fettuccine.
5. Fill a large pot full of water and bring to a boil. Add the olive oil and the fettuccine. Cook *al dente*. Drain and toss with the sauce.
6. Serve hot, add more pepper and nutmeg, if desired.

Makes fourteen 3½ oz/100 g servings.

Nutrition Facts: Calories 221, Fat 5 grams, Saturated Fat 3 grams, Cholesterol 14 mg, Protein 11 grams, Carbohydrate 438 grams, Sodium 562 mg

Active Wellness Portion Equivalents: 1½ Dairy and 1 Grain/Starches Serving.

Moroccan-Spiced Couscous

This couscous salad is a wonderful accompaniment with grilled fish or chicken. Or try serving it with some grilled vegetables and a light green salad for a satisfying vegetarian meal.

2 tsp (10 ml) vegetable oil
2 medium courgettes, cut into ½ in
  (1.25 cm) dice
1½ oz (45 g) thinly sliced spring onions
2 tsp (10 ml) curry powder
2 tsp (10 ml) ground cinnamon
1 tsp (5 ml) ground cumin

½ tsp turmeric
2 fl oz (60 ml) dry white wine
10 oz (300 g) Italian plum tomatoes,
  drained and finely chopped
8 oz (240 g) cooked chickpeas
1 oz (30 g) dried currants
1 tsp (5 ml) sugar

¼ tsp harissa or other hot pepper paste
  (optional)
16 fl oz (500 ml) vegetable stock
  or water

6 oz (170 g) wholemeal couscous
3 oz (90 g) cooked green peas
2 oz (60 g) chopped fresh parsley
1 tsp (5 ml) salt

1. Set a large deep frying pan over medium heat and add the oil. Add the courgettes and spring onions and cook 2 minutes. Stir in the curry powder, cinnamon, cumin, salt and turmeric and cook 30 seconds, stirring well to prevent spices from burning.
2. Add the wine and cook until the liquid has been reduced by half. Stir in the tomatoes, chickpeas, currants, sugar, salt and harissa paste, if desired.
3. Add the stock and bring to boil.
4. Take the frying pan off the heat, stir in the couscous, cover and let stand for 5 minutes, or until the couscous has absorbed the liquid.
5. Gently fluff the couscous with a fork and fold in the peas and parsley.

Makes six 6 oz (180 g) servings.

Nutrition Facts: Calories 357, Fat 3 grams, Saturated Fat 0 grams, Cholesterol 0 mg, Protein 12 grams, Carbohydrate 51 grams, Sodium 311 mg

Active Wellness Portion Equivalents: 4 Grains/Starches and ½ Fat Serving.

Sesame Noodles

Sauce

4 fl oz (125 g) plain non-fat yoghurt
2 fl oz (60 ml) low-sodium soy sauce
2 fl oz (60 ml) mirin (Japanese sweet
  rice wine)
2 tbsp (30 ml) reduced-fat peanut butter
1 tbsp (15 ml) fructose

1 tsp (5 ml) sesame oil
1 tsp (5 ml) minced fresh ginger
⅛ tsp hot pepper sauce or red chilli
  paste
1 clove garlic, minced

Noodles

8 oz (250 g) udon (Japanese wheat)
  noodles
1 large carrot, julienned
1 large cucumber, peeled, seeded and
  julienned

3 spring onions, sliced on the diagonal
1 oz (30 g) soya nuts, chopped

1. Combine all the sauce ingredients in a blender and blend until smooth and creamy.
2. Cook the noodles according to package directions and drain well. Add 4 fl oz (80 ml) of the sauce to the noodles. (Save extra sauce for later use.) Add the vegetables and toss lightly. Garnish with the soya nuts.

Serve immediately.

Sauce keeps refrigerated for 1 week.

Makes four 3½ oz (100g) servings.

Nutrition Facts: Calories 207, Fat 3 grams, Saturated Fat 1 gram, Cholesterol 0 mg, Carbohydrate 32 grams, Protein 10 grams, Sodium 873 mg

Active Wellness Portion Equivalents: 1 Grains/Starches, 1 Protein, 1 Fat and ½ Vegetable Serving.

MEAT MAIN COURSES

Meat can be a part of a healthy diet if you choose leaner cuts and smaller portions, and use cooking techniques that employ little or no additional fat. Try to include at least one or two fish main courses in your weekly menus because fish, particularly rich-fleshed types like salmon, is a marvellous source of the beneficial omega-3 fatty acids.

Chicken Breasts in Wine-Mustard Marinade

4 6½ oz (185 g) skinless, boneless chicken breasts, trimmed of fat

Wine-Mustard Marinade

4 fl oz (125 ml) white wine	1 shallot, minced
4 fl oz (125 ml) chicken or vegetable stock	1 tsp (5 ml) ground white pepper
	½ teaspoon fennel seed
2 fl oz (60 ml) Dijon mustard	½ teaspoon dried basil
2 tbsp (30 ml) olive oil	½ teaspoon dried thyme
1 clove garlic, minced	½ teaspoon dried rosemary

1. In a shallow dish, combine all the marinade ingredients, stirring well.
2. Add the chicken breasts and turn to coat. Cover with plastic wrap and refrigerate for 1 to 2 hours.
3. Preheat the oven to 350°F (175°C, gas mark 4).
4. Place a roasting pan in the oven for 5 to 10 minutes or until it is very hot. Put the chicken breasts in the pan with some of the marinade and roast until the chicken is done, about 10 to 12 minutes. If grilling: When the coals are white, place chicken on an oiled grill rack. Grill for 3 minutes then turn at a 45-degree angle to create a cross-hatch pattern and grill another 3 minutes.
5. Turn the breasts over and repeat on the second side until they are firm and the juices run clear.

Makes 4 servings.

Nutrition Facts for a Chicken Breast with Marinade: Calories 262, Fat 7 grams, Saturated Fat 1 gram, Cholesterol 112 mg, Protein 21 grams, Carbohydrate 2 grams, Sodium 109 mg

Nutrition Facts for Marinade Only per 4 tbsp (60 ml): Calories 95, Fat 0 grams, Saturated Fat 0 grams, Cholesterol 0 mg, Protein 0 grams, Carbohydrate 2 grams, Sodium 43 mg

Active Wellness Portion Equivalent: 5 oz (140 g) of a Protein Serving.

Chicken Roulade with Crumb-Nut Crust

This recipe can be made with turkey breast as well as any other type of flat fillet.

2 fl. oz (60 ml) pistachio nuts
2 fl. oz (60 ml) plain breadcrumbs
1 lb (450 g) spinach leaves, trimmed
   and washed
½ tsp freshly grated nutmeg
Cooking oil spray
10 oz (300 g) sliced button
   mushrooms
4 fl. oz (115 ml) white wine

½ small, sweet onion, sliced very thin
1 tsp (5 ml) dried thyme
1 tsp (5 ml) salt
1 tsp (5 ml) ground white pepper
4 boneless, skinless chicken breasts, about
   6 oz (180 g) each, trimmed of fat
2 egg whites
1 oz (30 g) plain flour

To Prepare the Filling

1. Grind the pistachios in the food processor or chop with a knife until finely ground. Set aside.
2. Steam the spinach or wilt it in a hot frying pan. Chop finely, sprinkle with nutmeg, and set aside.
3. Heat another frying pan, spray lightly with oil, and add mushrooms. Sauté mushrooms for 2 to 3 minutes and add 2 fl oz (60 ml) of the white wine. Cook until well browned and most of the juice has evaporated. Put mushrooms into the processor and blend until mixture resembles a coarse paste. Set aside.
4. Heat a small frying pan. Spray with oil and toss in sliced onions. Sear well, about 2 to 3 minutes, and add the remaining 2 fl oz (60 ml) white wine. Cover pan and cook until onion is soft and caramelized (browned). Set aside. If making on the same day, allow all the components to cool.

To Make the Roulades

1. Mix together in a small bowl the thyme, salt and white pepper.

2. Place each chicken breast between 2 sheets of plastic wrap and pound with the flat side of a meat pounder—from the centre out—so that the thickness is uniform, about ¼ inch (0.6 cm). Be careful not to tear the meat.

3. To assemble, remove the top layer of plastic and lay each breast flat. Sprinkle some of the thyme mixture on each breast.

4. For each breast, holding the breast so that it is at its longest vertically, place ¼ of the chopped spinach lengthwise on the bottom third of the breast.

5. Arrange ¼ of the mushroom mixture on top of the spinach, then ¼ of the onions. Roll the roulades carefully, lengthwise, pushing in on the top after each turn to secure a tight roll. Each roulade should have about two or three turns. Wrap in plastic wrap and roll each tightly to secure the sides. Refrigerate for about 20 minutes.

To Coat with the Pistachio Crust

1. Preheat the oven to 350°F (180°C, gas mark 4).

2. Place egg whites in a shallow bowl and flour in a separate bowl.

3. Combine plain breadcrumbs with pistachio nuts in a small bowl.

4. Unwrap roulades and dredge in flour and shake off excess.

5. Dip in egg white then in the pistachios to lightly cover on both sides.

6. Spray a roasting pan or baking sheet with oil spray. Place the roulades, folded side down, on the pan and bake until firm, about 15 to 20 minutes.

7. To serve, slice the ends off each roulade, then slice each roulade on the bias into thirds. Arrange decoratively on a plate. Suggested sides dishes are wild rice pilaf and roasted vegetables.

Makes 4 servings

Nutrition Facts: Calories 328, Fat 10 grams, Saturated Fat 2 grams, Cholesterol 90 mg, Protein 26 grams, Carbohydrate 32 grams, Sodium 811 mg

Active Wellness Portion Equivalents: 5 Proteins, 1 Fat and 1 Vegetable Serving.

Cajun Spice Rub

1½ oz (45 g) paprika	2½ tbsp (35 ml) ground black pepper
2½ tbsp (35 ml) onion powder	2 tbsp (30 ml) salt
2½ tbsp (35 ml) garlic powder	4 tsp (20 ml) dried thyme
2½ tbsp (35 ml) cayenne pepper	4 tsp (20 ml dried oregano
2½ tbsp (35 ml) ground white pepper	

1. Mix all the ingredients together in a bowl. Store in an airtight container for up to 1 month.

2. Use oil spray to coat the pan prior to cooking meat, poultry, soya or seafood. This dish can be prepared without salt.

Approximately 10 servings, 2 tbsp (30 ml) each.

Nutrition Facts per Serving: Calories 38, Fat 0 grams, Saturated Fat 0 grams, Cholesterol 0 mg, Protein 0 grams, Carbohydrate 8 grams, Sodium 1,281 mg, (without salt, Sodium 4 mg)

Active Wellness Portion Equivalent: Free Food

Crab Cakes

These crab cakes are baked, not fried, to significantly reduce the fat content. If you like, make little cakes (about 1 oz/30 g each) to serve as an appetizer or an hors d'oeuvre. Crab cakes freeze well and are great served sandwich-style on a whole-grain bun with coriander soured cream (see p. 274).

1 lb (450 g) fresh lump crabmeat
2 egg whites
1 small red pepper, finely diced
3 oz (90 g) sweetcorn kernels
2 fl. oz (60 ml) chopped flat leaf parsley
2 spring onions, chopped
2 tbsp (30 ml) fat-free mayonnaise

1 tsp (5 ml) Worcestershire sauce
1 tsp (5 ml) Dijon mustard
1 tsp (5 ml) fresh lemon juice
2 dashes Tabasco sauce
3 oz (90 g) panko (Japanese
   breadcrumbs) or fresh breadcrumbs

1. Preheat the oven to 375°F (190°C, gas mark 5).
2. Pick over the crabmeat to remove any bits of shell or cartilage. Do not shred the crabmeat, but let it remain in meaty chunks.
3. Beat the egg whites to soft peaks. Set aside.
4. In a mixing bowl, gently combine the crabmeat with the red pepper, sweetcorn, parsley, spring onions, mayonnaise, Worcestershire, mustard, lemon juice and Tabasco. Fold in the egg white mixture and ¼ to ½ of the breadcrumbs. Divide into 6 portions and form into rounded patties. These should just stick together and be somewhat delicate.
5. Roll each patty lightly in the panko or breadcrumbs, flatten slightly into a cake and place on a greaseproof paper-lined or non-stick baking sheet.
6. Bake for 12 to 15 minutes or until lightly puffed and brown.
7. Serve on top of fresh greens with fresh mango slices, soured cream or low-fat tartar sauce.
Makes six 3 oz (90 g) cakes, for 3 servings.

Nutrition Facts per Crab Cake: Calories 146, Fat 2 grams, Saturated Fat 1gram, Cholesterol 113mg, Protein 16.5 grams, Carbohydrate 15 grams, Sodium 500 mg

Active Wellness Portion Equivalents: 2½ Protein and ½ Grains/Starches Serving.

Coriander Soured Cream

8 fl. oz (235 ml) fat-free soured cream   ½ oz (15 g) chopped fresh coriander
2 dashes hot sauce, such as Tabasco   Juice of 1 lime (2 tsp/10 ml)

1. Combine all the ingredients in blender and blend until smooth. Add more lime juice, if necessary.
2. Refrigerate for at least 20 minutes.
Makes about 8 fl oz (235 ml), for 4 servings.

Nutrition Facts: Calories 36, Fat 0 grams, Saturated Fat 0 grams, Cholesterol 0 mg, Protein 2 grams, Carbohydrate 6 grams, Sodium 5.5 mg

Active Wellness Portion Equivalent: Free Food

Traditional Turkey Meat Loaf

2 slices whole-wheat bread   1 carrot, peeled and finely grated
8 fl oz (235 ml) skimmed milk   1 spring onion, thinly sliced
1 teaspoon vegetable oil   1 tsp (5 ml) salt
1 small onion, finely diced   1 tsp (5 ml) ground white pepper
3 mushrooms, minced   4 fl oz (125 ml) puréed canned
1 clove garlic, minced   tomatoes
2 tbsp (30 ml) chopped fresh parsley   1 tbsp (15 ml) dark brown sugar
½ teaspoon dried thyme   1 tbsp (15 ml) Dijon mustard
1½ lb (675 g) minced turkey (white meat)   1 tbsp (15 ml) balsamic vinegar
1 egg white

1. Preheat the oven to 375°F (190°C, gas mark 5).
2. Tear the bread into chunks and soak in the milk. Set aside.
3. Heat the oil in a non-stick frying pan over medium heat. Add the onion, mushrooms and garlic and sauté until vegetables are soft. Stir in the parsley and thyme.
4. In a large bowl, combine the turkey mince with the egg white, carrot, spring onion, sautéed vegetables, salt and pepper. Squeeze the excess milk from the bread and add the bread to the bowl. Mix the entire mixture with your fingers until lightly blended.
5. Transfer the mixture to an 8 x 4 in (20 x 10 cm) non-stick loaf pan and form into a smooth loaf.
6. In a small bowl, mix the tomatoes, brown sugar, mustard, and vinegar and pour the mixture over the top of the loaf.
7. Bake for about 1 hour or until a meat thermometer inserted into the centre of the loaf registers 160°F (91°C). Let stand for 5 minutes before slicing into 8 portions.

Makes 8 servings.

Nutrition Facts: Calories 152, Fat 4 grams, Saturated Fat 2 grams, Cholesterol 62 mg, Protein 17.5 grams, Carbohydrate 87 grams, Sodium 409 mg (without salt, Sodium 142 mg)

Active Wellness Portion Equivalents: 2 Protein and 1 Grains/Starches Serving.

Lite Paella

To make this a vegetarian recipe, just omit all the chicken and seafood and add a pound of sliced, baked tofu or seitan. Also, feel free to add some cooked chickpeas or white beans.

1 lb (450 g) boneless, skinless chicken breasts	½ tsp chopped fresh thyme
1 tsp (5 ml) paprika	2 bay leaves
1 lb (450 g) large prawns (about 16)	1 tsp (5 ml) sugar
16 large scallops	½ tsp salt plus more to taste
1½ lb (675 g) monkfish	1 tsp (5 ml) jalapeño powder (optional)
2 tsp (10 ml) mild chilli powder	6 tbsp (90 ml) chopped fresh coriander
1 tbsp (15 ml) vegetable oil	2 pints (1.2 litres) chicken or vegetable stock
2 medium onions, diced	½ tsp of saffron threads
1 jalapeño pepper, seeded and minced	20 oz (600 g) arborio rice
2 roasted red peppers, diced	2 fl oz (60 ml) white wine
2 cloves garlic, minced	6 oz (180 g) frozen peas
1 28-oz (800 ml) can chopped seeded tomatoes and their juice	2 medium spring onions, minced
½ tsp chopped fresh oregano	24 mussels, bearded, cleaned and rinsed
	2 tsp (10 ml) chopped fresh basil

1. Preheat the grill.
2. Sprinkle chicken pieces with paprika. Grill until just cooked, about 8 minutes. Do not overcook as chicken will be reheated later. When the chicken has cooled, cut each breast on the bias into thin slices and set aside.
3. Season prawns, scallops and monkfish with chilli powder. Cover with plastic wrap and set aside in the refrigerator.
4. Heat 2 tsp (10 ml) of the oil in a medium saucepan. Add onions, jalapeño peppers and garlic and sauté. Add tomatoes, oregano, thyme, bay leaves, sugar, salt and, if using, the jalapeño powder. Simmer, uncovered, until most of the liquid evaporates. Stir in 2 tbsp (30 ml) of the coriander.
5. Preheat the oven to 400°F (200°C, gas mark 6).
6. Bring the stock to a boil in a saucepan, add the saffron, and simmer over low heat. In a large frying pan, heat the remaining 1 tsp (5 ml) of oil, add the rice and stir constantly until rice is slightly toasted, or opaque, about 1 to 2 minutes. Add the wine and the tomato mixture and stir. Slowly add stock to the rice, 8 fl. oz (235 ml) at a time,

stirring constantly until liquid is almost absorbed. Add the peas and spring onions. Season to taste with salt. Remove pan from heat.

7. Arrange chicken, scallops, monkfish and prawns over rice mixture. Cover and bake for 7 minutes. Place mussels on top of rice and bake until mussels open, about 4 minutes. Sprinkle with basil and the remaining coriander, and serve.

Makes eight 10 oz/300 g servings.

Nutrition Facts: Calories 543, Fat 9 grams, Saturated Fat 1.9 grams, Cholesterol 185 mg, Carbohydrate 53 mg., Protein 58 grams, Sodium 694 mg, (without salt, sodium 560 mg)

Active Wellness Portion Equivalents: 3½ Grains/Starches, 4 Protein and 2 Vegetable Servings.

Yoghurt/Lime Marinade

This marinade is also a great dressing for a seafood salad.

2 fl oz (60 ml) honey	1 tbsp (15 ml) minced fresh ginger
2 fl oz (60 ml) fresh lime juice	1 tbsp (15 ml) minced fresh garlic
8 fl. oz (235 ml) non-fat yoghurt	1 tsp (5 ml) chopped fresh mint

1. Combine all the ingredients in a glass bowl and whisk well until creamy.
2. Marinate seafood or chicken in the marinade in the refrigerator for 1 to 2 hours. Grill.

Keeps for 3 to 4 days, refrigerated.

Makes approximately four 4 fl oz/125 ml servings.

Nutrition Facts: Calories 103, Fat 0 grams, Saturated Fat 0 grams, Cholesterol 1 mg, Protein 3.5 grams, Carbohydrate 23 grams, Sodium 45 mg

Active Wellness Portion Equivalents: ¼ Dairy and ½ Sweet Serving.

Spicy Indonesian Marinade

8 fl oz (250 ml) lite coconut milk	1 clove garlic, chopped
2½ oz (75 g) chopped fresh coriander	1 tsp (5 ml) grated fresh ginger
2 tbsp (30 ml) fructose	¼ tsp turmeric
1 tbsp (15 ml) curry powder	1 tsp (5 ml) vegetable oil
1 tbsp (15 ml) fresh lime juice	
1 jalapeño pepper, seeded and chopped	

1. Combine all the ingredients in a blender except oil. Blend until smooth. Pour into a bowl, add oil, and mix well.
2. Marinate seafood or chicken in the refrigerator for 1 to 2 hours. Grill.

Keeps for 5 days, refrigerated.

Makes about five 2 fl oz (60 ml) servings.

Nutrition Facts: Calories 62, Fat 4 grams, Saturated Fat 2 grams, Cholesterol 0 mg, Protein 0 grams, Carbohydrate 6 grams, Sodium 9 mg

Active Wellness Portion Equivalent: 1 Fat per Serving.

VEGETARIAN MAIN COURSES

Beans, grains and soya products not only provide good sources of protein for the vegetarian diet, they also offer a wealth of creative opportunities for the vegetarian cook. Even die-hard meat eaters will be tempted by the hearty offerings in this section, and everyone should consider making one or two meatless meals every week.

Black Bean and Spinach Burritos

Beans
1 tsp (5 ml) vegetable oil
1 onion, diced small
1 green pepper, diced small
2 tbsp (30 ml) fresh orange juice
2 cloves garlic, minced
1 tsp (5 ml) ground cumin
½ teaspoon chilli powder

8 fl oz (250 ml) chopped canned
   plum tomatoes with juice
2 15-oz (425 g) cans black beans,
   drained
2 tbsp (30 ml) fresh lime juice
2 tbsp (30 ml) chopped fresh coriander
Pinch of sugar or fructose

Rice
5 oz (150 g) brown rice
1 tsp (5 ml) ground cumin
½ tsp turmeric

16 fl oz (500 ml) water
½ tsp salt

2 lb (900 g) fresh spinach, stemmed
   and cleaned
12 fl. oz (355 ml) grated non-fat Cheddar or

soya cheese
6 large low-fat flour tortillas (12 in/30
   cm diameter)

≡ 277 ≡

Beans

1. Heat a large saucepan over high heat until very hot. Add the oil followed by the onion and sear for 30 seconds.
2. Add the peppers and sear for 30 seconds. Then add orange juice to deglaze and stir well.
3. Add the garlic, turn down the heat to medium, and add the cumin and the chilli powder. Stir vigorously for 15 seconds to release the flavours. Stir in the tomatoes with their juice. Cook for 2 minutes.
4. Add the black beans and lime juice, stir gently, and add water halfway up saucepan. Cook over low heat, uncovered, until the liquid is thick, about 15 minutes. Add the coriander and season to taste. An extra squeeze of lime juice and a pinch of sugar or fructose may be needed.

Rice

1. Put the rice, cumin and turmeric in a saucepan. Add the water and bring to the boil, uncovered, and turn down the heat.
2. Cook, covered, over low heat for 30 to 40 minutes, or until the liquid has been absorbed. Fluff the rice with a fork. Season with salt.

Spinach

1. Place the cleaned spinach with the water still clinging to its leaves in a frying pan and cook until just wilted. Let cool and squeeze out excess moisture.

ASSEMBLY:

1. Lay a tortilla on a work surface. Place 2 oz (60 g) cooked rice, a generous 4 oz (125 g) beans, 2 oz (60 g) spinach and 2 tbsp (30 ml) cheese on the bottom end of the tortilla. Fold over sides, then roll up neatly.
2. Burritos can be reheated in a microwave or warmed, seam side down, wrapped in foil, in a 325°F (160°C, gas mark 3) oven for 10 minutes.

Makes 6 servings.

Nutrition Facts: Calories 509, Fat 5 grams, Saturated Fat 1 gram, Cholesterol 0 mg, Protein 32 grams, Carbohydrate 68 grams, Sodium 385 mg

Active Wellness Portion Equivalents: 2½ Grains/Starches, 1 Protein, 2 Dairy (or if using soya cheese add another protein) and 1 Vegetable Serving.

Three-Bean Chilli with Bulgur

1 28-oz (800 g) can Italian plum tomatoes	2 green peppers, cut into ½ in (1.25 cm) dice
1 tsp (5 ml) vegetable oil	

2 medium onions, cut into ½ in
  (1.25 cm) dice
2 tsp (10 ml) dried basil
2 tsp (10 ml) ground cumin
1 tsp (5 ml) chilli powder
1 tsp (5 ml) dried oregano
¼ tsp cayenne or jalapeño powder
16 fl oz (500 ml) water
1 tsp (5 ml) salt

1 tsp (5 ml) sugar
4 oz (125 g) bulgur
1 15-oz (425 g) can black beans, drained
1 15-oz (425 g) can pinto beans,
  drained
1 15-oz (425 g) can kidney beans, drained
6½ oz (200 g) frozen sweetcorn kernels
½ oz (15 g) chopped fresh coriander

1. Blend the tomatoes in a blender or food processor until coarsely puréed. Set aside.
2. Add 1 tsp (5 ml) oil to a large pot and sear the peppers and onions over high heat.
Cook 2 minutes, stir in the basil, cumin, chilli powder, oregano and cayenne and cook
30 seconds. Add the tomatoes, water, salt and sugar.
3. Add the bulgur, stir well, lower the heat and simmer, covered, until the bulgur is
cooked, about 30 minutes. Stir in the beans, sweetcorn and coriander. Cook for 10
minutes.

Makes twelve 1-cup (8 fl oz/150 ml) serving.

Nutrition Facts: Calories 225, Fat 1.5 grams, Saturated Fat 0 grams, Cholesterol 0 mg,
Protein 23 grams, Carbohydrate 45 grams, Sodium 408 mg

Active Wellness Portion Equivalents: 3 Protein and 1 Grains/Starches Servings.

Vegetable Gratin Provençale

4 large ripe tomatoes
1 tsp (5 ml) olive oil
2 large onions, thinly sliced
2 cloves garlic, minced
2 fl oz (60 ml) vegetable stock
½ tsp dried thyme or 1½ tsp
  fresh
½ tsp dried oregano or 1½ tsp
  fresh

2 medium courgettes, sliced
  ¼ in (0.6 cm) thick
1 aubergine, peeled and sliced ¼ in
  (0.6 cm) thick
¼ tsp salt
¼ tsp ground black pepper
1 oz (30 g) fresh breadcrumbs
1 oz (30 g) grated Parmesan cheese

1. Preheat the oven to 375°F (190°C, gas mark 5).
2. Bring a large pot of water to a boil. With a sharp knife, score an 'x' on the stem ends
of the tomatoes. Drop the tomatoes into the boiling water for 10 to 15 seconds, then
remove and plunge into cold water. Remove the cores, and peel. Halve the tomatoes
and gently squeeze out the juice and seeds. Dice 2 of the tomatoes and set aside. Cut
the other 2 tomatoes into ¼ in (0.6 cm) slices.

3. Heat the oil in a large frying pan and add the onions and garlic. Sauté briefly until the onions are wilted and then add the stock. Cook until the onions are soft and the liquid has evaporated. Add the diced tomatoes, thyme and oregano. Cook for about 2 to 3 minutes.
4. Cover the bottom of a gratin dish or shallow baking dish with half of the onion-tomato mixture.
5. Layer the courgettes, sliced tomatoes and aubergine over the onion mixture. Season with salt and pepper. Top with the rest of the onion mixture. Sprinkle the breadcrumbs over the mixture, then top with the Parmesan cheese.
6. Cover with aluminium foil and bake for 20 minutes. Uncover and bake 10 to 15 minutes more, or until the top is golden brown and crispy and the mixture is bubbling. Serve warm.

Makes 6 servings.

Nutrition Facts: Calories 110, Fat 3 grams, Saturated Fat 1 gram, Cholesterol 3 mg, Protein 5 grams, Carbohydrate 18 grams, Sodium 150 mg.

Active Wellness Portion Equivalent: 4 Vegetable Servings.

SALADS & SIDE DISHES

Bright salad greens, sweet root vegetables, lively peppers, satisfying potatoes—nature packs more vitamins, carotenoids and phytochemicals into vegetables than any other group of foods. We at Active Wellness along with other health and nutrition professionals know that eating lots of vegetables will reduce your risk for heart disease and cancer. The Active Wellness combination of low-fat cooking methods and high-flavour seasonings ensures that you receive all the delicious benefits from these intrinsically healthy foods.

Fat-Free Balsamic Vinaigrette

This versatile vinaigrette will keep for 1 week in the refrigerator.

2 fl oz (60 ml) fat-free yoghurt
1 fl oz (30 ml) vegetable stock
1 fl oz (30 ml) balsamic vinegar
1 shallot, minced
1 clove garlic, minced
¼ tsp minced fresh thyme or
⅛ tsp dried

¼ tsp minced fresh parsley or
⅛ tsp dried
¼ tsp minced fresh basil or
⅛ tsp dried
Pinch of sugar
Pinch of freshly ground black pepper
Pinch of salt

1. Combine the yoghurt, broth, vinegar, shallot and garlic in a medium bowl. Whisk well.
2. Stir in the herbs and seasonings. Refrigerate until ready to serve.

Makes 6 servings, ½ fl. oz (15 ml) each.

Nutrition Facts: Calories 18, Fat 0 grams, Saturated Fat 0 grams, Cholesterol 0 mg, Protein 0 grams, Carbohydrate 4 grams, Sodium 97 mg

Active Wellness Portion Equivalent: Free Food

Honey Mustard Seed Dressing

Keeps for 1 week, covered, in the refrigerator.

4 fl. oz (125 ml) plain non-fat yoghurt
  or soft tofu
2 fl. oz (60 ml) fresh orange juice
2 fl. oz (60 ml) rice wine vinegar

2 tbsp (30 ml) honey
2 tbsp (30 ml) Dijon mustard
2 tsp (10 ml) mustard seed
¼ tsp ground white pepper

Combine all the ingredients in a blender until smooth. Refrigerate until ready to serve.

Makes 12 servings, ½ fl. oz (15 ml) each.

Nutrition Facts: Calories 21, Fat 0 grams, Saturated Fat 0 grams, Cholesterol 0 mg, Protein .5 gram, Carbohydrate 4.5 grams, Sodium 12.5 mg

Active Wellness Portion Equivalent: Free Food

Lite Caesar Dressing

Keeps for 1 week, covered, in the refrigerator.

8 fl. oz (125 ml) plain non-fat yoghurt
  or mayonnaise
2 tbsp (30 ml) grated Parmesan
1 tbsp (15 ml) fresh lemon juice
1 tsp (5 ml) Worcestershire sauce
1 tsp (5 ml) Dijon mustard

2 whole anchovies or 1 tsp (5 ml) anchovy
  paste
1 tsp (5 ml) ground black pepper
1 clove garlic, mashed
Pinch of cayenne pepper

Combine all the ingredients in a blender until smooth. Refrigerate until ready to use.

Makes 6 servings, ½ fl. oz (15 ml) each.

Nutrition Facts: Calories 24, Fat 1 gram, Saturated Fat 0 grams, Cholesterol 2 mg, Protein 2 grams, Carbohydrate 2 grams, Sodium 87 mg

Active Wellness Portion Equivalent: Free Food

Raspberry Vinaigrette

Keeps for 1 week, covered, in the refrigerator.

6 oz (180 g) fresh or frozen
  raspberries
¼ tsp chopped fresh thyme
¼ tsp ground black pepper
3 tbsp (45 ml) raspberry vinegar

2 fl. oz (60 ml) water
2 tsp (10 ml) vegetable oil
1½ tsp (7 ml) low-sodium soy sauce
1 tbsp (15 ml) fructose

Combine all the ingredients in a blender until smooth. Refrigerate until ready to use.

Makes 16 servings, ½ fl. oz (15 ml) each.

Nutrition Facts: Calories 28, Fat 1 gram, Saturated Fat 0 grams, Cholesterol 0 mg, Protein 0 grams, Carbohydrate 5 grams, Sodium 64 mg

Active Wellness Portion Equivalent: Free Food

Fat-Free Coleslaw

If you'd like to simplify, you can buy prepared coleslaw ingredients in the supermarket in the produce section, which is usually a mixture of sliced cabbage and carrots.

½ medium green cabbage
3 carrots

Dressing
4 fl. oz (115 ml) fat-free mayonnaise
2 tbsp (30 ml) cider vinegar
2½ tbsp (35 ml) honey or fructose
1 tsp (5 ml) Dijon mustard (optional)

¼ tsp salt
1 tsp (5 ml) celery seed
Pinch of ground white pepper

1. Finely cut the cabbage into thin slices.
2. Peel the carrots and shred by using a hand grater or with the shredder disk of a food processor
3. Combine all the dressing ingredients and whisk well to blend.
4. Add the dressing to the slaw and toss well.
5. Refrigerate until ready to serve.

Keeps for 3 days, covered, in the refrigerator.

Makes five 6 oz (185 g) servings

Nutrition Facts: Calories 60, Fat 0 grams, Saturated Fat 0 grams, Cholesterol 0 mg, Protein 1 gram, Carbohydrate 16 grams, Sodium 278 mg

Active Wellness Portion Equivalent: 1 Vegetable Serving.

Wheatgrain Salad with Raspberry Vinaigrette

7 oz (210 g) wheatgrain (Ebly)
1 medium onion, peeled and finely diced
1 clove garlic, chopped
1 bay leaf
2 tsp (10 ml) dried thyme
1 tsp (5 ml) grated lemon zest
1 medium carrot, peeled and cut into
  ½ in (1.25 cm) dice

1 stalk celery, thinly sliced
8 oz (240 g) chopped raw fennel
3 oz (90 g) chopped dried fruits such
  as cherries, cranberries or coarsely
  chopped apricots
1 tbsp (15 ml) minced fresh parsley
4 fl. oz (115 ml)Raspberry Vinaigrette (see
  opposite page)

1. Place 32 fl. oz (945 ml) water in a large saucepan and bring to the boil. Add the wheatgrain. Cook for 2 minutes. Remove from the heat and let stand for 1 hour. Add enough water to cover by 1 in (2.5 cm).
2. Stir in the onion, garlic, bay leaf, thyme, and lemon zest. Cover and simmer for 15 minutes until berries are slightly puffed and softened. Remove from the heat, transfer to a large bowl, and let cool. Remove and discard the bay leaf.
3. Add the carrot, celery, fennel, dried fruits and parsley. Toss with the Raspberry Vinaigrette.

Makes four 6½ oz (200 g) servings.

Nutrition Facts: Calories 90, Fat 0 grams, Saturated Fat 0 grams, Cholesterol 0 mg, Protein 3 grams, Carbohydrate 21 grams, Sodium 36 mg

Active Wellness Portion Equivalents: 1 Grains/Starches Serving.

Wild and Brown Rice Pilaf

1 tsp (5 ml) vegetable oil
2 oz (60 g) finely chopped onions
5 oz (150 g) wild rice

5 oz (150 g) brown rice
35 fl. oz (1 litre) vegetable stock
2 oz (60 g) dried cranberries

Juice and zest of 1 medium orange
1 small red pepper, diced
1 small yellow pepper, diced
1 bunch spring onions, sliced

1 oz (30 g) chopped fresh parsley
1 tsp (5 ml) salt
1 tsp (5 ml) freshly ground black pepper

1. Heat the oil in a large saucepan over medium heat. Add the wild rice and brown rice and stir to coat with the oil. Add onions and cook until soft. Pour in the stock and bring to the boil. Reduce the heat to medium-low and simmer for 30 to 40 minutes, until the stock has been absorbed and the rice is tender.
2. While the rice is cooking, soak the cranberries in the orange juice.
3. When the rice is done, combine it with the soaked cranberries and juice, the peppers, spring onions, orange zest, parsley, salt and pepper. Serve warm or cold.

Makes eight 3½ oz (100 g) servings.

Nutrition Facts: Calories 124, Fat 1 gram, Saturated Fat 0 grams, Cholesterol 0 mg, Protein 4 grams, Carbohydrate 26 grams, Sodium 275 mg

Active Wellness Portion Equivalents: 1 Grains/Starches and 1 Vegetable Serving.

Mashed Potatoes

4 large potatoes, peeled
   and cut into large dice
8 fl. oz (250 ml) skimmed milk or
   low-fat buttermilk

1 tsp (5 ml) salt
½ tsp ground white pepper

1. Place the potatoes in a saucepan and cover with cold water. Bring the water to a boil and cook the potatoes until soft.
2. Simmer the milk in a small saucepan.
3. Run potatoes through a food mill, add the hot milk and, with a whisk or wooden spoon, mix well until the potatoes are creamy and smooth. Add more milk for desired consistency.
4. Season with salt and white pepper.

Makes four 4 oz (115 g) servings

Nutrition Facts: Calories 72, Carbohydrate 15 grams, Protein 34 grams, Fat 0 grams, Saturated Fat 0 grams, Cholesterol 0 mg, Sodium 582 mg

Active Wellness Portion Equivalent: 1 Grains/Starches Serving.

Hoummus

Serve with vegetables as a dip or make a sandwich with hoummus as the spread.

1 10-oz (300 g) can chickpeas
2 oz (60 g) plain non-fat yoghurt
2–3 tbsp (30–45 ml) fresh lemon juice
2 tbsp (30 ml) chopped fresh parsley
1 tsp (5 ml) ground cumin

½ tsp allspice
1 large clove garlic, minced
Salt to taste
Freshly ground black pepper to taste
¼ tsp cayenne pepper

1. Rinse and drain the chickpeas.
2. Combine the chickpeas with the remaining ingredients in a food processor and purée until smooth. Add a little water if the mixture is too thick. Season with salt and pepper to taste.

Makes eight 2 oz (60 g) servings.

Nutrition Facts: Calories 80, Fat 1.5 grams, Saturated Fat 0 grams, Cholesterol 0 mg, Protein 1 gram, Carbohydrate 6 grams, Sodium 70 mg

Papaya Peach Salsa

If peaches and papayas are not in season, feel free to substitute other fruits, such as pineapple, bananas or strawberries. Serve with grilled chicken, fish or meat. It is also good with toasted pita or tortilla crisps.

10 oz (300 g) diced papaya (about
   1½ small papayas)
10 oz (300 g) diced peaches (about
   3 peaches)
1 red pepper, diced
1 green pepper, diced
1 small, mild green chilli, minced

2 fl oz (60 ml) vegetable stock
2 tbsp (30 ml) chopped fresh coriander
2 tsp (10 ml) white wine vinegar
Dash of Tabasco sauce, or to taste
½ tsp sugar

1. Gently combine all the ingredients in a small mixing bowl.
2. Cover and refrigerate until ready to serve.

Makes 14 servings, 2 fl. oz (60 ml) each.

Nutrition Facts: Calories 20, Fat 0 grams, Saturated Fat 0 grams, Cholesterol 0 mg, Protein 0 grams, Carbohydrate 5 grams, Sodium 36 mg

Active Wellness Portion Equivalent: ½ Fruit Serving

Roasted Red Pepper and Aubergine Dip

2 medium aubergines
Sea salt
1 head garlic
3 tsp (15 ml) (approximately) olive oil
Cooking oil spray
2 red peppers
2 tsp (10 ml) fresh lemon juice

½ oz (15 g) chopped fresh basil
2 tbsp (30 ml) chopped fresh parsley
1 tsp (5 ml) chopped fresh thyme or
½ tsp (2.5 ml) dried thyme
¼ tsp freshly ground black pepper
Pinch of cayenne

1. Peel the aubergines, cut into ½ in (1.25 cm) slices, and sprinkle generously with salt. Let drain in a colander for 40 minutes. Rinse and pat dry.

2. Preheat the oven to 350°F (175°C, gas mark 4). Slice off the top ¼ in (0.6 cm) of the garlic head, to reveal the cloves. Season lightly with salt and sprinkle with 1 tsp (5 ml) of the oil. Wrap the head completely in aluminium foil.

3. Spray a baking sheet with cooking oil spray or line with greaseproof paper. Place the aubergine, red peppers and the garlic on the baking sheet. Roast until the aubergine is soft and golden, the peppers are completely roasted and the garlic is caramelized, or soft and golden, about 40 to 50 minutes. The garlic might need a little more time to become soft.

4. Transfer the peppers to a bowl and cover with plastic wrap. Allow the peppers to steam for 10 minutes, then remove the wrap. When the peppers are cool, peel and seed them. The skin should come off easily.

5. When the garlic is cool, squeeze the cloves into a food processor. Add the red peppers, aubergine, lemon juice, basil, parsley, and thyme. Pulse until coarsely blended—do not purée. Season with salt, black pepper and cayenne.

Makes about 32 fl. oz (1 litre).

Nutrition Facts per 2 Tablespoons: Calories 32, Fat 0 grams, Saturated Fat 0 grams, Cholesterol 0 mg, Protein 0 grams, Carbohydrate 2 grams, Sodium 28 mg

Active Wellness Portion Equivalent: 1 Vegetable Serving.

DESSERTS

Once you make the choice to follow an Active Wellness plan, it doesn't mean saying goodbye to chocolate and other sweet treats. As long as those goodies are low in fat and are made from wholesome ingredients—and consumed in moderation, of course—desserts can be a part of your weekly menus. Keep in mind, also, that fruit desserts are a fine way to work more beneficial fruits into your diet.

Apple Crisp

Use this all-purpose topping for other fruits such as pears, peaches, berries or rhubarb. Dried cherries or cranberries make a flavourful addition.

Filling

4 large apples	2 tbsp (30 ml) maple syrup
1 tbsp (15 ml) fresh lemon juice	1 tbsp (15 ml) plain flour (optional)
1 tsp (5 ml) cinnamon	

Topping

1 oz (30 g) walnuts	2 tbsp (30 ml) maple syrup
2 tbsp (30 ml) wholemeal flour	1 tbsp (15 ml) butter
2 tbsp (30 ml) dark brown sugar	12 oz (350 g) low-fat museli
2 tsp (10 ml) ground cinnamon	1 egg white

1. Preheat the oven to 375°F (190°C, gas mark 5). To make the filling, peel and core the apples and cut into diced pieces. Toss the apple pieces with lemon juice, cinnamon and flour, if using. Spread the mixture evenly in 4 individual ramekins or in a shallow gratin dish.

2. To make the topping, combine the nuts, flour, brown sugar and cinnamon in a food processor and pulse briefly. Add the maple syrup and butter and pulse until grainy. Add the museli and process briefly. Add the egg white, a little at a time, until mixture starts to clump. Do not let the mixture get too wet or it will turn soggy.

3. Using your hands, spread the topping over the apples. Bake 15 minutes or until the apples are simmering and the topping is brown and crisp. Cool slightly before serving. Makes 4 servings.

Nutrition Facts: Calories 238, Fat 3 grams, Saturated Fat 1 gram, Cholesterol 8 mg, Protein 1 gram, Carbohydrate 42 grams, Sodium 52 mg

Active Wellness Portion Equivalents: 1 Fruit, 1 Sweet, 1 Grains/Starches Serving.

Low-Fat Fudge Brownies

The better the quality of the chocolate and cocoa powder, the better the brownie.

Cooking oil spray	coarsely chopped
7 oz (150 g) plain flour	1 tbsp (15 ml) vegetable oil
8 oz (250 g) icing sugar	2 tsp (10 ml) unsalted butter
2 oz (60 g) unsweetened cocoa powder	4 tbsp (60 ml) light corn syrup
1 tsp (5 ml) baking powder	2 tsp (10 ml) pure vanilla extract
Pinch of salt	4 large egg whites
2 oz (60 g) plain chocolate,	

1. Preheat the oven to 350°F (175°C, gas mark 4). Line an 8 in (20 cm) square baking pan with aluminium foil. Spray with cooking oil spray.
2. In a medium bowl, sift together the flour, sugar, cocoa, baking powder and salt.
3. In a heavy, medium saucepan, combine the chocolate, oil and butter and heat over very low heat, stirring until melted and smooth. Do not let the chocolate burn. Remove from the heat and stir in the corn syrup and vanilla. Mix in the egg whites.
4. Stir the dry ingredients into the chocolate mixture until the batter is smooth and dense. Transfer the batter to the prepared baking pan and spread evenly. Bake for 20 minutes, or until the centre top is almost firm.
5. Cool the pan on a wire rack.
6. Remove the foil from the pan and peel off foil from the bottom of the brownies.
7. Cut the brownies into 12 bars, trimming off the edges if dry. Store in an airtight container or wrap each one in plastic wrap and refrigerate.

Makes 12 brownies.

Nutrition Facts: Calories 196, Fat 3 grams, Saturated Fat 1.5 grams, Cholesterol 0 mg, Protein 2 grams, Carbohydrate 36 grams, Sodium 50 mg

Active Wellness Portion Equivalents: 1 Sweet and 1 Grains/Starches Serving.

'I Can't Believe It's Fat-Free' Cheesecake

Crust
Cooking oil spray

6 oz (180 g) plain digestive biscuit crumbs

Cheesecake
16 oz (450 g) fat-free cream cheese
6½ oz (200 g) sugar
8 oz (240 ml) egg substitute
    or 8 egg whites

2 tbsp (30 ml) fresh lemon juice
2 tsp (10 ml) grated lemon zest
1½ tsp (7 ml) pure vanilla extract
¼ tsp salt
1 lb (450 g) fat-free or low-fat soured cream

Topping
12 oz (375 g) dried California apricots
10 fl. oz (300 ml) water
4 fl. oz (115 ml) sugar

2 tsp (10 ml) Grand Marnier or other
    orange liqueur
1 tsp (5 ml) fresh orange juice

1. Preheat the oven to 350°F (175°C, gas mark 4). Spray an 8 in (20 cm) springform pan with oil spray and coat the bottom with the digestive biscuit crumbs.
2. In a food processor or with an electric mixer, beat the cream cheese and sugar until very smooth, about 3 minutes. Blend in the egg substitute or egg whites. Add the

lemon juice, lemon zest, vanilla and salt. Blend until well mixed. Beat in the soured cream, just until blended.

3. Pour the batter into the prepared pan. Wrap the bottom of the pan with foil to prevent seepage. Set the pan in a larger pan and surround it with 1 in (2.5 cm) of very hot water. Bake for 45 minutes. Turn off the oven without opening the door and let the cake cool for 1 hour.

4. Place the apricots and water in a saucepan, cover tightly, and simmer for 20 minutes over a medium heat until the apricots are soft. Add the sugar and Grand Marnier and simmer for 5 more minutes. Purée the mixture in a food processor or blender. Press through a fine strainer. Stir in the orange juice. Spread the topping over the cheesecake and refrigerate.

5. When ready to serve, run a thin metal spatula around the sides of the cake and release the sides of the springform pan.

Makes 8 servings.

Nutrition Facts: Calories per slice 237, Fat 0 grams, Saturated Fat 0 grams, Cholesterol 0 mg, Protein 8 grams, Carbohydrate 92 grams, Sodium 304 mg

Active Wellness Portion Equivalents: 1 Sweet, 1 Dairy and ½ Fruit Serving.

Quick and Easy Low-Fat Lemon Curd

This recipe is very versatile. It can become an added ingredient for a low-fat fruit tart, a mille feuille or simply enjoyed with fresh berries or a slice of fairy cake.

1 egg	½ tsp (2.5 ml) grated lemon zest
5 oz (150 g) sugar or fructose	2½ oz (85 ml) water
5 tsp (25 ml) corn flour	2½ oz (85 ml) fresh lemon juice

1. Lightly beat the egg in a small bowl and set aside
2. Combine sugar, corn flour and lemon zest in a small saucepan. Stir well.
3. Add the water and lemon juice, and blend well with a whisk.
4. Bring to a boil over medium heat; cook for 1 minute, stirring constantly.
5. Gradually add, stirring, a small amount of hot lemon mixture into the beaten egg; add it back to the remaining lemon mixture in the saucepan, whisking constantly.
6. Cook over a medium heat until thickened, about 1 minute.
7. Remove from the heat and strain into a small bowl. Cover the lemon curd with plastic wrap and refrigerate.

Keeps for 3 days, covered, in the refrigerator.

Makes four 2 fl. oz (60 ml) servings.

Nutrition Facts: Calories 171, Fat 1 gram, Saturated Fat 0 grams, Cholesterol 53 mg, Protein 2 grams, Carbohydrate 42 grams, Sodium 17 mg

Active Wellness Portion Equivalents: 1 Sweet and 1 Grains/Starches Serving.

APPENDIX

Starter Eating Plans
General Eating Plan and Vegetarian Eating Plan for Women and Men
(Please note, additional servings are given for men.)

Breakfast

1 Grains/Starches	8 fl. oz (235 ml) dry flake cereal or hot cereal
1 Fruit	2 tbsp (30 ml) raisins or 6 fl. oz (175 ml) berries
½ Dairy Equivalent	4 fl. oz (115 ml)skimmed milk or soya bean milk
Water Equivalent	8–16 fl. oz (235–475 ml) of herbal tea or water
Other	Vitamins
Other	Sprinkle flaxseeds on cereal or mix in flax oil with milk
Men add: 1 Grains/Starches	1 slice of whole-grain toast
Men add:	1 tbsp(15 ml) of nuts for cereal (e.g. walnuts), or 4 pecan halves or 2 tsp(10 ml) of natural peanut butter for your toast or 1 tbsp (15 ml) low-fat cream cheese

Lunch

1 Grains/Starches	4 fl. oz (115 ml) cooked beans (e.g. chickpeas, kidney and black beans, lentils) or 8 fl. oz (235 ml) of bean soup.
Men add: 1 Grains/Starches	8 fl. oz (235 ml) bean soup or 4 fl. oz (115 ml)bean salad (if oil is added to the salad—count a fat and omit a fat later) or 4 fl. oz (115 ml) pasta salad or potato salad with fat-free or low-fat dressing, or 1 oz. (30 g) popcorn or low-fat or fat-free crisps
1½ Dairy Equivalent	1½ oz (45 g) low-fat cheese, or 4 fl. oz (115 ml) low-fat cottage cheese or 8 fl. oz (235 ml) yoghurt
1 Fat	2 tbsp (30 ml) low-fat salad dressing
Vegetables (Free) Equals about 3 servings	At least 8 fl. oz (235 ml) dark green lettuce or spinach, 4 fl. oz (115 ml) of any other vegetable that is unlimited—can include carrots, tomatoes, plus any other vegetables you would like.
1 Sweet	4 fl. oz (115 ml) low-fat or fat-free frozen yoghurt
Water Equivalent	16 fl. oz (475 ml) herbal tea, water or sparkling water

Snack

1 Fruit	1 small apple or orange
Water Equivalent	8 fl. oz (235 ml) herbal tea

Dinner

3 servings of lean protein equivalent Men add: 2 servings to make a total of 5 servings	3 oz (85 ml) lean poultry, fish, beef, pork, or 4½ oz (130 g) shellfish, 1 low-fat veggie burger, or 6 oz (170 g) of baked tofu
2 Grains/Starches Men add: 2 Grains/Starches	8 fl. oz (235 ml) any cooked grain: brown rice, couscous, barley 8 fl. oz (235 ml) bean soup plus extra serving of cooked grain (4 fl. oz/115 ml) or 2 slices of bread or 8 fl. oz (235 ml) of cooked grain
1 Vegetable	4 fl. oz (115 ml) steamed broccoli
2 Vegetables	Mixed salad (16 fl. oz/475 ml raw vegetables)
2 Fat Men add: 1 Fat	2 tbsp (30 ml) low-fat salad dressing and 1 tsp (5 ml) olive oil for cooking) 1 tsp (5 ml) of olive oil for cooking
1 Alcohol *If you do not drink, you can trade alcohol for an extra grain or fruit serving	1 alcoholic beverage equivalent (e.g. 6 oz/175 ml wine), or 1 serving of fruit or grain (e.g. ⅓ melon or add an extra 4 fl. oz/115 ml of cooked grain to your meal or 8 fl. oz/235 ml bean soup)
Water Equivalent Men add: 1 Fruit	16 fl. oz (475 ml) sparkling water or herbal tea 8 fl. oz (235 ml) berries or other fruit

Snack

Water Equivalent	8 fl. oz (235 ml) of herbal tea
Men add: 1 Grains/Starches	1 oz (30 g) wholemeal pretzels or low-fat or fat-free popcorn

Insulin Resistance/Carbohydrate Cravings

Breakfast

1 Grains/Starches	8 fl. oz (235 ml) dry flake cereal or hot cereal
1 Fruit	2 tbsp (30 ml) raisins or 6 fl. oz (175 ml) berries
½ Dairy Equivalent	4 fl. oz (115 ml) skimmed milk or soya bean milk
Water Equivalent	8–16 fl. oz (235–475 ml) of herbal tea or water
Other	Vitamins
Other	Sprinkle flaxseeds on cereal or mix in flax oil with milk
Men add: 1 Fat	1 tbsp (15 ml) of nuts for cereal (e.g, walnuts), or 4 pecan halves

Lunch

1 Grains/Starches	4 fl. oz (115 ml) cooked beans (e.g. chickpeas, kidney beans, lentils) or 8 fl. oz (235 ml) of bean soup
1½ Dairy or dairy equivalent	1½ oz (45 g) of low-fat cheese or soya cheese, or 8 fl. oz (235 ml) low-fat cottage cheese or 8 fl. oz (235 ml) yoghurt or soya custard
1 Fat	2 tbsp (30 ml) low-fat salad dressing
Vegetables (Free) Equals about 3 servings of vegetables	At least 8 fl. oz (235 ml) dark green letuce or spinach, 4 fl. oz (115 ml) of any other vegetable that is unlimited—can include carrots, tomatoes, plus any other vegetables you would like
1 Sweet	4 fl. oz (115 ml) low-fat or fat-free frozen yoghurt
Water Equivalent	16 fl. oz (475 ml) herbal tea, water or sparkling water

Snack

1 Fruit	1 small apple or orange
Water Equivalent	8 fl. oz (235 ml) herbal tea

Dinner

3 servings of lean protein equivalent. Men add: 3 servings (to make 6)	3 oz (85 g) lean poultry, fish, beef, pork, or 4½ oz (130 g) shellfish, 1 low-fat veggie burger, or 6 oz (170 g) of baked tofu

2 Grains	8 fl. oz (235 ml) any cooked grain: brown rice, wholemeal couscous, barley, buckwheat
1 Vegetables	4 fl. oz (115 ml) steamed broccoli
1 Vegetables	8 fl. oz/235 ml mixed green salad with toasted nuts—see below for servings
2½ Fat Men add: ½ tablespoon more of fat	2½ tbsp (35 ml) toasted nuts (e.g. walnuts, pine nuts, pumpkin seeds) Add ½ tbsp (7 ml) more of nuts or seeds to fat serving
2 Fat Men add: 1 Fat	2 tbsp (30 ml) low-fat salad dressing and 1 tsp (5 ml) olive oil for cooking 1 tsp (5 ml) of olive oil for cooking
1 Alcohol *If you do not drink, you can trade alcohol for an extra grain or fruit serving	1 alcoholic beverage equivalent (e.g. 6 oz/175 ml wine), or 1 serving of fruit or grain (e.g. ⅓ melon or add an extra 4 fl. oz/115 ml of cooked grain to your meal or 8 fl. oz/235 ml of bean soup)
Water Equivalent	16 fl. oz (475 ml) sparkling water or herbal tea
Men add: 1 Dairy	8 fl. oz (235 m) low-fat or fat-free yoghurt

Osteoporosis

Breakfast

1 Grains/Starches	8 fl. oz (235 ml) dry flake cereal or hot cereal
1 Fruit	2 tbsp (30 ml) raisins or 6 fl. oz (175 ml) berries
½ Dairy Equivalent	4 fl. oz (115 ml) skimmed milk or soya bean milk
Water Equivalent	8–16 fl. oz (235–475 ml) of herbal tea or water
Other	Vitamins
Other	Sprinkle flaxseeds on cereal or mix in flax oil with milk
Men add: 1 Grains/Starches	1 slice of whole-grain toast
Men add: 1 Fat	1 tbsp (15 ml) nuts for cereal (e.g. walnuts), or 4 pecan halves or 2 tsp (10 ml) natural peanut butter for your toast or 1 tbsp (15 ml) low-fat cream cheese

Lunch

1 Grains/Starches Men add: 1 Grains/Starches	4 fl. oz (115 ml) cooked beans (e.g. chickpeas, kidney beans, lentils) or 8 fl. oz (235 ml) of bean soup 8 fl. oz (235 ml) bean soup or 4 fl. oz (115 ml) bean salad (if oil is added to the salad, count a fat and omit a fat later), 4 fl. oz (115 ml) pasta salad or potato salad with fat-free or low-fat dressing, or 1 oz. (30 g) of popcorn or low-fat or fat-free crisps
1½ Dairy Equivalent	1½ oz (45 g) low-fat cheese, or 8 fl. oz (235 ml) low-fat cottage cheese or 8 fl. oz (235 ml) yoghurt
1½ Fat Men add: ½ Fat	3 tbsp (45 ml) low-fat salad dressing Men add an extra tablespoon of dressing
Vegetables (Free) Equals about 2 servings	At least 8 fl. oz (235 ml) dark green lettuce or spinach, 8 fl. oz (235 ml) of any other vegetable that is unlimited—can include carrots, tomatoes, plus any other vegetables you would like.
1 Sweet	4 fl. oz (115 ml) low-fat or fat-free frozen yoghurt
Water Equivalent	16 fl. oz (475 ml) herbal tea, water or sparkling water

Snack

1 Fruit	1 small apple or orange
1 Dairy Equivalent	1 oz (30 g) low-fat or fat-free cheese and 1 low-fat yoghurt
Water Equivalent	8 fl. oz (235 ml) herbal tea

Dinner

2 servings of lean protein equivalent Men add: 4 servings	2 oz (60 g) lean poultry, fish, beef, pork, or 3 oz (85 g) of shellfish, 1 low-fat veggie burger or 4 oz (115 g) of baked tofu
1 Dairy Equivalent	1 oz (30 g) of low-fat cheese or 4 fl. oz (115 ml)cottage cheese—can be used as a topping for cooked vegetables, protein, or mixed in with grains
2 Grains/Starches	8 fl. oz (235 ml) any cooked grain: brown rice, wholemeal couscous, barley, buckwheat
1 Vegetables	4 fl. oz (115 ml) steamed broccoli
1 Vegetables	Mixed green salad (8 fl. oz/235 ml)
2 Fat	2 tbsp (30 ml) low-fat salad dressing and 1 tsp olive oil for cooking

Men add: 1 Fat	1 tsp (5 ml) of olive oil for cooking
1 Alcohol *If you do not drink, you can trade alcohol for an extra grain or fruit serving	1 alcoholic beverage equivalent (e.g. 6 fl. oz/175 ml wine), or 1 serving of fruit or grain (e.g. ⅓ melon or add an extra 4 fl. oz/115 ml of cooked grain to your meal or 8 fl. oz/235 ml of bean soup)
Water Equivalent	16 fl. oz (475 ml) sparkling water or herbal tea
Men add: 1 Fruit	8 fl. oz (235 ml) berries or other fruit

Snack

Water Equivalent	8 fl. oz (235 ml) herbal tea
Men add: 1 Grains/Starches	1 oz (30 g) wholemeal pretzels or low-fat or fat-free popcorn

Cardiovascular

Breakfast

1 Grains/Starches	8 fl. oz (235 ml) dry flake cereal or hot cereal
1 Fruit	2 tbsp (30 ml) raisins or 6 fl. oz (175 ml) berries
½ Dairy	4 fl. oz (115 ml) skimmed milk or soya bean milk
Water Equivalent	8–16 fl. oz (235–475 ml) of herbal tea or water
Other	Vitamins
Other	Sprinkle flaxseeds on cereal or mix in flax oil with milk
Men add: 1 Grains/Starches	1 slice of wholemeal toast
Men add: 1 Fat	1 tbsp (15 ml) of nuts for cereal (e.g. walnuts), or 4 pecan halves or 2 tsp (5 ml) of natural peanut butter for your toast or 1 tbsp (15 ml) low-fat cream cheese

Lunch

1 Grains/Starches	4 fl. oz (115 ml) cooked beans (e.g. chickpeas, kidney beans, lentils) or 8 fl. oz (235 ml) of bean soup
Men add the following foods: 1 Grains/Starches	8 fl. oz (235 ml) bean soup or 4 fl. oz (115 ml) bean salad (if oil is added to the salad, count a fat and omit a fat later), 4 fl. oz (115 ml) pasta salad or potato salad with fat-free or low-fat dressing, or 1 oz (30 g) of popcorn or low-fat or fat-free crisps
1 Dairy Equivalent	1½ oz (45 g) low-fat cheese, or 8 fl. oz (235 ml) low-fat cottage cheese or 8 fl. oz (235 ml) yoghurt
Foods to use sparingly	2–3 tbsp (30–45 ml) of fat-free salad dressing for salad
Vegetables (Free) Equals about 2 servings	At least 8 fl. oz (235 ml) dark green lettuce or spinach, 8 fl. oz (235 ml) of any other vegetable that is unlimited—can include carrots, tomatoes, plus any other vegetables you would like
1 Sweet	4 fl. oz (115 ml) low-fat or fat-free frozen yoghurt
Men add: 1 Fruit	1 small banana (4 in/10 cm) or other fruit
Water Equivalent	16 fl. oz (475 ml) herbal tea, water or sparkling water

Snack

1 Fruit	1 small apple or orange
Water Equivalent	8 fl. oz (235 ml) herbal tea

Dinner

3 servings of lean protein equivalent Men add: 2 servings	3 oz (85 g) lean poultry, fish, beef, pork, or 4½ oz (125 g) shellfish, 1 low-fat veggie burger, or 6 oz (170 g) of baked tofu
2 Grains/Starches	8 fl. oz (235 ml) any cooked grain: brown rice, wholemeal couscous, barley, buckwheat grain pasta
Men add: 2 Grains/Starches	8 fl. oz (235 ml) of bean soup plus an extra serving of cooked grain (4 fl. oz/115 ml) or 2 slices of bread or 8 fl. oz (235 ml) of cooked grain
1 Vegetables	4 fl. oz (115 ml) steamed broccoli
2 Vegetables	Mixed salad (16 fl. oz/475 ml raw vegetables)

1 Alcohol *If you do not drink, you can trade alcohol for an extra grain or fruit serving	1 alcoholic beverage equivalent (e.g. 6 fl. oz/175 ml wine), or 1 serving of fruit or grain (e.g. ⅓ melon or add an extra 4 fl. oz/115 ml cooked grain to your meal or 8 fl. oz/235 ml of bean soup)
Water Equivalent	16 fl. oz (475 ml) sparkling water or herbal tea
Men add: 1 Fruit	8 fl. oz (235 ml) berries or other fruit

Snack

Water Equivalent	8 fl. oz (235 ml) herbal tea
Men add: 1 Grains/Starches	1 oz (30 g) wholemeal pretzels or low-fat or fat-free popcorn

Cancer

Breakfast

1 Grains/Starches	8 fl. oz (235 ml) dry flake cereal or hot cereal
1 Fruit	2 tbsp (30 ml) raisins or 6 fl. oz (175 ml) berries
½ Dairy Equivalent	4 fl. oz (115 ml) skimmed milk or soya bean milk
Water Equivalent	8–16 fl. oz (115 –235 ml) of herbal tea or water
Other	Vitamins
Other	Sprinkle flaxseeds on cereal or mix in flax oil with milk
Men add: 1 Grains/Starches	1 slice of wholemeal toast
Men add: 1 Fat	1 tbsp (15 ml) of nuts for cereal (e.g. walnuts), or 4 pecan halves or 2 tsp (10 ml) of natural peanut butter for your toast or 1 tbsp (15 ml) low-fat cream cheese

Lunch

1 Grains/Starches	4 fl. oz (115 ml) cooked beans (e.g. chickpeas, kidney beans, lentils) or 8 fl. oz (235 ml) of bean soup
Men add: 1 Grains/Starches	8 fl. oz (235 ml) bean soup or 4 fl. oz (115 ml) bean salad (if oil is added to the salad, count a fat and omit a fat later), 4 fl. oz (115 ml) pasta salad or potato salad with fat-free or low-fat dressing, or 1 oz (30 g) of popcorn or low-fat or fat-free crisps
1½ Dairy Equivalent	1½ oz (45 ml) of low-fat cheese, or 8 fl. oz (235 ml) low-fat cottage cheese or 8 fl. oz (235 ml) yoghurt
1 Fat	2 tbsp (30 ml) low-fat salad dressing
Vegetables (Free) Equals about 2 servings	At least 8 fl. oz (235 ml) dark green lettuce or spinach, 8 fl. oz (235 ml) of any other vegetable that is unlimited—can include carrots, tomatoes, plus any other vegetables you would like
1 Sweet	4 fl. oz (115 ml) low-fat or fat-free frozen yoghurt
1 Fruit	1 small apple, pear, orange or other fruit
Water Equivalent	16 fl. oz (475 ml) herbal tea, water or sparkling water

Snack

1 Fruit	1 small apple or orange
Water Equivalent	8 fl. oz (235 ml) herbal tea

Dinner

4 Servings of lean protein equivalent	4 oz (115 g) lean poultry, fish, beef, pork, or 6 oz (170 g) shellfish, 2 low-fat veggie burgers or 8 oz (225 g) of baked tofu or 16 fl. oz (475 ml) of cooked beans
1 Grains/Starches	4 fl. oz (115 ml) of any cooked grain: brown rice, wholemeal couscous, barley, buckwheat
Men add: 1 Grain/Starches	8 fl. oz (235 ml) of bean soup or 1 slice of bread or 8 fl. oz (235 ml) of cooked grain soup or 8 fl. oz (235 ml) of minestrone soup (which has beans and grains)
1 Vegetables	4 fl. oz (115 ml) steamed broccoli
2 Vegetables	Mixed salad (16 fl. oz/475 ml raw vegetables)
2 Fat	2 tbsp (30 ml) low-fat salad dressing and 1 tsp (5 ml) olive oil for cooking
Men add: 1 Fat	1 tsp (5 ml) of olive oil for cooking

1 Alcohol *If you do not drink, you can trade alcohol for an extra grain or fruit serving	1 alcoholic beverage equivalent (e.g. 6 fl. oz/175 ml wine), or 1 serving of fruit or grain (e.g. ⅓ melon or add an extra 4 fl. oz (115 ml) of cooked grain to your meal or 8 fl. oz/235 ml of bean soup)
Water Equivalent	16 fl. oz (475 ml) sparkling water or herbal tea
1 Fruit	8 fl. oz (235 ml) of berries or other fruit
Water Equivalent	8 fl. oz (235 ml) herbal tea
Men add: 1 Grains/Starches	1 oz (30 g) wholemeal pretzels or low-fat or fat-free popcorn

Starter Exercise Plans

Aerobic Programme—Light Activity			
Week	Warm Up	Aerobic Activity aiming to reach your Target Heart Rate (Exercise Time) Activities = walking, light biking, walking up stairs. Remember, you can break up your exercise time into shorter sessions that total the recommended time allotment.	Frequency (Days/Week)
1-2	10 minutes (walking or walking up stairs)	10 minutes week one 15 minutes week two	3 days/week
3-4	10 minutes (walking or walking up stairs)	20 minutes week one 25 minutes week two	3 days/week
5-6	10 minutes (walking or walking up stairs)	30 minutes week one 35 minutes week two	4 days/week
7-8	10 minutes (walking or walking up stairs)	40 minutes week one 45 minutes week two	4 days/week
9-10	10 minutes (walking or walking up stairs)	50 minutes week one 60 minutes week two	5 days/week
11-12	10 minutes (walking or walking up stairs)	60 min. week; then increase distance (pick up your pace, but stay within target heart rate)	5 days/week
13-14	10 minutes (walking or walking up stairs)	60 min. week; then increase distance (pick up your pace, but stay within target heart rate)	5 days/week
15-16	10 minutes (walking or walking up stairs)	60 min. week; then increase distance (pick up your pace, but stay within target heart rate)	5 days/week

Aerobic Programme—Moderate Activity

Week	Warm Up 10 minutes (e.g. walking, light jogging in place, cycling)	Aerobic Activity at your Target Heart Rate Duration (Exercise Time) Activities = brisk walking, cycling, beginner-intermediate aerobic classes. Remember, you can break up your exercise time into two sessions.	Cool Down with light aerobic activity (e.g. brisk walking) and stretching	Frequency (Days/ Week)
1-2	10 minutes	20 to 30 minutes/day	5 min. lower intensity aerobic 5 min. stretching	3-4 days/ week
3-4	10 minutes	25 to 35 minutes/day	5 min. lower intensity aerobic 5 min. stretching	3-4 days/ week
5-6	10 minutes	35 to 40 minutes/day	5 min. lower intensity aerobic 5 min. stretching	4-5 days/ week
7-8	10 minutes	45 to 50 minutes/day	5 min. lower intensity aerobic 5 min. stretching	4-5 days/ week
9-10	10 minutes	50 to 60 minutes/day	5 min. lower intensity aerobic 5 min. stretching	4-5 days/ week
11-12	10 minutes	60 min. week; then increase distance (pick up pace, but stay within target heart rate) or increase time by 5-10 min.	5 min. lower intensity aerobic 5 min. stretching	4-5 days/ week
13-14	10 minutes	60 min. week; then increase distance (pick up pace, but stay within target heart rate) or increase time by 5-10 min.	5 min. lower intensity aerobic 5 min. stretching	4-5 days/ week
15-16	10 minutes	60 min. week; then increase distance (pick up pace, but stay within target heart rate) or increase time by 5-10 min.	5 min. lower intensity aerobic 5 min. stretching	4-5 days/ week

Aerobic Programme—High Activity

Week	Warm Up 10 minutes (e.g. walking, light jogging in place, cycling)	Aerobic Activity at your Target Heart Rate Duration (Exercise Time) Activities = jogging (5mph), cycling (15 mph), advanced aerobic classes (e.g. step, spinning). Remember, you can break up your exercise time into two sessions.	Cool Down with light aerobic activity (e.g. brisk walking) and stretching	Frequency (Days/ Week)
1-2	10 minutes	15 to 20 minutes/day	5 min. lower intensity aerobic 5 min. stretching	3-4 days/ week
3-4	10 minutes	25 to 30 minutes/day	5 min. lower intensity aerobic 5 min. stretching	3-4 days/ week
5-6	10 minutes	35 to 40 minutes/day	5 min. lower intensity aerobic 5 min. stretching	4-5 days/ week
7-8	10 minutes	45 to 50 minutes/day	5 min. lower intensity aerobic 5 min. stretching	4-5 days/ week
9-10	10 minutes	55 to 60 minutes/day	5 min. lower intensity aerobic 5 min. stretching	4-5 days/ week
11-12	10 minutes	60 min. week; then increase distance (pick up pace, but stay within target heart rate) or increase time by 5-10 min.	5 min. lower intensity aerobic 5 min. stretching	4-5 days/ week
13-14	10 minutes	60 min. week; then increase distance (pick up pace, but stay within target heart rate) or increase time by 5-10 min.	5 min. lower intensity aerobic 5 min. stretching	4-5 days/ week
15-16	10 minutes	60 min. week; then increase distance (pick up pace, but stay within target heart rate) or increase time by 5-10 min.	5 min. lower intensity aerobic 5 min. stretching	4-5 days/ week

General Strength Training Programme—Light Activity
Refer to Strength Training in Step 5

Week	Weight/Resistance	Repetitions	Frequency (Days/Week)
1-2	No weight or resistance	5-10 repetitions of each exercise without strain	1-2 sessions/week
3-4	No weight or resistance	8-12 repetitions of each exercise without strain	2 sessions/week
5-6	Light weight or light resistance	8-12 repetitions of each exercise without strain	2 sessions/week
7-8	Light weight or light resistance	5-10 repetitions of each exercise without strain. Increase to two sets of 8-12 repetitions of each exercise.	2 sessions/week
9-10	Increase resistance by 5 per cent if you are achieving your current resistance level with ease	5-10 repetitions of each exercise without strain. Increase to two sets of 8-12 repetitions of each exercise.	2-3 sessions/week

Resistance Note: Do not increase resistance until you are achieving the recommended number of repetitions comfortably. Also, remember to breathe during each exercise.

Repetition Note: The goal is to achieve 10 to 12 repetitions of each exercise per set. If you are working toward this goal, begin with the number of repetitions you can complete comfortably without strain and increase this number by 2 repetitions each week until you reach the goal of 12 repetitions for each exercise.

General Strength Training Programme—Moderate Activity
Refer to Strength Training in Step 5

Week	Weight/Resistance	Repetitions	Frequency (Days/Week)
1-2	Light weight or light resistance	8-12 repetitions of each exercise without strain	2-3 sessions/ week
3-4	Light weight or light resistance	8-12 repetitions of each exercise without strain. Increase to 2-3 sets of 8-12 repetitions of each exercise	2-3 sessions/ week
5-6	Light weight or light resistance	8-12 repetitions of each exercise without strain. Increase to 2-3 sets of 8-12 repetitions of each exercise	2-3 sessions/ week
7-8	Increase resistance by 5 per cent if you are achieving your current resistance level with ease	8-12 repetitions of each exercise without strain. Increase to 2-3 sets of 8-12 repetitions of each exercise	2-3 sessions/ week
9-10	Maintain resistance level from week 8	8-12 repetitions of each exercise without strain. Increase to 2-3 sets of 8-12 repetitions of each exercise	2-3 sessions/ week

Resistance Note: Do not increase resistance until you are achieving the recommended number of repetitions comfortably. Also, remember to breathe during each exercise.

Repetition Note: The goal is to achieve 10 to 12 repetitions of each exercise per set. If you are working toward this goal, begin with the number of repetitions you can complete comfortably without strain and increase this number by 2 repetitions each week until you reach the goal of 12 repetitions for each exercise. Increase the number of sets up to three per exercise; when you achieve this comfortably, increase resistance by 5 per cent.

General Strength Training Programme—High Activity
Refer to Strength Training in Step 5

Week	Weight/Resistance	Repetitions	Frequency (Days/Week) Take at least one rest day between each session
1-2	Adequate weight or resistance to achieve 8-12 repetitions with some effort, but no strain	10-12 repetitions of each exercise without strain. Two sets.	3 sessions/ week
3-4	Maintain weight/ resistance level during week 2.	10-12 repetitions of each exercise without strain. Two sets.	3 sessions/ week
5-6	Increase resistance by 5 per cent if you are achieving your current resistance level with ease	10-12 repetitions of each exercise without strain. Two sets.	3 sessions/ week
7-8	Maintain weight/ resistance level during week 6.	10-12 repetitions of each exercise without strain. Two sets.	3 sessions/ week
9-10	Increase resistance by 5 per cent if you are achieving your current resistance level with ease	10-12 repetitions of each exercise without strain. Two sets.	3 sessions/ week

Resistance Note: Do not increase resistance until you are achieving the recommended number of repetitions comfortably. Also, remember to breathe during each exercise.

Repetition Note: The goal is to achieve 10 to 12 repetitions of each exercise per set. If you are working toward this goal, begin with the number of repetitions you can complete comfortably without strain and increase this number by 2 repetitions each week until you reach the goal of 12 repetitions for each exercise. Increase the number of sets up to three per exercise; when you achieve this comfortably, increase resistance by 5 per cent.

General Stretching Programme—All Flexibility Levels

Week	Warm Up (at your current intensity level)	Duration (Time) of Stretch	Repetitions	Frequency in Days/Week and Minutes/ Day
1-2	10 minutes	20 seconds/stretch	2-5 repetitions/ exercise	1-2 sessions/week 15-30 minutes/day
3-4	10 minutes	20 seconds/stretch	2-5 repetitions/ exercise	1-2 sessions/week 15-30 minutes/day
5-6	10 minutes	20 seconds/stretch	2-5 repetitions/ exercise	2 sessions/week 20-40 minutes/day
7-8	10 minutes	20 seconds/stretch	2-5 repetitions/ exercise	2-3 sessions/week 25-45 minutes/day
9-10	10 minutes	20 seconds/stretch	2-5 repetitions/ exercise	3 sessions/week 30-60 minutes/day

Repetition Note: See specific exercises in Stretching Exercises in Step 5 to guide you with the number of repetitions for each movement. When holding the stretch do not bounce, aim for a sustained comfortable stretch. Also, remember yoga can count as a stretch routine and a stress management routine. If you are very flexible, start at your current level and aim for a goal to increase your frequency (days/week) or duration (minutes/session). Remember, stretching can be done every day without harming your body.

BIBLIOGRAPHY

American College of Sports Medicine. *Resource Manual for Guidelines for Exercise Testing and Prescription,* 2nd ed. Philadelphia: William and Wilkins, 1993.

American College of Sports Medicine. *Fitness Book.* Champaign, Ill: Leisure Press, 1992.

American Council on Exercise. *Personal Trainer Manual.* Boston: Reebok University Press, 1991.

Anderson, B. *Stretching.* Bolinas, CA: Shelter Publications, Inc., 1980.

Birkedahl, N. *The Habit Control Workbook.* Oakland, CA: New Harbinger Publications, Inc., 1990.

Christensen, A. *The American Yoga Association Beginner's Manual.* New York: Simon & Schuster, 1997.

Clark, N. *Sports Nutrition Guidebook.* Champaign, Ill: Leisure Press, 1990.

Coleman, E. *Eating for Endurance,* 3rd ed. Palo Alto, CA: Bull Publishing Co., 1992.

Corriher, S. *Cookwise.* New York: William Morrow & Co., Inc., 1997.

Craig, S., J. Haigh, and S. Harrar. *The Complete Book of Alternative Nutrition.* Emmaus, PA: Rodale Press, 1997.

Culinary Institute of America. *Culinary Orientation for Dietitians.* New York, 1996.

Dalton, S. *Overweight and Weight Management.* Maryland: Aspen Publishers, Inc., 1997.

Daviglus, M. L., et al. 'Fish Intake and Risk of Myocardial Infarction.' *The New England Journal of Medicine* Vol. 336, 1997.

Dietz, W. H., and S. L. Gortmaker. 'Do We Fatten Our Children at the Television Set? Obesity and Television Viewing in Children and Adolescents.' *Pediatrics* Vol. 75, 1985.

Drummond, K., and J. F. Vastano. *Cook's Healthy Handbook.* New York: John Wiley & Sons, Inc., 1993.

Duerr, M. *Above and Below the Belt.* Canyon Ranch, Arizona: 1989.

Edwards, B. *America's Favorite Drug—Caffeine.* Berkeley, CA: Odian Press, 1992.

Environmental Nutrition: The Newsletter of Food, Nutrition, and Health. 1997-April 1998.

Erasmus, U. *Fats That Heal and Fats That Kill.* Canada: Alive Books, 1993.

Eriksson, J., et al. 'Aerobic Endurance Exercise or Circuit-Type Resistance Training for Individuals with Impaired Glucose Tolerance.' *Hormone and Metabolic Research* Vol. 30, 1998.

Fescanich, D., et al. 'Protein Consumption and Bone Fractures in Women.' *American Journal of Epidemiology* Vol. 143, 1996.

Foreyt, J., and K. Goodrick. 'The Ultimate Triumph of Obesity.' *Lancet* Vol. 346, 1995.

Fried, R. E., et al. 'The Effect of Filtered Coffee Consumption on Plasma Lipid Levels: Results of a Randomized Clinical Trial.' *JAMA* Vol. 267, 1992.

Groppel, J., N. Hall, and J. Loehr. *Optimal Health.* Niles, IL: Nightingale Conant Corporation. Audiocassette, 1996.

Indiana Soybean Development Council. *Soy Facts for Dietitians, 1996.*

Jones, S. *How To Meditate.* New Canaan, CT: Keats Publishing, Inc., 1997.

Kabat-Zinn, J. *Full Catastrophe Living: Using the Wisdom of Your Body and Mind to Face Stress, Pain, and Illness.* New York: Delacorte Press, 1990.

Kannel, W. B., and R. C. Ellison. 'Alcohol and Coronary Heart Disease: The Evidence for a Protective Effect.' *Clinica Chimica Acta* Vol. 246, 1996.

Kline, D. A. *Nutrition & Immunity—Part I: Immune Components and Nutrients,* 3rd ed. Nutrition Dimension, Inc., 1995.

Kuczarmanski, R. J., et al. 'Increasing Prevalence of Overweight Among U.S. Adults: The National Health and Nutrition Examination Surveys, 1960-1991.' *JAMA* Vol. 272, 1994.

LaForge, R. 'Mind-Body Fitness: Encouraging Prospects for Primary and Secondary Prevention.' *Journal Cardiovascular Nursing* 1997.

Lagatree, K. *Feng Shui.* New York: Villard, 1996.

Lazarus, R., and S. Folkman. *Stress, Appraisal, and Coping.* New York: Springer Publishing Co., 1984.

Mahan, K., and M. Arlin. *Krause's Food, Nutrition, and Diet Therapy,* 8th ed. Philadelphia: W. B. Saunders and Company, 1992.

Marcus, B. H., and L. H. Forsyth. 'The Challenge of Behavior Change.' *Medicine and Health, Rhode Island,* Sept., 1997.

Margen, S. *The Wellness Nutrition Counter.* New York: Rebus, 1997.

University of CA at Berkeley, *The Wellness Encyclopedia of Food and Nutrition.* New York: Rebus, 1992.

McConnaughy, E., et al. 'Stages of Change in Psychotherapy: A Follow-up Report.' *Psychotherapy* Vol. 4, 1989.

Miles, E. *Tune Your Brain—Using Music to Manage Your Mind, Body, and Mood*. New York: Berkley Books, 1997.

Moore, K. A., and J. A. Blumenthal. 'Exercising Training as an Alternative Treatment for Depression Among Older Adults.' *Alternative Therapies in Health and Medicine* Vol. 77, 1998.

Moore, M. *How to Master Change in Your Life*. Minneapolis, MN: Eckankar, 1997.

Nutrition Action Newsletter. Washington D.C., 1997.

Nutrition and the MD. 'Is Stored Iron a Risk for Heart Disease or Cancer?' University of California, San Diego Vol. 7, 1997.

Nutrition and the MD. 'Dietary Factors Controlling Homocystine and Cardiovascular Risk.' University of California, San Diego Vol. 9, 1997.

Ornish, D. *Dr. Dean Ornish's Program for Reversing Heart Disease*. New York: Ballantine Books, 1990.

Ornstein, R, and D. Sobel. *Healthy Pleasures*. New York: Addison-Wesley, 1989.

'Physical Activity and Cardiovascular Health.' *JAMA* Vol. 276, 1996.

Remen, R. *Open Your Heart Retreat*. Berkeley, CA: Conference Recording Services. Audio-cassette, 1993.

Rock, C. L., R. A. Jacob, and P. E. Bowen. 'Update on the Biological Characteristics of the Antioxidant Macronutrients: Vitamin C, Vitamin E, and Caretenoids.' *Journal American Dietetic Association* Vol. 96, 1996.

Rossman, M. *Healing Yourself*. New York: Pocket Books, 1989.

Sapolsky, R. *Why Zebras Don't Get Ulcers*. New York: W. H. Freeman & Co, 1994.

Schwartz, B. *Diets Don't Work*. Houston, TX: Breakthrough Publishing, 1985.

Segar, M. L., et al. 'The Effect of Aerobic Exercise on Self-Esteem and Depressive and Anxiety Symptoms Among Breast Cancer Survivors.' *Oncology Nursing Forum* Vol. 25, 1998.

Seligman, M. *Learned Optimism*. New York: Simon & Schuster, 1990.

Simopoulos, A., V. Herbert, and B. Jacobson. *Genetic Nutrition*. New York: MacMillan Publishing Co., 1993.

Strecher, V. J., et al. 'Goal Setting as a Strategy for Health Behavior Change.' *Health Education Quarterly* Vol. 22, 1995.

Sutherland, V., and C. Cooper. *Understanding Stress: A Psychological Perspective for Health Professionals.* New York: Chapman and Hall, 1990.

Tufts University Health and Nutrition Letter. June 1996-April 1998.

UCLA Berkeley School of Public Health. *The Wellness Supermarket Shopper's Guide.* USA: Health Letter Associates, 1997.

United States Department of Agriculture, Human Nutrition Information Service, Leaflet No. 572 August 1992.

University of California Berkeley Wellness Letter. December 1996-August 1997.

Vayda, W. *Mood Foods.* Berkeley, CA: Ulysses Press, 1995.

Venolia, C. *Healing Environments.* Berkeley, CA: Celestial Arts, 1988.

Wallberg-Henriksson, H., J. Rincon, and J. R. Zierath. 'Exercise in the Management of Non-Insulin Dependent Diabetes Mellitus.' *Sports Medicine* Vol. 25, 1998.

Webb, D., and S. Smith. *Foods for Better Health: Prevention and Healing of Disease.* Linwood, IL: Publications International, Ltd., 1994.

Williams, P. T., 'Relationship of Heart Disease Risk Factors to Exercise Quantity and Intensity.' *Archives of Internal Medicine* Vol. 158, 1998.

Willis, J., ed. 'FDA Consumer: Focus on Food Labeling.' USDA: 1993.

Willis, P. *Visualization.* Chicago, IL: NTC Publishing Group, 1994.

ACKNOWLEDGEMENTS

The realization of a vision requires love, respect, attention, and time. Giving birth to Active Wellness as a healthy and vital book required all this and more. Each person involved in the Active Wellness programme has made an important contribution to the book you hold in your hands. Although this list will seem comprehensive, I will not be able to mention everyone. Therefore, I would first like to thank all those who have been a part of Active Wellness and who have contributed to its development.

Active Wellness evolved from my meeting Paula Glaser, whose belief and enthusiasm became the catalyst that helped launch this project. Our fortuitous meeting led me to Dorie Simmonds, my literary agent. Dorie's tremendous expertise made it possible for the book to become a reality by finding it a home with the team of professional and talented people at Time Life.

Working closely with Time Life has been a pleasure. I applaud the team at Time-Life, a group of people who are delightful and excellent at what they do: Kate Hartson, Executive Editor, for her vision, foresight, and expertise in creating and directing the team of writers, editors, and artists; Linda Bellamy, Editor, for her co-ordinating, editing, writing, and wonderfully cheerful disposition during deadline time; Olga Vezeris; and the copy editors, line editors, proofreaders, designers, and marketers. For the cover, a big thank you to Frierson Mee + Kraft.

Also, a special thanks to the team of professionals who work with the Active Wellness programme and who helped make this book possible: Leslie Passaro, R.D., 'my right hand' for the programme, and a wonderful teacher and manager; Susan Jakubowicz Psy.D., psychoanalyst and specialist in behaviour and group therapy; Luis F. Sierra, for his expertise in yoga and stress management; and Marie Scioscia, M.S., R.D., A.C.E. certified trainer/instructor, for her knowledge of movement and the human body. To the Active Wellness Gourmet team: Chef Deborah Cohen, for her culinary savvy and support, and the staff—Hillary Cooper, Jill Feibusch, Kate Molnar, Ed Olbrych, Sharon Richter, and Jennifer Rosenfeld.

To those who have inspired me and served as my teachers and supporters: Sharron Dalton, R.D., Ph.D., Dr. Steven Horowitz, Dr. James Kennedy, Marion Nestle Ph.D, M.P.H., Dr. Dean Ornish, Marilyn Majchrzak R.D., and Lisa Powell R.D.

A thank you to all the others who have contributed to Active Wellness through their effort and support of the programme and the book, including Amy Beim, Jane Ubell & Jane Berk of The Jane Group, Megan E. Furey, Tamara M. Ketler, the Wharton Team, NBC, including Art Finkelstein, Linda Langer, Dr. Paul Shank, Andy Smith, and Dr. Philip Weintraub, Susan Bishop and Alice Austin at the American Heart Association, New York City, Marianne Forsyth Bee at Sony Music and Laurie Pollock at Ogilvy & Mather. And to those who are invaluable for their ongoing love and support of all that

I do, my extended family: The Bassetts, Berzacks, Friedmans, Kortens, Knudsens, and Salzers; and my dear friends: Karen Angel, Amanda Bell & Dr. Joel Kirson, Laurel Iverson, Lee Dannay, Teri Dubeck, Denise Goodbar, Laurie Green, Mark E. Greenwald, Amy and Richard Land, Janice & Gary Levinson, Risa Mish, Peter Miller, Melanie Stein, Allegra Themmen, and Dan Weber. To those who help me to continue to expand and grow: Anita Menfi, M.Ed., Elliot M. Zeisel, Ph.D., P.C., and 'The Group'.

And last but definitely not least, a special heartfelt thanks to Doug Mazlish, for his love, patience, support, understanding, and encouragement.

INDEX

away from home, 212-29
calories in, 45-47, 52-53, 55-58, 134-36
designing, 47-54
energy requirements in, 47
food and nutrition guidelines, 73-84
food as energy and, 45-47
food groups in, 59-72, 93
nutrients in, 45-46, 55-58
for special needs, 55-58
weight-loss goal and, 48-53
See also Active Wellness Eating Plans; kitchen
personal physical fitness plan, 128-61
aerobics/cardiovascular workout, 137, 141-49, 230
away from home, 229-30
beginning, 130-36
benefits of exercise, 128-29
cool-downs in, 149-50
designing, 136-39
goals in, 137-39, 145-46
habits and, 46-47, 130
shoes and, 155-56
for special needs, 154-55
strength training in, 137, 150-53, 157-58, 230
stretching in, 137, 153-54, 159-60, 201-5, 230, 231-32
warm-ups in, 140-41
phenylalanine, 167-68
phytochemicals, 78
phyto-oestrogens, 87
pickled foods, 95
pizza, 224
planning, 29-38
assessment in, 32-36, 37-38, 43, 131-34
for dining away from home, 217, 218, 228
See also goals
polyunsaturated fats, 69, 81
portion sizes, 62, 63-72
positive reinforcement, 236
potassium, 76, 91
poultry. *See* meat and poultry
pregnancy, 55-56
priorities, 39
proteins, 45, 59-61, 65-66, 87-88. *See also specific proteins*

R
relaxation techniques, 192-210
renal disease, 57
renin, 90-91
restaurants, 213-22
rewards, 235, 239
rice, 64, 107
rubs, 254
Cajun Spice Rub, 272-73

S
salad(s), 250-51
Fat-Free Coleslaw, 282-83

Wheatgrain Salad with Raspberry Vinaigrette, 283
salad bars, 224-25
salad dressings, 70, 72, 108, 216, 250, 280-82
Fat-Free Balsamic Vinaigrette, 280-81
Honey Mustard Seed Dressing, 281
Lite Caesar Dressing, 281-82
Raspberry Vinaigrette, 282
saturated fats, 80
sauces, 108, 216, 253
Papaya Peach Salsa, 285
Sesame Sauce, 286-87
seafood, 66, 74, 82, 90, 103
Crab Cakes, 273
Lite Paella, 275-76
sedentary habits, 46-47, 130
seitan, 259
selenium, 73, 78
self-appraisal, 236-37
self-care, 235
self-help groups, 240
self-talk, 114-17, 172
serotonin, 163, 165-66, 167
serving sizes, 62, 63-72
setbacks, handling, 172-82
shoes, 155-56
sleeping problems, 76
smoked foods, 95
snacks, 65, 106, 110
sodium/salt, 76, 87-88, 90-91, 102, 104, 219
soups, 107, 216, 249-50, 264-66
Basic Vegetable Stock, 264
Hearty Vegetable Soup, 265
White Bean Soup, 265-66
soured cream, 68, 102, 216
Coriander Soured Cream, 274
soya-based foods, 64, 66, 87, 88, 102, 110, 255, 258
special occasions, 226-27
spreads, 71, 102-3, 108, 216
strength training, 137, 150-53, 157-58, 230
stress, 75, 76, 153, 165-66, 182, 184-210, 230-32
stretching, 137, 153-54, 159-60, 201-5, 230, 231-32
stroke, 78, 82, 89-92
supermarkets, 99-111, 223
support groups, 240
sweets/desserts, 59-61, 70, 74, 75, 79-80, 94, 105, 109-10, 163-64, 220, 227, 263
Apple Crisp, 287-88
'I Can't Believe It's Fat-Free' Cheesecake, 288
Low-Fat Fudge Brownies, 287
Quick and Easy Low-Fat Lemon Curd, 289

T
Target Heart Rate (THR), 142-44
time, 38-41, 146
travel, 227-32
triggers, 162-82. *See also* feelings
triglycerides, 33, 76, 79, 81, 90, 92